Post Mortem CT for Non-Suspicious Adult Deaths

Ayeshea Shenton • Peter Kralt
S. Kim Suvarna

Post Mortem CT for Non-Suspicious Adult Deaths

An Introduction

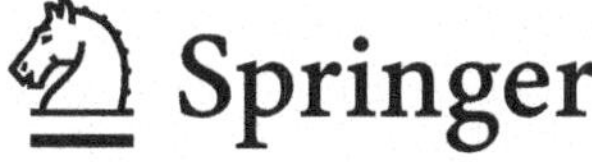

Ayeshea Shenton
Department of Radiology
iGene London Ltd.
Sheffield
UK

Peter Kralt
Department of Radiology
iGene London Ltd.
Sheffield
UK

S. Kim Suvarna
Department of Histopathology
Royal Hallamshire Hospital
Sheffield
UK

ISBN 978-3-030-70831-3 ISBN 978-3-030-70829-0 (eBook)
https://doi.org/10.1007/978-3-030-70829-0

This Springer imprint is published by the registered company Springer Nature Switzerland AG
The registered company address is: Gewerbestrasse 11, 6330 Cham, Switzerland

Preface

Post mortem computed tomography (PMCT) is an evolving diagnostic arena dealing with autopsy practice. It has only been the last decade or so that has seen it gaining traction in the United Kingdom although it has a more established role elsewhere in the world.

This book was written to address a need for an introductory text for those entering the world of post mortem imaging. It is based upon the cases encountered during the authors' first few years of PMCT practice and their learning experiences. As principally a radiology text, it is populated with many examples of both normal appearances and structural pathology on PMCT. We hope that it addresses the needs of the trainee in radiology, through to the established practitioner starting PMCT work and others working in mortuaries. We also envisage that it will be a ready resource for autopsy pathologists and Coroners in the United Kingdom.

We are extremely grateful to our many colleagues who have helped us with images and provided critical commentary. We are particularly indebted to the dedicated radiographers, administrative and information technology staff at iGene, without whom this work would not have been possible. We also are conscious of the support given by the mortuary and medicolegal staff at multiple sites across the country, and to the pathologists who have validated our scans and occasionally shown the limitations of radiology of the deceased. We are lucky to have had the support and understanding of Springer, as a publishing team, and lastly salute our families for their significant understanding while this project progressed.

We would like this text to be a positive-step forward for further research and understanding in the field of PMCT and that it may serve the needs of the deceased and their families into the future.

Sheffield, UK — Ayeshea Shenton
Sheffield, UK — Peter Kralt
Sheffield, UK — S. Kim Suvarna

Contents

1 Introduction to the Investigation of Death and Post Mortem Computed Tomography

Introduction

Post mortem computed tomography (PMCT, Fig. 1.1) has an evolving role in the investigation of non-suspicious adult death and offers the potential to avoid open autopsy in many cases. Although this book is written from the perspective of working within the medicolegal coronial system of England and Wales, many of the issues are common elsewhere within the United Kingdom and in many parts of world. The methodology and considerations of PMCT should be fully understood by involved medicolegal parties, radiologists, pathologists, relatives and society.

What Is an Autopsy?

In England and Wales, the majority of deaths are expected and fully understood, allowing a cause of death to be provided by the family/hospital doctor. These cases do not require any investigation, having often had numerous investigations in life which would confirm the disease/s responsible for the death of the individual.

Currently, most autopsy cases, at the behest of HM Coroner ('coronial cases'), proceed because there is no clear cause of death or where there are issues of a medicolegal nature. This latter group includes deaths during surgery/anaesthesia, maternal deaths, deaths in custody or in relation to occupational dust exposures—to name but a few [1].

Of the deaths registered in 2018, 41% (220,600 deaths) were reported to coroners [2], mostly being referred by a family or hospital doctor or, less commonly, the police. The coroner decides if, and when, a post mortem examination of the body is needed [1]. The coroner also has the power to decide what type of investigation is most appropriate, whether by open dissection or whether to consider imaging solutions, where available and suitable. The ability of imaging to wholly provide the post mortem examination result is dependent on the circumstances of death [3], so

A. Shenton et al., *Post Mortem CT for Non-Suspicious Adult Deaths*, https://doi.org/10.1007/978-3-030-70829-0_1

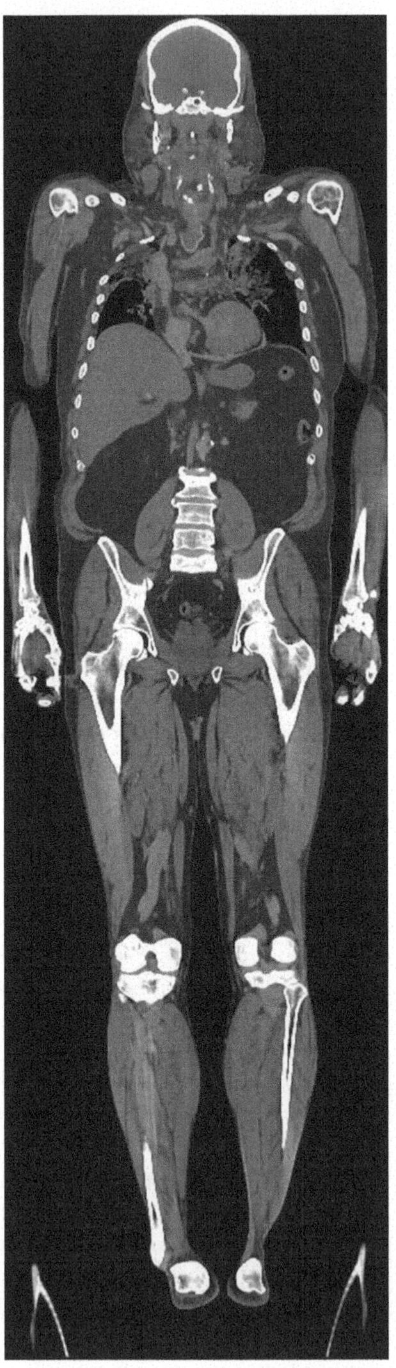

Fig. 1.1 Coronal PMCT on soft tissue windows offers a comprehensive cross-sectional examination of the whole body

cases should ideally be assessed on an individual basis, although some centres prefer to scan all bodies as a first-line assessment [4].

There are also (non-coronial) consent/hospital autopsies, being hospital-based investigations, requested by the clinical team to further consider the pathology involved in the deceased. These investigations often revolve around the efficacy of therapies applied. They may seek to investigate unusual findings seen before death which did not achieve a clear answer in life. The relatives can agree to, or deny, the opportunity for this autopsy investigation. Once being the majority of autopsies in the United Kingdom, these consent examinations have declined in number over recent decades. Reasons include a higher diagnostic performance during life due to increasing use of clinical imaging and possibly also increasing public concerns about the nature of an autopsy [5].

The last type of autopsy considered here is that of the forensic examination, which is normally performed by specialist autopsy pathologists with training in medicolegal and criminal pathologies. These cases deal with possible homicides, manslaughter and other criminal acts.

Of all the autopsies currently performed in England and Wales, the majority are within the coronial medicolegal framework, which will be the substrate for the cases considered in this chapter and onwards in the book.

The coroner's investigation covers four basic questions. The first three are relatively straightforward, posing little difficulty for those considering the case. They include the (rarely disputed) following questions:

1. who has died
2. where the individual died
3. when the individual died

It is the fourth question, namely *how* they died, which is variably complex to answer.

In some cases, the triangulation of ante mortem data and conversations with those who attended the deceased provide reassurance as to the case being a natural death. However, if the circumstances and information do not provide sufficient confidence in terms of the cause of death being natural, or merit an autopsy examination automatically (as above), these will come to further coronial investigation.

There is insufficient space in this book to fully describe the variable methods of conducting an open autopsy examination, in the traditional style that has been practiced in the United Kingdom for more than 150 years. However, if asked, the general population would consider an autopsy examination to involve direct knife incisions into the body and examination of the internal tissues. This examination can be a matter of direct inspection only, with the results simply being written into a report. In some cases, specialist investigations will also be applied, with these variably including toxicology, microscope examination of tissues, microbiology, serology, photography and other specialist tests [6]. A brief description of techniques and approach used for the individual body cavities is given from the pathologist's perspective in each relevant chapter.

In 2018, post mortem examinations were carried out in 39% of cases referred to the coroner [2] amounting to 85,600 deaths. Legally, the coroner does not require family or other consent to order a post mortem examination, but, where possible, the relatives' religious and cultural beliefs will always be considered [7].

The purpose of the autopsy could be argued to revolve solely around finding the medical cause of death. However, this could be argued as too simplistic, as the autopsy will look at the body as a whole, attempting to rationalise all the pathological disorders and factors that led to the death of the individual. This analysis, traditionally provided by pathologists, allows the coroner to ascertain whether the death was natural, or not, and thereby enables accurate registration of the death.

In some circumstances, the investigation may highlight aspects of imperfect social, nursing or clinical care, with legal directions subsequently being made, or could influence future health policies. Yet, the coroner may not be seen to directly criticise the witnesses, or any institution, where later legal considerations are possible.

On an individual level, the identification of diseases with a particular genetic risk within the family can allow recommendation of clinical assessment of close family members, for example those with a risk of sudden cardiac death [8].

In England and Wales, the leading cause of death for older adults (age over 80) in 2018 was dementia (often described as Alzheimer's disease), although this covers a variety of degenerative and neurovascular pathologies. For men aged 50–80, the leading cause remained ischemic heart disease, and for women aged 50–80, malignancies of the breast, trachea, bronchus or lung were cited. Younger adults (generally under the age of 50) tended to die through other mechanisms such as suicide, injury or other unexpected acute organic pathology [9].

In the investigation of a coronial non-suspicious death, the cause of death must be ascertained on the '*balance of probabilities*'. This is a legal test that may be summarised as being 'more probable than not'! Thus, one might regard it as *only just* over the 50:50 likelihood ratio. This is clearly a lesser legal test than that required in criminal cases (and probably less certainty than required in most clinical practice) but has been both pragmatic and realistic in terms of managing the coronial caseload for many decades.

Looking at coronial-directed autopsy examinations, most cases are found to be natural deaths and non-suspicious in nature, allowing appropriate paperwork to be completed with no further medicolegal consideration. However, some cases will require a court-based discussion, commonly described as the inquest. This non-adversarial court room investigation (inquisition) has the opportunity to question the relatives, the pathologist, medical practitioners and other parties (potentially including the radiologist) in order to derive a cause of death. The inquest may involve a jury, but the majority are managed by the coroner alone.

The Arrival of Post Mortem Imaging

Diagnostic imaging has become extremely important in the routine clinical management of the living, particularly with the advent of computed tomography and magnetic resonance imaging. Indeed, the results of the various scans performed during life, mapped against other investigations, will often show the patterns of disease and permit a clear cause of death to be defined later.

It also has to be understood that imaging has had a role in autopsy investigations performed for many decades now. This has been relatively basic, generally revolving around plain radiograph identification of foreign objects (e.g. bullets) and fractures. It is also noted that the drive towards more modern radiological techniques being used in autopsy examinations has actually been increasing across the United Kingdom for the last two to three decades.

The proportions of current radiology autopsy examinations vary greatly by jurisdiction [2], originally driven by faith groups in Manchester and other areas. By 2018, the proportion of post mortem examinations involving less-invasive techniques such as PMCT was rising (3326 cases), compared to the prior year (1671 cases), [2] and more centres are planning to adopt imaging techniques in the next few years.

In the hospital setting, PMCT can improve diagnosis of the cause of death over clinical diagnosis alone [10, 11]. Potentially coupled with image-guided biopsy, the radiology-centred autopsy may be argued to provide similar diagnoses to open autopsy [12, 13]. Such biopsy techniques could be incorporated into PMCT imaging with additional resource. This is not currently a common practice but could perhaps be one of the aspirations for autopsy examinations in the next decades.

The demand for non-invasive or minimally interactive post mortem imaging has increased in recent years for many reasons. There has been some public concern about open autopsy with ethical and religious objections, possibly furthered by organ retention scandals [14]. Furthermore, the numbers of autopsy pathologists available to perform routine open autopsies are diminishing, with more pathologists opting for less stressful surgical pathological disciplines.

Once radiological autopsy (PMCT) investigations started, it was quickly evident that additional benefits could be realised. These include the permanent record of anatomical findings, which unlike open autopsy with its necessarily destructive technique means that pathological concerns can be seen by many without ongoing tissue degradation [15]. Furthermore, the common use of radiological techniques means that there is an instant familiarity with the technique, with this potentially being of benefit when discussing cases with relatives or the court.

Broadly speaking, PMCT is particularly good at finding internal haemorrhage, bony injury, foreign bodies, gas patterns and calcification (e.g. in coronary arteries). It is therefore generally suited to investigate the relevant pathologies of adult deaths.

PMCT is particularly effective in the investigation of sudden death, where a catastrophic structural event such as aortic rupture or intracranial haemorrhage is confidently visualised. By contrast, for example when used to investigate hospital deaths, where a cause of death was not already clinically or radiologically apparent, PMCT is often less definitive.

PMCT can be supplemented with angiography, a vascular infusion of radiopaque contrast which may be 'whole body' or targeted locally. Typical indications for post mortem CT angiography (PMCTA) are trauma, vascular pathologies [16] and deaths after medical interventions [17]. In our practice of this technique, we have used targeted CT coronary angiography in selected cases (see Chap. 8).

Very few centres use post mortem magnetic resonance (PMMR) as the mainstay for autopsy investigation, despite the advantages in assessing soft tissue, such as detecting oedema in the setting of myocardial infarction [15]. Minimally invasive autopsy with PMMR has proven to be as accurate as invasive autopsy to detect major pathological findings in paediatric cases (fetus, neonate and infant) [18]. The investigation of paediatric death by post mortem imaging techniques is beyond the scope of this book, with the reader being directed to specialist texts [19].

It would be fair to say that the facilities for PMMR in the autopsy arena are limited, being relatively more costly and time-consuming to perform. It is therefore not widely practiced in the United Kingdom. Yet, a combined (PMCT, PMCTA and PMMR) approach may be most comprehensive as has been used with the Virtopsy® technique in Switzerland [20].

It has been suggested that a two-thirds reduction in the number of invasive coronial autopsies may be achieved by the use of PMCT, possibly augmented by coronary angiography [21]. Within the United Kingdom, one service reports a cause of death could be given on the 'balance of probabilities' following PMCT (with coronary angiography and ventilation) in 97.1% of cases [22], although it should be understood that these examinations are mostly preselected for suitability. In another centre, where all (i.e. no-selected) cases entering the mortuary are scanned, it has been possible to achieve a cause of death in 55.6% of cases by PMCT alone [4].

Coronial guidance recognises that post mortem imaging is a developing field, and therefore the results from PMCT should be used cautiously [23]. The role of PMCT radiologist is primarily to indicate pathologies leading to a medical cause of death. Collaborative working with the pathologist is considered of paramount importance in order to establish and run a post mortem imaging service. Generally, both the pathologist and the radiologist prepare a report for the coroner, with the radiology data usually being available first. The pathologist then performs an external examination and considers the results of the radiology, balanced against the previous medical history and circumstances surrounding the death of the individual. At present, the UK Chief Coroner has recommended that the pathologist states the cause of death or (if the cause of death cannot be defined) instructs the pathologist to proceed to full or focussed autopsy [4, 23].

The Emerging Subspecialty of PMCT

As described, plain film radiography has long been used in post mortem and forensic imaging, with cross-sectional imaging practice growing for several decades in coronial and forensic cases [24]. What was initially an extrapolation of image interpretation, derived from the radiologists' experience of scans in the living, post mortem radiology is now a rapidly growing and distinct subspecialty [25], evidenced by the increase in scientific publications that deal with this subject [26].

PMCT is well established in many countries such as Switzerland, Japan and Australia. The widespread introduction of a non-invasive (or minimally invasive) alternative to open autopsy is a realistic concept in the United Kingdom. This is well underway, although the United Kingdom has been variably slow to follow this uptake [27]. Proposals for national implementation have been made, as it is recognised that there may no longer be the need for invasive examination in certain types of death [28].

As can be predicted, change is not easy and may be hindered by a lack of scanners, radiologists, and financial constraints. For imaging to become routine, cultural adaptation will be required, especially for pathologists [13]. Resistance has variably been encountered although this could serve to challenge advocates of PMCT to develop a clear understanding and justification for the service [27] and increase the wealth of relevant scientific evidence available.

Interpretation of PMCT

The technique and equipment required for the radiological autopsy are the same as those used in hospital medicine. Yet, it should be understood from the start that PMCT is different to clinical imaging. There are a wide range of post mortem changes that evolve from the time immediately after death onward, to those seen in the days and weeks following the cessation of life. It is apparent that the radiologist cannot simply move from reporting cases of the living to describing the pathology of the dead in one easy step. There are a variety of changes that reflect processes of normal decomposition, which have to be mapped against the variable pathologies that have caused the death of the individual. Consequently, appropriate training and exposure to a range of cases is required if one wishes to achieve a good understanding of PMCT [29].

As is often seen in the elderly, multiple structural comorbidities may be present. For example, it is vital that the radiologist does not simply focus on the presence of coronary artery calcification/stenosis or pneumonia. Such pathologies can be present in the deceased and yet not be part of the pathophysiology of death. For example, one might see a case who has died from significant cranial injury with coincidental significant coronary disease. Of course, there is a possibility that the coronary artery disease was involved in the circumstances leading up to the head trauma. The presence of pneumonia is also common in the final stages of life. In this regard, it may be a readily expected process rather than the primary disease. It may be commonly seen in cases of disseminated malignancy or cerebrovascular disease, where the final stage of the patient's journey involves several days of palliative bed rest.

Conversely, in other cases, there may be little pathology to find on imaging, despite there being a strong hint from the circumstances. One example could be a history of drug misuse and the finding of the deceased in the presence of drug paraphernalia, but the PMCT does not show any significant structural pathology and might be considered 'inconclusive', although the absence of structural findings is an expected reality.

It is recognised that radiology is somewhat limited in terms of identifying conditions such as drug overdose, metabolic derangement, sepsis, various dementias and a variety of abdominal disorders that lead to death. In these cases, the role of PMCT is mainly to exclude other structural pathologies, with this being of general help for potential subsequent invasive autopsy.

This leaves a group of other inconclusive PMCT scans, which may be frustrating for the radiologist as well as the pathologist. Scans with non-specific structural changes and minor variations in terms of architecture are found regularly in PMCT. They are generally more likely to be encountered in younger population (i.e. less than 50 years). In these cases, without a diagnostic radiological pathology, it may be impossible to state the definite cause of death from PMCT without supplementary investigations. These possibilities range from progressing to an invasive autopsy, toxicology investigations, sampling for microbiology, accessing spleen for DNA studies and so on. This is not a failure of the PMCT technique. Rather, PMCT can help streamline the further steps in the process of the investigation, thereby decreasing the use of resources and time taken, alongside limiting the extent of autopsy investigation from the relatives' perspective.

Some centres request the radiologist to arrive at a defined cause of death, whereas others simply request the radiologist to list any relevant findings, there is no single best process. Care should be taken when defining the cause of death to separate the cause of death from the 'mode' of dying (e.g. an abnormal physiological state such as cardiac or respiratory arrest, syncope or coma) [30]. The cause of death should not indicate a mode of death, but should be precise with regard to the pathology that has ended the life of the person (e.g. cerebral infarction, pneumonia). It goes without saying that the radiologist should be cautious about independently offering any commentary that might take a cause of death assessment from the natural into the realm of non-natural death (e.g. homicide, suicide, accident).

There are established guidelines in England and Wales for completing medical certificates of cause of death [31], and these are useful in providing examples of how medical causes of death are written.

One should always be mindful that deaths referred to the coroner, which have been declared non-suspicious, may still include *unnatural* causes (such as accidental trauma, suicide or interaction with other parties). Pathologists are trained specifically to look at all cases with a view to suspicious circumstances, although this is perhaps not something that comes automatically to the radiologist through their training [32].

It is important for the radiologist to keep an open mind about the possibility of concealed third-party involvement or negligence in care and discuss concerns—if needed. Clearly, any findings that may be interpreted as signs of a violent or non-natural death could change the nature of the case investigation. The radiologist should not feel inhibited from reporting any concerns directly to the pathologist or coroner who instructed the PMCT. In some circumstances, a forensic investigation may immediately follow.

Even if, after PMCT, an open autopsy is needed, a clear interpretation of the absence of pathology in certain body regions has an advantage, as it allows a 'limited autopsy' of the remaining parts. The PMCT images would serve as a permanent record of the body before dissection or further decomposition and can be used to 'cross-reference' findings. Overall, a combination of PMCT, especially when augmented with targeted PMCTA and a limited autopsy, is becoming accepted as the 'gold standard' in death investigation rather than a full open (traditional or invasive) autopsy alone [3, 11, 14, 21, 33–35].

In time, with experience and collaboration between pathologists and radiologists, the true extent of the role of PMCT in death investigation will certainly further evolve and improve.

Collaborative Working

Ideally, direct case discussion between the radiologist and the pathologist would allow the best degree of collaboration [25]. It would also allow each to understand the techniques and limitations of both imaging and open autopsy [36]. This communication is comparable to the relationship between physician and radiologist in a clinical setting [36]. However, it is clear that the variable pressures upon radiologists, pathologists, and other staff means that text (e.g. written reports and email) communication of data is often the medium utilised. Overall, the guidance from the UK Chief Coroner and Royal Medical Colleges suggests that the pathologist should retain a central coordinating role in the investigation of deaths [37], although this could potentially change in the future.

It remains a challenge to develop effective communication when in a remote working setting, without face-to-face professional discussion, as perhaps would happen in a clinical multidisciplinary team meeting, although multiple platforms to facilitate this have been introduced in recent times. When the pathologist's report is available sometime after the radiologist's report, alternative arrangements to provide case feedback may also need to be made to enhance interprofessional communication and improve learning and diagnostic outcomes. These can also be augmented by subsequent reviews and ongoing audit.

As has been pointed out, radiologists with little experience in reporting PMCT are at risk of misinterpretation of cases if they rely on their clinical experience of the living alone [25]. This could have significant medicolegal implications and potentially adversely impact on their personal professional accreditation. It is imperative that appropriate training is provided if the radiologist wishes to begin reporting PMCT given that there are differences in image analysis and a new scope of 'normal' to appreciate. Furthermore, any training will have to deliver an understanding of the appearances of those dying with a range of progressive disorders that are seen in community death investigations as well as those dying in hospitals (which may also be in fields outside of the radiologist's normal clinical practice). Learning should therefore be sought from both radiology and pathology colleagues in this respect.

It is equally possible for autopsy pathologists to learn and undertake PMCT analysis independently. This process is being pushed by some forensic pathologists [38]. Yet, a radiologist still adds particular value to the team because of their general cross-sectional and three-dimensional anatomic understanding, knowledge of CT technique, anatomical/other artefacts and image pattern recognition skills.

The Future of PMCT

It is likely that the relatively new technique of PMCT investigation may alter death statistics in autopsy cases. For example, currently PMCT has a relative lack of sensitivity in diagnosing pulmonary emboli, which may see a decrease in these registered as the cause of death. By contrast, it may uncover other pathologies (hip fractures for example) that might have previously gone unrecognised.

Apart from a 'routine' non-contrast–enhanced PMCT, there are various additional techniques such as angiography, ventilation, PMMR and image-guided biopsies that could find a place in post mortem and forensic imaging. Similar to the concept of personalised clinical medicine, one may expect to see a more tailored approach to the deceased in post mortem investigation. Indeed, it is likely that a combination of these techniques may become the norm in UK deaths, although the publicly funded coronial service may find it challenging to meet the additional cost.

One evolving technique that may benefit PMCT is dual-energy CT (DECT). Images are acquired at different energy levels, allow differentiation of materials and better tissue characterisation. Applications that might be useful include metallic dental artefact reduction to improve the image quality of dental CT used for identification purposes [39]. Various other possible applications have also been suggested, more relevant to the coronial setting, for example differentiation of arterial and venous clots, improved characterisation of coronary artery plaques and detection of foreign bodies [40].

Successful evaluation and implementation of any new techniques, mapped to the collaboration between radiologist and pathologist, is likely to be the best way forward. Yet, it is certain that further change lies ahead...

References

1. Dorries C. Coroners' courts: a guide to law and practice [Internet]. 3rd ed. Oxford: Oxford University Press; 2014. https://global.oup.com/academic/product/coroners-courts-9780199566112.
2. Ministry of Justice. Coroners statistics annual 2018 England and Wales [Internet]. 2019. https://assets.publishing.service.gov.uk/government/uploads/system/uploads/attachment_data/file/810303/Coroners_Statistics_Annual_2018.pdf.
3. Morgan B, Rutty GN. How does post-mortem imaging compare to autopsy, is this a relevant question? J Forensic Radiol Imaging [Internet]. 2016;4:2–6. https://linkinghub.elsevier.com/retrieve/pii/S2212478015300277.
4. Suvarna SK, Kitsanta P, Burton JL. The effects of postmortem CT scanning all cases entering a UK public mortuary: a 3-month pilot. J Clin Pathol [Internet]. 2017;70(10):903–5. http://jcp.bmj.com/lookup/doi/10.1136/jclinpath-2017-204505.
5. Turnbull A, Osborn M, Nicholas N. Hospital autopsy: endangered or extinct? J Clin Pathol [Internet]. 2015;68(8):601–4. http://jcp.bmj.com/lookup/doi/10.1136/jclinpath-2014-202700.
6. Burton J, Rutty G. In: Burton JL, Rutty G, editors. The hospital autopsy [Internet]. 3rd ed. London: CRC Press; 2010. https://www.routledge.com/The-Hospital-Autopsy-A-Manual-of-Fundamental-Autopsy-Practice-Third-Edition/Burton-Rutty/p/book/9780340965146.
7. Ministry of Justice. Guide to coroner services for bereaved people. [Internet]. 2020. https://assets.publishing.service.gov.uk/government/uploads/system/uploads/attachment_data/file/859076/guide-to-coroner-services-bereaved-people-jan-2020.pdf.
8. Suvarna SK. National guidelines for adult autopsy cardiac dissection and diagnosis—are they achievable? A personal view. Histopathology [Internet]. 2008;53(1):97–112. http://doi.wiley.com/10.1111/j.1365-2559.2008.02993.x.
9. Office for National Statistics. Deaths registered in England and Wales: 2018 [Internet]. 2019. https://www.ons.gov.uk/peoplepopulationandcommunity/birthsdeathsandmarriages/deaths/bulletins/deathsregistrationsummarytables/2018.
10. Inai K, Noriki S, Kinoshita K, Sakai T, Kimura H, Nishijima A, et al. Postmortem CT is more accurate than clinical diagnosis for identifying the immediate cause of death in hospitalized patients: a prospective autopsy-based study. Virchows Arch [Internet]. 2016;469(1):101–9. http://link.springer.com/10.1007/s00428-016-1937-6.
11. Sonnemans LJP, Kubat B, Prokop M, Klein WM. Can virtual autopsy with postmortem CT improve clinical diagnosis of cause of death? A retrospective observational cohort study in a Dutch tertiary referral centre. BMJ Open [Internet]. 2018;8(3):e018834. http://bmjopen.bmj.com/lookup/doi/10.1136/bmjopen-2017-018834.
12. Blokker BM, Wagensveld IM, Weustink AC, Oosterhuis JW, Hunink MGM. Non-invasive or minimally invasive autopsy compared to conventional autopsy of suspected natural deaths in adults: a systematic review. Eur Radiol [Internet]. 2016;26(4):1159–79. http://link.springer.com/10.1007/s00330-015-3908-8.
13. Blokker BM, Weustink AC, Wagensveld IM, von der Thüsen JH, Pezzato A, Dammers R, et al. Conventional autopsy versus minimally invasive autopsy with postmortem MRI, CT, and CT-guided biopsy: comparison of diagnostic performance. Radiology [Internet]. 2018;289(3):658–67. http://pubs.rsna.org/doi/10.1148/radiol.2018180924.
14. Roberts ISD, Benamore RE, Benbow EW, Lee SH, Harris JN, Jackson A, et al. Post-mortem imaging as an alternative to autopsy in the diagnosis of adult deaths: a validation study. Lancet [Internet]. 2012;379(9811):136–42. https://linkinghub.elsevier.com/retrieve/pii/S0140673611614839.
15. Smith AP, Traill ZC, Roberts IS. Post-mortem imaging in adults. Diag Histopathol [Internet]. 2018;24(9):365–71. https://linkinghub.elsevier.com/retrieve/pii/S1756231718301208.
16. Grabherr S, Egger C, Vilarino R, Campana L, Jotterand M, Dedouit F. Modern post-mortem imaging: an update on recent developments. Forensic Sci Res [Internet]. 2017;2(2):52–64. https://www.tandfonline.com/doi/full/10.1080/20961790.2017.1330738.

17. Heinemann A, Vogel H, Heller M, Tzikas A, Püschel K. Investigation of medical intervention with fatal outcome: the impact of post-mortem CT and CT angiography. Radiol Med [Internet]. 2015;120(9):835–45. http://link.springer.com/10.1007/s11547-015-0574-5.
18. Thayyil S, Sebire NJ, Chitty LS, Wade A, Chong W, Olsen O, et al. Post-mortem MRI versus conventional autopsy in fetuses and children: a prospective validation study. Lancet [Internet]. 2013;382(9888):223–33. https://linkinghub.elsevier.com/retrieve/pii/S0140673613601348.
19. Cohen MC, Scheimberg I. The pediatric and perinatal autopsy manual [Internet]. Cambridge: Cambridge University Press; 2014. http://ebooks.cambridge.org/ref/id/CBO9781139237017.
20. Thali MJ, Dirnhofer R, Vock P. In: Thali M, Dirnhofer R, Vock P, editors. The virtopsy approach [Internet]. 1st ed. Boca Raton: CRC Press; 2009. https://www.taylorfrancis.com/books/9780849381898.
21. Roberts ISD, Traill ZC. Minimally invasive autopsy employing post-mortem CT and targeted coronary angiography: evaluation of its application to a routine coronial service. Histopathology [Internet]. 2014;64(2):211–7. http://doi.wiley.com/10.1111/his.12271.
22. Robinson C, Deshpande A, Richards C, Rutty G, Mason C, Morgan B. Post-mortem computed tomography in adult non-suspicious death investigation—evaluation of an NHS based service. BJR Open [Internet]. 2019;1(1):20190017. https://www.birpublications.org/doi/10.1259/bjro.20190017.
23. Chief Coroner. Guidance No 1. The use of post-mortem imaging (adults) [Internet]. 2016. https://www.judiciary.uk/wp-content/uploads/2013/09/guidance-no-1-use-of-port-mortem-imaging.pdf.
24. Bolliger SA, Thali MJ, Ross S, Buck U, Naether S, Vock P. Virtual autopsy using imaging: bridging radiologic and forensic sciences. A review of the virtopsy and similar projects. Eur Radiol [Internet]. 2008;18(2):273–82. http://link.springer.com/10.1007/s00330-007-0737-4.
25. O'Donnell C, Woodford N. Post-mortem radiology—a new sub-speciality? Clin Radiol [Internet]. 2008;63(11):1189–94. https://linkinghub.elsevier.com/retrieve/pii/S0009926008002122.
26. Baglivo M, Winklhofer S, Hatch GM, Ampanozi G, Thali MJ, Ruder TD. The rise of forensic and post-mortem radiology—analysis of the literature between the year 2000 and 2011. J Forensic Radiol Imaging [Internet]. 2013;1(1):3–9. https://linkinghub.elsevier.com/retrieve/pii/S2212478012000044.
27. Rutty JE, Morgan B, Rutty GN. Managing transformational change: implementing cross-sectional imaging into death investigation services in the United Kingdom. J Forensic Radiol Imaging [Internet]. 2015;3(1):57–60. https://linkinghub.elsevier.com/retrieve/pii/S2212478014001191.
28. NHS Implementation Sub-Group of the Department of Health. Can cross-sectional imaging as an adjunct and/or alternative to the invasive autopsy be implemented within the NHS? [Internet]. 2012. https://www.aaptuk.org/downloads/Cross-Sectional-Imaging-October-2012.pdf.
29. Roberts I, Traill Z. The radiological autopsy. In: Suvarna SK, editor. Atlas of adult autopsy [Internet]. Cham: Springer International Publishing; 2016. p. 362. http://link.springer.com/10.1007/978-3-319-27022-7_13.
30. Saukko P, Knight B. Knight's forensic pathology [Internet]. 4th ed. Boca Raton: CRC Press; 2015. https://www.routledge.com/Knights-Forensic-Pathology/Saukko-Knight/p/book/9780340972533.
31. HM Passport Office. Guidance for doctors completing medical certificates of cause of death in England and Wales [Internet]. 2018. https://assets.publishing.service.gov.uk/government/uploads/system/uploads/attachment_data/file/757010/guidance-for-doctors-completing-medical-certificates-of-cause-of-death.pdf.
32. Leadbeatter S, Lucas S, Lowe J. Standards for coroners' pathologists in post-mortem examinations of deaths that appear not to be suspicious [Internet]. The Royal College of Pathologists, London; 2014. https://www.rcpath.org/uploads/assets/1b02cfb9-000a-4b2f-b6b80256b719a5ee/Standards-for-Coroners-pathologists-in-post-mortem-examinations-of-deaths-that-appear-not-to-be-suspicious.pdf.

33. Rutty GN, Morgan B, Robinson C, Raj V, Pakkal M, Amoroso J, et al. Diagnostic accuracy of post-mortem CT with targeted coronary angiography versus autopsy for coroner-requested post-mortem investigations: a prospective, masked, comparison study. Lancet [Internet]. 2017;390(10090):145–54. https://linkinghub.elsevier.com/retrieve/pii/S0140673617303331.
34. Le Blanc-Louvry I, Thureau S, Duval C, Papin-Lefebvre F, Thiebot J, Dacher JN, et al. Post-mortem computed tomography compared to forensic autopsy findings: a French experience. Eur Radiol [Internet]. 2013;23(7):1829–35. http://link.springer.com/10.1007/s00330-013-2779-0.
35. Clarke M, McGregor A, Robinson C, Amoroso J, Morgan B, Rutty GN. Identifying the correct cause of death: the role of post-mortem computed tomography in sudden unexplained death. J Forensic Radiol Imaging [Internet]. 2014;2(4):210–2. https://linkinghub.elsevier.com/retrieve/pii/S2212478014001075.
36. Flach PM, Thali MJ, Germerott T. Times have changed! Forensic radiology—a new challenge for radiology and forensic pathology. Am J Roentgenol [Internet]. 2014;202(4):W325–34. http://www.ajronline.org/doi/10.2214/AJR.12.10283.
37. Maskell G, Wells M. RCR/RCPath statement on standards for medico-legal post-mortem cross-sectional imaging in adults [Internet]. The Royal College of Radiologists and The Royal College of Pathologists, London; 2012. https://www.rcr.ac.uk/system/files/publication/field_publication_files/FINALDOCUMENT_PMImaging_Oct12.pdf.
38. Bedford PJ. Should pathologists be reporting forensic CT scans? Acad Forensic Pathol [Internet]. 2012;2(2):198–201. http://journals.sagepub.com/doi/10.23907/2012.028.
39. Alkadhi H, Leschka S. Dual-energy CT: Principles, clinical value and potential applications in forensic imaging. J Forensic Radiol Imaging [Internet]. 2013;1(4):180–5. https://linkinghub.elsevier.com/retrieve/pii/S2212478013000956.
40. Persson A, Jackowski C, Engström E, Zachrisson H. Advances of dual source, dual-energy imaging in postmortem CT. Eur J Radiol [Internet]. 2008;68(3):446–55. https://linkinghub.elsevier.com/retrieve/pii/S0720048X08002507.

Practical Considerations of Post Mortem Computed Tomography and Report Writing

2

Introduction

With the increasing use of post mortem computed tomography (PMCT), there will be more call to commission services in bulk fashion, often as part of a service contract rather than an intermittent or ad hoc service, or paid for by relatives. There are many considerations, some of which will be familiar to those working in a clinical imaging department. Others will be specific to the post mortem setting and may therefore be unfamiliar unless appropriate training has been delivered. Some aspects of practice will interface with national or local guidelines, that need to be applied. Of note, there are the standards for medicolegal post mortem cross-sectional imaging in adults, written by the UK Royal College of Pathologists and the Royal College of Radiologists [1]. At the time of writing this book, new guidelines are being developed.

Factors Governing the Choice of PMCT

Case selection and how PMCT fits into death investigations should be an agreed process with the relevant medicolegal authorities, the pathologists, the mortuary and the relatives of the deceased. The process of using PMCT should be procured in stages. The first question is whether the case is suitable for PMCT, or whether a standard open autopsy without PMCT is the solution. It is noted that PMCT is a useful tool to confirm many specific pathological lesions and to exclude certain findings, but it is neither perfect nor all-encompassing. Some aspects of industrial lung disease, sepsis and metabolic processes may require open autopsy investigation, with the argument applied that adding in a PMCT study is just delaying matters. Others argue that knowledge from a scan before considering an open autopsy is always valuable [2].

A. Shenton et al., *Post Mortem CT for Non-Suspicious Adult Deaths*,
https://doi.org/10.1007/978-3-030-70829-0_2

Based on local preferences, and also given that there is some variation in coronial decision-making and different realities for the procurator fiscal, the case mix of PMCT studies can differ between services in different parts of the country. In some jurisdictions, all cases entering the mortuary will be scanned, including hospital deaths. In other centres, hospital deaths are excluded because the yield of PMCT to provide a cause of death is lower in this patient group. In some other jurisdictions, the progress towards PMCT is based upon the willingness and ability of the family or state to pay a fee for the radiological investigation. In short, there is no current standard rule or system of which case should progress to PMCT.

The coroner (or other medicolegal party) often has a specific set of cases that require active autopsy consideration. It also has to be understood that the information available to those considering these cases is often limited. This can make the decision of whether PMCT might be a suitable type of autopsy examination quite difficult. Examples of cases that almost always require some form of investigation include:

- The adult found deceased with no overt cause of death or appropriate supportive history, whether in hospital, nursing home or community.
- Witnessed collapse in an individual with no significant preceding history of illness or similar collapse events.
- Trauma, whether of a non-suspicious nature or non-natural type, including workplace injuries, road traffic incidents, injuries whilst inebriated and so on.
- Those not seen alive in the hospital or emergency department but certified deceased upon arrival at hospital in a state of cardiorespiratory arrest.
- In-hospital deaths, particularly in cases undergoing medical, obstetric, anaesthetic or surgical interaction, and where the underlying pathophysiology is unclear.
- Suicides, including hanging, drug overdose, various self-directed trauma, etc.
- Drowning in sea and fresh water.
- Industry-related deaths with these commonly implicating asbestos, coal, silica dust exposures, although this is not an exclusive list.
- Cases that have complaints and/or concerns regarding the medical/nursing care afforded to the deceased beforehand.

When PMCT is being offered and discussed with the relatives, the bereaved family should be informed of the potentials and limitations of imaging. This might mean that if no clear diagnosis is achieved, a traditional open autopsy may still be required [3]. It is worth noting that cases with areas of concern will often merit additional open autopsy procedures anyway. In many other cases, however, the radiological information obtained will allow a cause of death to be defined by the pathologist and to permit appropriate registration of death paperwork.

PMCT Scanning Facility Options

There are both advantages and disadvantages of using dedicated rather than public health service facilities. Co-located mortuary and CT facilities offer easy body transfer from storage fridges to the scanner and reduces scan turnaround times. The benefit of having experienced mortuary staff is vital when learning how to handle bodies and when angiography techniques are being employed. The mortuary staff can also assist with the timely aspiration of toxicology samples for any cases that might require this investigation (Figs. 2.1, 2.2, and 2.3).

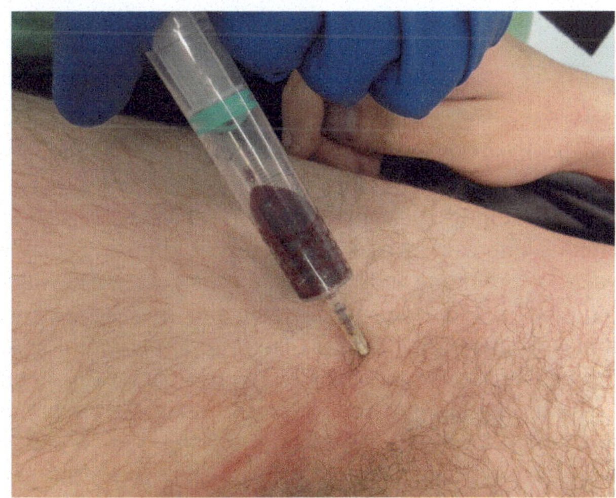

Fig. 2.1 Post mortem sampling of blood can be accomplished by direct needle aspiration from the femoral vessels

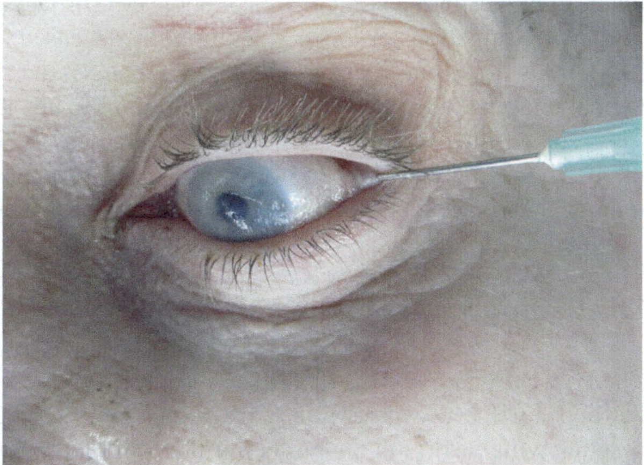

Fig. 2.2 The vitreous can be sampled by needle aspiration of fluid from the eye, with subsequent re-filling of the eye afterwards with water

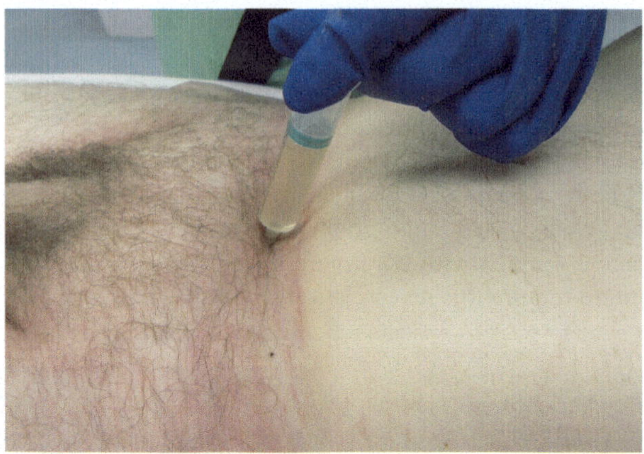

Fig. 2.3 The bladder is usually easy to sample by needle passed centrally just above the pubis, although this requires the bladder to contain some urine. The PMCT can be used to assess bladder filling prior to aspiration

The disadvantages of this co-location are that there will likely be an initial set-up capital investment and (probably) no opportunity to use the scanner for potentially profitable clinical activity to offset running costs. Radiographic staff will need to be employed to work in co-located units. Radiologists may work on-site with the added value of providing individualised protocols, reviewing images before the body is returned from the scanner and being directly available for case discussions. However, it may be more practical for a larger group of radiologists to be remotely accessible through teleradiology, email and equivalent on-line communications.

Using local health service facilities for PMCT by special arrangement may be more simple and cheaper overall, but this should not conflict with imaging of the living. Radiographers might then be more accessible throughout the day, but some will need to be trained and available for angiogram procedures or other appropriate personnel be available if required. Another factor is the sensitivity element of bringing dead bodies into a clinical area, where staff (or visitors) may not be accustomed to such investigations or indeed handling the deceased.

There is no requirement by the UK Human Tissue Authority (HTA) that radiological imaging of a body (including angiography) needs to occur on licensed premises. This contrasts with traditional open autopsy where tissue sampling would likely occur. Imaging sites do however need to be licensed if there is any potential removal of tissue, such as blood for toxicology or needle biopsy.

The Radiographer in the PMCT Unit

The conventional practice of PMCT requires a trained radiographer working with the body of the deceased in a CT scanner unit. The radiographer undertakes the imaging with the digital images being stored for later consideration, or rarely immediate reporting by a radiologist or imaging-trained pathologist. Internationally, other systems exist with mortuary staff or forensic technologists being trained to provide day to day use of equipment [4, 5].

An experienced radiographer can also offer a wealth of knowledge when setting up services and how to use the equipment to achieve the best images possible. They will be able to find solutions to 'work around' difficult patient positioning, deal with various post mortem artefacts and compensate for scanner limitations. If the scanned images are sent remotely to the radiologist, then a more autonomous role of the radiographer will be necessary to undertake additional image series, perhaps as per agreed protocols or as judged appropriate to the circumstances. Any PMCT service will be dependent on the quality of images produced. In the United Kingdom, the Society of Radiographers has published standards of radiographic practice [6].

One early worry was the potentially distressing nature of the service, dealing with the dead, with possible psychological risks to the staff involved. Appropriate education and support should be made available for any staff working in this environment if they have never interacted with the deceased beforehand [6]. However, our experience to date is that the radiographers adapt well with appropriate and ongoing support.

Scanning Technique

There are many options for scanning technique, and these will be tailored to local facilities and preferences. One option is to scan the whole body, from head-to-toes in one acquisition, capturing all the data, rather than potentially having to return the body to the scanner for additional assessment (Fig. 2.4).

The total body scan depends on the scanner available; factors that should be considered include the room size, gantry bore size and table length. If scanning rooms have size limitations, then body handling will be an issue, which has implications for the radiographer as well as the mortuary staff.

Alternative protocols split the body into sections such as head and neck, chest to pelvis and pelvis to toes. Not all PMCT protocols include full leg length imaging, as this part of the body (thigh downwards) rarely has any unexpected pathology of significance in terms of the cause of death.

Suggested scan parameters will vary for different machines although they do not differ much from clinical applications to ensure the best images. Dose reduction techniques are not an essential consideration. However, it does not automatically mean that increasing the radiation dose will result in better pictures. Scans may be reconstructed to variable slice thicknesses, but to make best use of multi-planar reconstructions (MPR), 1 mm slices are recommended. When scanning thin slices over such a length, however, X-ray tube overload may become an issue, particularly if numerous cases are being examined in a relatively short period of time.

If whole-body scanning is required but technically not possible on the available scanner, then two acquisitions may be undertaken. This solution involves moving the body from head-first to feet-first, although this has significant time and manual handling implications. Rarely, only one area of body scanning is required, such as the head. In these cases, there is often cross-sectional imaging available taken in hospital shortly before death.

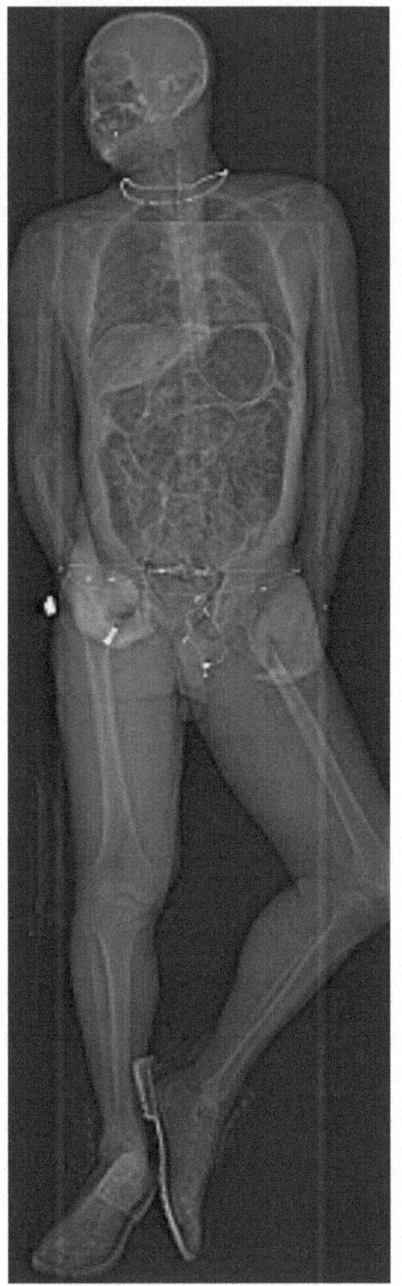

Fig. 2.4 Scanogram/scout image of a whole body with clothing, shoes and jewellery still in place. The body is positioned with knee flexed and head turned due to rigor mortis

The issues of radiation dose, renal function (for contrast administration) and subject movement artefact do not apply in the PMCT setting, but there are other issues to consider. Contrast administration (angiography) into a non-flowing vascular system, body positioning problems and decomposition factors may be present.

Looking at the safety requirements surrounding use of ionising radiation [7], there are regulations governing radiation protection, equipment maintenance and calibration, also health and safety for handling the deceased, infection control and cleaning factors to be considered, notwithstanding the practical aspects of manual handling. These matters will need careful evaluation by those working in the mortuary and PMCT suite, with potential variations to solutions compared to clinical settings.

Wherever the scan takes place, it is imperative that image acquisition is of a high standard, ideally being performed as soon as practicable so that any decomposition change is minimised. The process of imaging should not delay the investigation and progression of the body towards funeral arrangements. Factors of privacy and dignity should always be preserved at all times when providing this sensitive service.

Body Handling and Positioning

During transportation to the mortuary and within the building itself, the body will normally remain within a body bag (Fig. 2.5). This bag protects mortuary staff, the radiographer and the scanner from potential leakage of body fluids. The scan can be performed without opening the bag, which is advisable in cases of decomposition (Fig. 2.6), severe trauma with body fluid leakage or in cases which have a potential infection risk. One is also mindful of the reality that radiographers are not generally used to direct inspection or interaction with deceased bodies, and it is an aesthetic principle to keep the bag closed during the interaction with the scanner suite on most occasions.

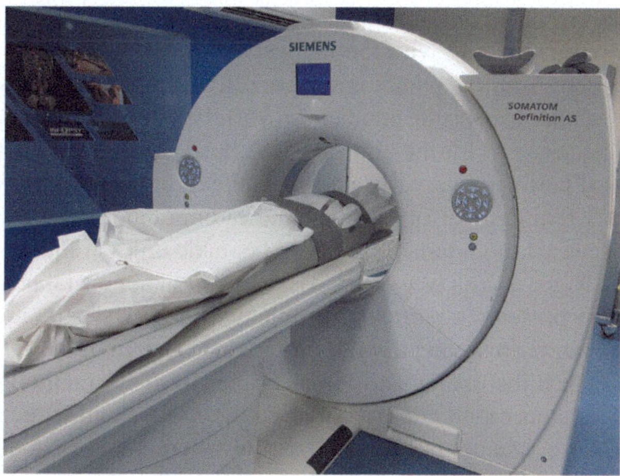

Fig. 2.5 A PMCT scanner with a body awaiting scan. The body is enclosed in a securely sealed bag for safe and hygienic case transfer

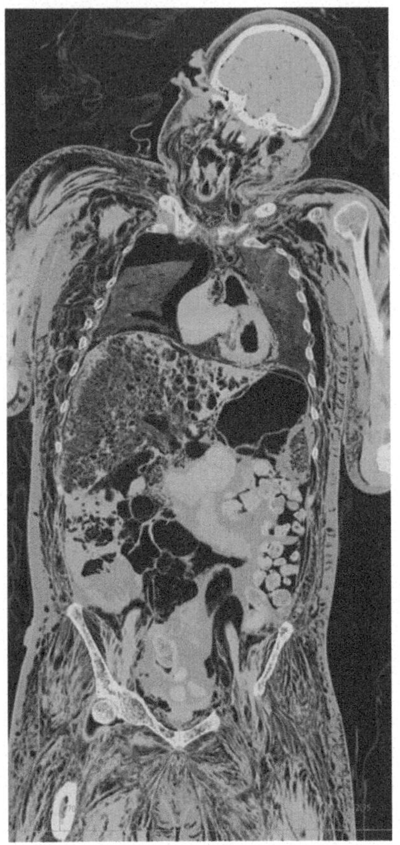

Fig. 2.6 Coronal view of the head to pelvis on lung windows shows extensive soft tissue gas due to decomposition

If possible, body bags should be free from metallic or other items, as this may cause artefacts. This does not mean that the body will arrive in an unclothed state or covered solely by a shroud. It follows that, on occasion, the bag may require opening to permit removal of such items if this will enhance the scan or prevent artefacts from interfering with the images obtained. Permission for this interaction may be sought from the pathologist or medicolegal representative instructing the scan.

Other aspects of interaction with the body may include better positioning in the scanner or to lift the arms over the head when scanning the torso. The radiographer may perform such tasks, although the mortuary staff may be better placed to deliver this requirement or to assist the radiographer. As always when dealing with the deceased, no interaction should be made unless requested and providing it is safe.

Rigor mortis (see Chap. 3) can result in abnormal positioning (Figs. 2.4 and 2.7). This presents a particular problem when body parts are positioned in such a way that they do not readily fit through the aperture of the CT scanner. It may be suitable to teach the operator to 'break' rigor mortis (a method of firmly stretching the tissues adjacent to a joint to realign the limb) to allow better positioning of the body. A large scanner bore size is helpful when scanning bodies in such nonconventional positions, either due to rigor or other pathology (Fig. 2.8). Such scanners are also useful in dealing with those bodies with a raised body mass index (Fig. 2.9).

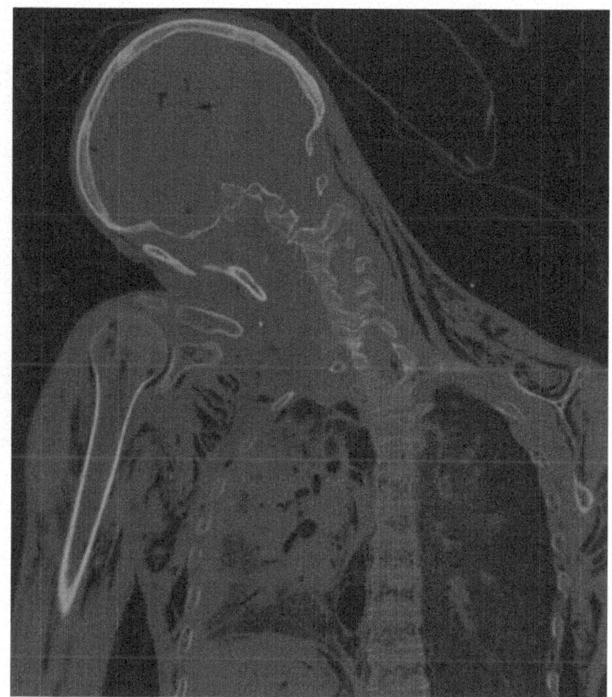

Fig. 2.7 Coronal view of the head, neck and chest on bone windows shows abnormal body positioning due to rigor mortis

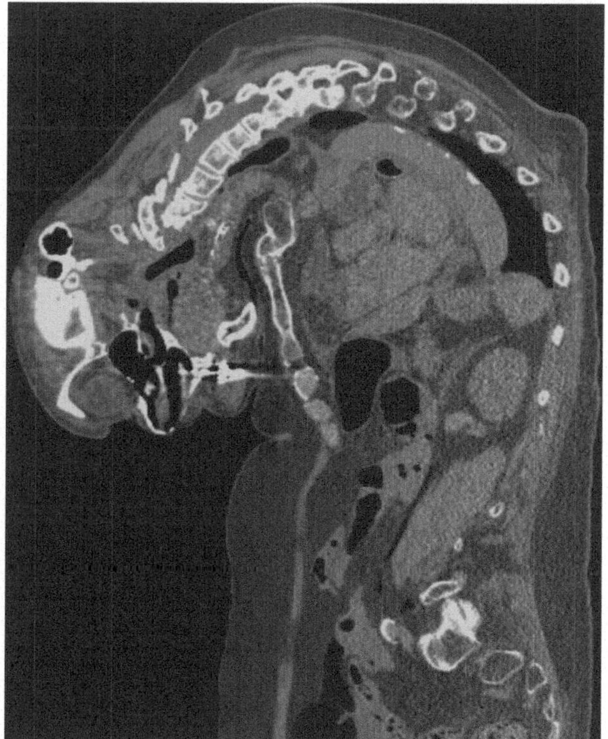

Fig. 2.8 Sagittal view of the head to pelvis on soft tissue windows shows non-conventional positioning due to fixed flexion deformities in a patient with multiple sclerosis

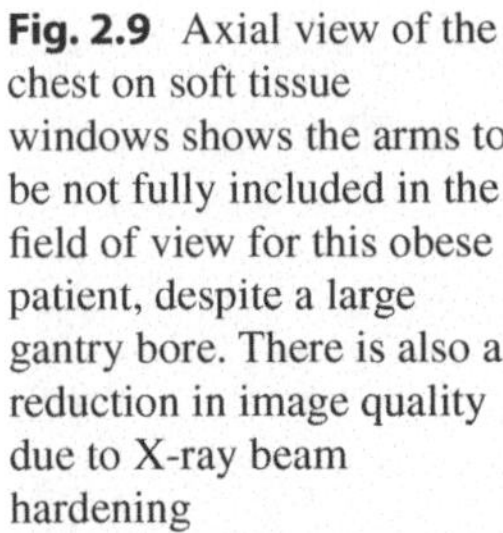

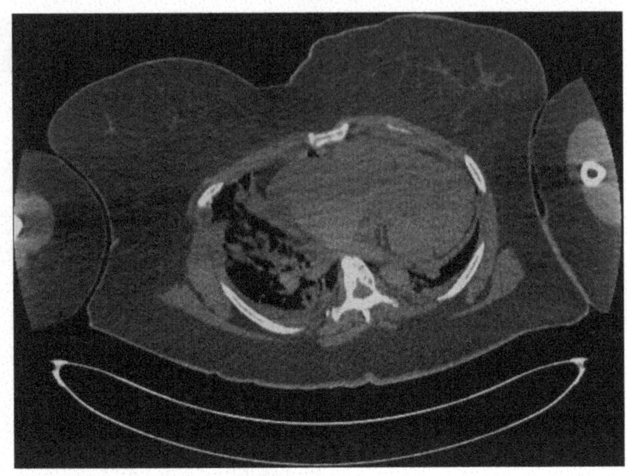

Fig. 2.9 Axial view of the chest on soft tissue windows shows the arms to be not fully included in the field of view for this obese patient, despite a large gantry bore. There is also a reduction in image quality due to X-ray beam hardening

Contrast Media and PMCT Angiography

In general, one knows that clinical CT without contrast is more limited in the detail it can offer, particularly regarding the vascular system and soft tissues. The same reality applies to PMCT examinations, although plain CT is the norm for PMCT in the United Kingdom.

The use of contrast may potentially increase the yield of the examination [8, 9], assuming it is successfully placed into the vasculature. However, one must appreciate that it automatically changes the nature of the test from non-invasive to minimally invasive. Some centres may prefer to have a decision algorithm for when to progress to angiography, whereas others have devolved this decision to either the radiologist and/or the pathologist.

For PMCT with angiography, cannulation of the deceased is commonly undertaken by a mortuary technician or pathologist. It may prompt consideration of whether toxicology, microbiology, and other tests are required at this point. The use of targeted contrast has not been shown to affect subsequent toxicology analysis, but medicolegal considerations usually mandate that all removal of samples for toxicological analysis (Figs. 2.1, 2.2, and 2.3) and other tests should occur prior to angiography to avoid any potential legal challenge to test results.

There are different options for post mortem CT angiography (PMCTA), such as whole-body or targeted techniques [10], which will be chosen according to the preceding history, the question being asked and local skill set of the radiographer and facilities available. The technique and application of targeted coronary angiography are discussed further in Chap. 8.

Ventilated PMCT

The collapse of lung tissue following death and the secondary pooling of blood into the pulmonary circulation may limit radiological assessment of the lung parenchyma of the deceased. Consequently, methods of artificially ventilated PMCT have been developed in order to improve the diagnostic quality of lung imaging using a number of different techniques [11]. The technique of inflating the lung can mimic inspiration, thereby clearing some post mortem atelectasis and hypostasis without altering any true pathology [11]. As will be appreciated, any such technique requires additional time and resource. It should certainly not be used where there is risk of transmitting any respiratory infection.

When already present (e.g. following resuscitation attempts) an existing airway can be used. However, if none is present, an airway can be introduced or instead lung inflation can be achieved by using a continuous positive airway pressure (CPAP) mask. In adults, the airway pressure can be provided and maintained by a portable ventilator. If rigor mortis prevents oral airway insertion, a tracheostomy can be performed, although this is clearly an invasive procedure that should not occur without due consideration and appropriate permission.

The Radiologist and PMCT

The radiological skills required to interpret PMCT are broadly the same as those required to interpret cross-sectional imaging in the living [1] although the subject knowledge differs. The interpretation should be undertaken by either a qualified radiologist or a medical practitioner with equivalent competencies in cross-sectional imaging. However, even for radiologists with many years of experience, it is clear that some training is required when dealing with the deceased, as there are different considerations to be made if one wishes to avoid significant image misinterpretation.

It is recommended that specific training is supplied by an experienced practitioner, rather than the ad hoc method of simply learning 'as one goes along'. For example, a knowledge of the wide range of normal appearances after death and particularly the appearance of decomposition is required from the beginning. This is not always obvious and cannot be extrapolated solely from knowledge of scanning the living or a few post mortem cases. Post mortem changes vary greatly depending on the time since death occurred and many other factors.

Most clinical radiologists will also require some training in the mechanisms and language of death used in the medicolegal arena and by pathologists. They will require some understanding of how the process of death investigation takes place. This has particular pertinence, as many of the cases will ultimately be debated in court. It should be understood that lawyers and other medicolegal practitioners may take particular interest in the wording of a radiology report, particularly if it is at variance with the preceding clinical history or any open post mortem pathology.

There is currently no mandatory training or examination in PMCT, although many radiology training centres are now starting to teach this method of investigation as part of standard radiology learning. In the United Kingdom, there are also several groups providing dedicated teaching for established practitioners. There is a wealth of scientific literature available [12]. It is noted that the UK Royal College of Pathologists autopsy exam now has questions dealing with PMCT cases. However, the pathologists are not required to read the radiological images but rather to interpret the radiology reports and to debate possible causes of death.

If the radiologist has no prior experience of working in the autopsy arena, then going to see open autopsies, if possible, with local pathologists that use PMCT in their practice, is invaluable for understanding the examination. Alternatively, there are books that describe and illustrate the open autopsy procedure [13, 14]. The converse is true for pathologists, with their practice being enhanced if they develop an understanding of the methodology of imaging and how reports are produced. This will benefit from targeted teaching and reading relevant texts. This enhanced understanding between the different disciplines will naturally benefit both the radiologist and the autopsy pathologist.

The PMCT Report

There is no single, fixed and perfect way to write a PMCT report. There are many different models that are used across the United Kingdom and indeed further afield. However, all reports start in the same way, with the referral of the case for examination, usually with accompanying information. The request for imaging will come from the coroner's office (or equivalent) and will be accompanied by a medicolegal report and/or clinical history from the general practitioner or hospital clinicians. The full medical history should always be made available for use.

As ever, the history is of paramount importance to the interpretation of any imaging findings. Any circumstantial information surrounding the death or medical history will need to be set against whether the death was expected or not; whether it was sudden or prolonged; witnessed or un-witnessed. The history data must be considered against the known past medical history for the individual whilst appreciating that any previous medical history may actually be irrelevant to the cause of death. How and where the body was found may also have bearing upon the interpretation of findings. The data provided may also guide the need for additional tests, such as toxicology and microbiology.

In addition to this background data, it can be helpful to know the time since death (post mortem interval or PMI), as this may affect the interpretation of appearances/decomposition. Knowledge of whether cardiopulmonary resuscitation (CPR) was attempted is important, particularly in the context of broken ribs from chest compressions. The reporter should read any information made available but bear in mind that sometimes the information is incomplete or preliminary in its nature and on occasion almost completely wrong!

The PMCT scan should be reviewed in the same systematic manner as any clinical examination. The analysis needs to be undertaken with appropriate time being available, without distractions and with the opportunity to interact with other parties as deemed appropriate. Unlike an open autopsy, in PMCT there exists the opportunity for further independent review of unaltered images and therefore possible future case debate and challenges. The reporter needs to be mindful that adversarial criticism of the report may occur later in court. However, looking at this from a positive perspective, the ability to store images and have additional opinion later also allows for quality improvement and learning, such as from double reporting and audit. It is also relevant in terms of case discussion between colleagues before any PMCT report is issued to the pathologist.

In general, it is important to document all existing pathology that may, or may not, have contributed to death. It is only by taking a holistic perspective on the case that any determination can be made. However, not all cases have a clear interpretation or diagnosis. The radiologist's conclusion in terms of the likely cause of death might cross quite a range of possibilities and probabilities. These might be expressed as 'definite', 'probable' or 'possible' causes of death.

When reporting PMCT as an adjunctive technique, (such that full or limited open autopsy follows), the report should allow the pathologist to plan the autopsy. Perhaps the most useful aspect of an 'inconclusive' PMCT analysis is permitting the pathologist to focus on one part of the body. Arbitrarily, the body compartments may be divided into the cranial cavity, the neck, the chest, the abdomen and the pelvis. Information as to the normality of tissues in these regions may avoid time being wasted on unnecessary dissection, which would have no pathology or relevance to the cause of death. In addition, limiting the dissection may also improve the acceptability of the open autopsy to the relatives.

The PMCT analysis should also provide information with regard to any potential open autopsy hazards (e.g. bony fragments) as well as the position of any foreign bodies (orthopaedic implants, pacemakers, bullets etc.). The scan may also provide important information about anatomic anomalies such as aberrant vessels and any suspicion of infection risks such as tuberculosis. Furthermore, the consequences of any surgical intervention previously may be apparent on PMCT, acting to guide a specific dissection approach during an invasive autopsy.

Turning to the substance of the report, one is mindful that this depends on various factors. The first is the time available to produce the report, which is often reflected in the length of the report data presented. This includes whether focal or whole-body studies are reviewed, along with any additional series or angiography. Then, there is the amount of detail provided. Overall, the quality of the report is not to be measured by the word count but rather by the data presented and the content/style of discussion. It is accepted that different radiologists will work at different paces and in different ways, reflecting the individual reporter's experience and confidence. Therefore, the time taken to write a report, and its structure, will inevitably be variable.

Broadly speaking, straightforward cases with catastrophic findings and a history commensurate with the radiological views can be dealt with quite promptly by an experienced reporter. Rapid reporting is possible, particularly when using structured reports or proformas, along with voice dictation software. These reports will take considerably less time than complex cases with multiple comorbidities, which often have competing pathophysiological events prior to death. Nevertheless, it is reasonable to expect a PMCT report to be provided within 4–24 h of the scan being completed. There may need to be some very fast progression of reporting, where religious or family social issues prompt urgent case completion for funeral purposes. One should be as helpful as possible in these cases but always within acceptable professional standards.

As with all autopsy matters, unless authorised by the coroner, the person making a post mortem radiological examination must not communicate the full, or part of their report, to any person other than the coroner, their officers or the pathologist [15]. This confidentiality is mandated by medicolegal realities, and inappropriate release of information may be tested in court. The very basic level of confidentiality is at least equivalent to clinical practice. Yet, it is also worth noting that the family may later be given copies of the final post mortem report by the coroner or procurator fiscal, which may include a copy or full transcript of the PMCT report.

It should be remembered that pathologists are required to specifically mention negative findings when reporting a post mortem examination [16]. The same is advised for the radiological report. Important negatives should be included to a standard and structure agreed between radiologist and pathologist to aid in report confidence and understanding. However, as with clinical imaging, wasting time detailing multiple irrelevant findings whilst missing important data results in a report that is often of little practical use. Any limitations of PMCT study, if these apply, should always be made clear. A thorough and useful report is always required, as the pathologist may cite the radiological report as reason for their conclusions when formulating a cause of death. It is currently usual practice for the pathologist to retain a central coordinating role in the establishment of the cause of death [1] although in the future other arrangements may develop.

Now turning to the report construct itself, one appreciates that all reporters (trainees and established specialists/consultants) will usually, or at least initially, benefit from a defined report structure. This often uses a systematic approach to the body compartments and organs, which should avoid missing important findings. The use of a proforma template can be adapted and refined to local and/or personal preference.

One may then choose to follow a free text style of structured reporting, or potentially follow a sequential checklist of items, to be assessed as present or absent. This latter approach is favoured in the forensic setting [17, 18]. Both are acceptable. When assembling the data for the report, the following items are normally required to achieve a full summary. Not all need to be present on every occasion, but (serving as an example checklist) they are there to remind the reporter of the totality of the examination:

- *General introduction*
  - Background information, from the coroner, and occasionally from the ambulance service or police.
  - Past medical history, including medications of relevance to the case.
  - Whether resuscitation was attempted.
- *External findings*
  - Vascular lines, drainage tubes and implanted devices.
  - Ligatures or clothing affecting the imaging.
  - External trauma.
- *Internal findings*
  - Decomposition assessment, indicating if the quality of the study is not satisfactory.
  - Head (brain, cranial bones and local soft tissues).
  - Neck (soft tissues, cervical spine, airway, thyroid).
  - Chest (soft tissues, lungs, pleural tissues, mediastinum, heart, bones).
  - Coronary artery calcification, possibly augmented by the Agatston calcium score.
  - CT coronary angiography findings if applicable.
  - Abdomen and pelvis (soft tissues, major organs, the bowel, the pelvic tissues, bones).
  - Retroperitoneum (aorta, kidneys, soft tissues).
  - Musculoskeletal/limbs (soft tissues, bones).
- *Clinicoradiological correlation*
  - Free text description.
  - Cause of death (definite, probable, possible, unascertained or defined in standard format: 1a, 1b, 1c; and contributory factor/s 2)
  - Potential autopsy hazards such as fractures, foreign bodies and aberrant vessels.

As indicated at the start of the chapter, there is no single solution to reporting a PMCT scan. However, for the benefit of the beginner, one example of a complete report might be as given below:

Clinical Data

This 75-year-old male had a history of emphysema and lung basal scarring, along with recurrent chest infections. There was a history of previous myocardial infarction 2 years ago, and hyperlipidaemia. There had been a previous hip replacement and history of osteoporosis. He was found deceased at home. CPR attempts were unsuccessful.

External Findings

No pacemaker or other implanted device.
Minimal expected post mortem decomposition changes.

Brain, Head and Neck
Normal ventricular system and extra-axial spaces. Diminished differentiation between grey and white matter is a normal post mortem finding. No intracranial haemorrhage, acute large vessel infarct or space-occupying lesion. Background of periventricular small vessel ischemic changes.
Normal skull vault and cervical spine.
Normal soft tissues of the neck. Normal intra-orbital contents.

Thorax
No supraclavicular, axillary or mediastinal lymphadenopathy.
Heart enlarged with a cardiothoracic ratio of 0.63. No haemopericardium. Significant coronary calcification (Agatston score total 2238). Marked mitral valve annulus calcification. Normal sedimentation in the pulmonary arteries. Normal calibre thoracic aorta.
Small volume bilateral pleural effusion. Background of centrilobular and paraseptal emphysema. Symmetrical ground-glass opacities displaying a dependent gradient in keeping with normal fluid hypostasis. No focal air-space consolidation to suggest pneumonia.

Abdomen and Pelvis
No free fluid. No free gas. Normal post mortem appearances of the liver and gallbladder. Normal pancreas. Normal spleen. Bilateral, uncomplicated cysts up to 2.0 cm in both kidneys. Normal urinary bladder. Enlarged prostate measures 5 cm transverse.
Incidental right adrenal adenoma measuring 1.5 cm. Normal left adrenal gland.
Sigmoid diverticulosis with no acute feature. No focal bowel mass or obstruction.
No abdominal or pelvic lymphadenopathy.
Incidental aneurysm of the abdominal aorta—4.0 cm. No retroperitoneal haematoma.

Musculoskeletal
There is generalised osteopenia. Acute, bilateral, inner cortex rib fractures are judged consistent with attempted cardiopulmonary resuscitation. Superior endplate fractures of L3 and L4 appear old. There is generalised peripheral vascular atherosclerosis.

Clinicoradiological Correlation

1. *Extensive atherosclerosis of the coronary arteries (calcium score of 2238 equates to a high risk of a significant coronary artery stenosis). In the absence of another demonstrated pathology, an acute cardiac event is considered a possible cause of death.*
2. *Background of paraseptal and centrilobular lung emphysema. No features of (superimposed) chest infection.*
3. *No acute or suspicious intracranial/intra-abdominal findings.*

[Note: Some PMCT centres provide a cause of death, with the radiologist stating the cause of death as per medical certificate of cause of death (MCCD) format at this point. Many pathologists prefer not to have such analysis provided in case there is any disparity that could provoke confusion in a court setting.]

When coming to conclusions, the radiologist should always remain mindful that many pathologies can be identified on the scans that might have no bearing upon the cause of death. For example, there is a high prevalence of coronary artery calcification seen on PMCT images. Coronary artery disease is a common reality (reflecting the Western diet and other risk factors), but this does not mean that it is the cause of death, unless there is other corroborative data and the clear absence of alternate pathologies.

The authors would recommend using a common lexicon to define level of certainty in a diagnosis or the suggested cause of death, for example the term 'probable' being a certainty above 75% and 'possible' above 50% [19]. An agreed manner of describing pathology to assist those instructing the autopsy and/or the pathologist will also aid case analysis.

Nevertheless, despite high-quality imaging and experienced interpretation, in some cases, and especially when there is a lack of clinical history, the cause of death may remain unclear or, in medicolegal terminology, 'unascertained'.

Quality Assurance and Audit

All services providing post mortem imaging data and diagnoses should be subject to review of findings and audit [1] in the same manner as would be expected in a clinical setting. Local arrangements may also include occasional double reporting by radiologists, discussion of diagnoses and potential review of the radiology by the pathologists and analysis correlation of PMCT results against the final cause of death provided. These review policies will naturally benefit the family, medicolegal representatives and society. Ultimately, multidisciplinary working and review can be invaluable for discussion of findings, learning, continuous professional development and decision-making. This is unfortunately not always practical or achievable with the differing and complex working patterns of radiologists and pathologists, particularly if working in separate locations. As with any aspect of clinical practice, continuing professional development (CPD), in the form of literature, courses and online resources, is important for appraisal and revalidation.

References

1. Maskell G, Wells M. RCR/RCPath statement on standards for medico-legal post-mortem cross-sectional imaging in adults [Internet]. The Royal College of Radiologists and The Royal College of Pathologists, London; 2012. https://www.rcr.ac.uk/system/files/publication/field_publication_files/FINALDOCUMENT_PMImaging_Oct12.pdf.
2. Roberts I, Traill Z. The radiological autopsy. In: Suvarna SK, editor. Atlas of adult autopsy [Internet]. Cham: Springer International Publishing; 2016. p. 362. http://link.springer.com/10.1007/978-3-319-27022-7_13.
3. Chief Coroner. Guidance no. 1. The use of post-mortem imaging (adults) [Internet]. 2016. https://www.judiciary.uk/wp-content/uploads/2013/09/guidance-no-1-use-of-port-mortem-imaging.pdf.
4. Bedford PJ, Oesterhelweg L. Different conditions and strategies to utilize forensic radiology in the cities of Melbourne, Australia and Berlin, Germany. Forensic Sci Med Pathol [Internet]. 2013;9(3):321–6. http://link.springer.com/10.1007/s12024-013-9424-8.
5. Bedford PJ. Should pathologists be reporting forensic CT scans? Acad Forensic Pathol [Internet]. 2012;2(2):198–201. http://journals.sagepub.com/doi/10.23907/2012.028.
6. Standards of radiographic practice for post-mortem cross-sectional imaging (PMC-SI) [Internet]. The Society and College of Radiographers and the International Association of Forensic Radiographers, London; 2015. https://www.sor.org/Learning-advice/Professional-body-guidance-and-publications/Documents-and-publications/Policy-Guidance-Document-Library/Standards-of-Radiographic-Practice-for-Post-Mortem.
7. The ionising radiations regulations 2017 no. 1075 [Internet]. http://www.legislation.gov.uk/uksi/2017/1075/contents/made.
8. Ross SG, Bolliger SA, Ampanozi G, Oesterhelweg L, Thali MJ, Flach PM. Postmortem CT angiography: capabilities and limitations in traumatic and natural causes of death. RadioGraphics [Internet]. 2014;34(3):830–46. http://pubs.rsna.org/doi/10.1148/rg.343115169.
9. Grabherr S, Heinemann A, Vogel H, Rutty G, Morgan B, Woźniak K, et al. Postmortem CT angiography compared with autopsy: a forensic multicenter study. Radiology [Internet]. 2018;288(1):270–6. http://pubs.rsna.org/doi/10.1148/radiol.2018170559.
10. Grabherr S, Grimm J, Dominguez A, Vanhaebost J, Mangin P. Advances in post-mortem CT-angiography. Br J Radiol [Internet]. 2014;87(1036):20130488. http://www.birpublications.org/doi/10.1259/bjr.20130488.
11. Rutty GN, Morgan B, Germerott T, Thali M, Athurs O. Ventilated post-mortem computed tomography—A historical review. J Forensic Radiol Imaging [Internet]. 2016;4:35–42. https://linkinghub.elsevier.com/retrieve/pii/S2212478016300028.
12. Baglivo M, Winklhofer S, Hatch GM, Ampanozi G, Thali MJ, Ruder TD. The rise of forensic and post-mortem radiology—analysis of the literature between the year 2000 and 2011. J Forensic Radiol Imaging [Internet]. 2013;1(1):3–9. https://linkinghub.elsevier.com/retrieve/pii/S2212478012000044.

13. Burton JL and Rutty G. The hospital autopsy [Internet]. 3rd ed. London: CRC Press; 2010. https://www.routledge.com/The-Hospital-Autopsy-A-Manual-of-Fundamental-Autopsy-Practice-Third-Edition/Burton-Rutty/p/book/9780340965146.
14. Suvarna SK, editor. Atlas of adult autopsy [Internet]. 1st ed. Cham: Springer International Publishing; 2016. http://link.springer.com/10.1007/978-3-319-27022-7.
15. The coroners rules 1984 No. 552 PART III rule 10 [Internet]. http://www.legislation.gov.uk/uksi/1984/552/article/10/made.
16. Leadbeatter S, Lucas S, Lowe J. Standards for coroners' pathologists in post-mortem examinations of deaths that appear not to be suspicious [Internet]. The Royal College of Pathologists, London; 2014. https://www.rcpath.org/uploads/assets/1b02cfb9-000a-4b2f-b6b80256b719a5ee/Standards-for-Coroners-pathologists-in-post-mortem-examinations-of-deaths-that-appear-not-to-be-suspicious.pdf.
17. Schweitzer W, Bartsch C, Ruder TD, Thali MJ. Virtopsy approach: structured reporting versus free reporting for PMCT findings. J Forensic Radiol Imaging [Internet]. 2014;2(1):28–33. https://linkinghub.elsevier.com/retrieve/pii/S2212478013001251.
18. Reporting forensic PMCT cases [Internet] (accessed 2019 Nov 22). https://virtopsy.com/virtopsy-education-2-cas/.
19. Panicek DM, Hricak H. How sure are you, doctor? A standardized Lexicon to describe the radiologist's level of certainty. Am J Roentgenol [Internet]. 2016;207(1):2–3. http://www.ajronline.org/doi/10.2214/AJR.15.15895.

Death, Post Mortem Changes and Decomposition on Post Mortem Computed Tomography

3

Introduction

This chapter sets out to consider 'death' and the terminology used in assessing bodies after death. These are specified with the various pathology terms and features, explained in chronological sequence to aid the appreciation of related radiology changes. Factors that may increase the rate of body decay (decomposition) are presented along with some artefacts affecting bodies, which are not seen in the radiology of the living.

Death and its Broad Causes

It is reasonable to first consider what is meant by 'death'. One could look at it simply as the endpoint of life, but in most cases, death is said to have occurred after cessation of cardiac and respiratory effort. Alternatively, in hospital settings, one might regard death as having occurred after loss of higher brain function [1], or one might define it as somatic and cellular death [2]. However, even if one addresses this matter from a scientific/medical standpoint, one should be aware that society, religion and the relatives often have varying views on this matter [3]. These are beyond the scope of this chapter, although various literary and online texts on the subject exist.

There are a variety of reasons why death may occur. Many are natural in type, reflecting standard pathological deaths in the community and in hospitals. Indeed, these cases will make up the majority of the post mortem computerised tomography (PMCT) service workload. Put simply, most autopsy radiology is concerned with natural death processes, such as ageing and complications of various metabolic and structural diseases. Examples would include cardiovascular disease, chest infections, cancers and so on [4]. The radiologist should remember that many cases, at the point of death, have had a period of attempted resuscitation, usually involving

A. Shenton et al., *Post Mortem CT for Non-Suspicious Adult Deaths*,
https://doi.org/10.1007/978-3-030-70829-0_3

chest compressions and ventilatory support—which may also have effects on the ultimate PMCT appearances.

However, one must be aware that death can also follow an episode of intoxication, starvation, dehydration, suicide or trauma. Any and all of these may cause an individual to be admitted to hospital or may cause death within a medically supervised background, rather than in the community. There are also deaths that are the consequence of adverse nursing and/or medical (iatrogenic) interactions. These may involve errors of diagnosis and treatment, aspects of neglect and potentially negligence. Far less common are deaths caused by physical assaults, poisoning, homicides and animal predation. Suspicious deaths are covered in forensic pathology texts [2].

Society places great importance on the date and time of death, yet one is aware that the physical body persists after this event. The body no longer remains stable, as it did until the point of death, losing its various homeostatic biochemical and physiological processes. After death these reactions stop, the cells start to autolyse (break down) and the characteristic post mortem (decomposition) features start to develop. In addition, there is microbial interaction enhancing tissue breakdown, usually beginning in the gut (Fig. 3.1) and leading to putrefaction. Decomposition,

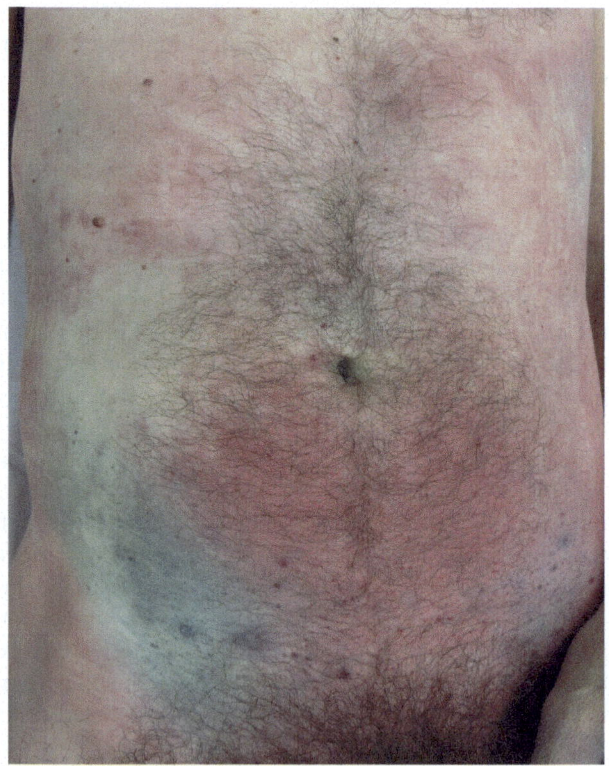

Fig. 3.1 Early-stage decomposition shows as green discolouration of the abdomen near the caecum

the overall body process of autolysis, is a progressive (yet variable) process often reflecting ambient temperature. Consequently, interpretation of post mortem imaging requires an appreciation of the range of possible appearances of the decaying body.

All of the broad causes of death and factors surrounding the deceased may have bearing on how the body is seen on PMCT, with this being complicated by tissue autolysis and breakdown of the body. An understanding and appreciation of normal/expected post mortem changes is crucial to avoid erroneous interpretation of any structural pathological changes [5], as it can be more difficult to define true pathology in and among the ongoing decomposition realities.

Nevertheless, there is still a role for scanning even in cases of moderate and advanced decomposition and putrefaction, as PMCT may reveal significant pathology such as trauma, cerebral or other haemorrhage [6, 7]. If no catastrophic event is demonstrated, a scan can also be complementary to invasive autopsy in demonstrating foreign bodies/devices and bony findings (e.g. fractures). Comparison of PMCT with clinical imaging can also play a role in body identification [8], particularly from dental assessment.

Post Mortem Interval

The date and time of death should ideally be provided in any supporting information by the person/s requesting the PMCT scan. If death was not witnessed or recorded, this may be an estimate of the likely time of death or just the time and date when the body was discovered.

The time between death and another timepoint such as the scan is known as the post mortem interval (PMI). It is sometimes a useful datum, as it allows some anticipation of the variable post mortem decomposition changes, although decomposition is often more reflective of the local circumstances. Thus, a death in hospital, with prompt refrigeration of the corpse, will have had a stable ambient temperature applied in a sealed environment. The degree of post mortem autolysis will be different for this body when compared to another body left at room temperature for several days or when the body is in an exposed environment. One should also be aware that it is possible for quite florid decomposition to be present even with a known short PMI, as may be seen in cases that involve sepsis.

Determination of an unknown PMI by PMCT is a forensic application, beyond the scope of the routine coronial workload and this text. It is a difficult task, reflecting the numerous factors involved [9–12]. At present, there is general consensus that there is no reliable and consistent imaging method for this task.

It is generally accepted that there are a variety of stages that follow death, mostly in sequential pattern. These are dealt with in the following section.

Initial Changes Seen After Death

Pallor Mortis

This is the earliest change identified following cessation of breathing, circulation and neurological function. Pallor mortis reflects the external skin colour change, whereby the body appears to lose its normal colour density. This process reflects the loss of blood circulating to the skin. Often the body will still be warm, flexible at the joints and potentially may be mistaken for one still in life. One should always be aware that shock, significant cardiac failure and neurological dysfunction could mimic this state. However, pallor mortis is not an issue for PMCT, as cases are not usually taken for scanning immediately after death—reflecting time for paperwork issues, etc. It is plainly evident that pallor mortis cannot be detected by PMCT.

Algor Mortis

The next stage seen after death, with loss of normal catabolism, is the gradual cooling of the body. This progressive decrease (depending on climate) in body temperature is known as algor mortis. Ultimately, the body will come into equilibrium with the surrounding environment, whether this be temperate, polar or tropical. It also cannot be defined by PMCT.

The difference in the body temperature and the ambient room/surrounding temperature will determine how fast the body may cool and has been used to give a guide to PMI (i.e. establishing the time of death). There is often a misconception that the time of death can be accurately predicted from such body/vicinity temperature observations, but this is generally accepted as imprecise at best. Clearly, if a body has been discovered long after death, then the body temperature calculations will not assist.

If the body has been actively refrigerated, at about 4 °C in a mortuary, then defining the PMI may be entirely unrealistic.

Livor Mortis or Hypostasis

Over time, the non-circulating blood and other fluids will settle with gravity towards the dependent parts of the body. Soon after death the position of this livor mortis/hypostasis can be affected by moving the body; however, at around 6–8 h after death, it becomes fixed [13]. This may be of particular forensic interest in cases where bodies have been moved following death.

The settling of blood is a readily determined feature (Fig. 3.2). It may help assess the PMI, being a commonly visible early post mortem change [14]. It occurs throughout the body, the various tissues appearing darker at open autopsy when in more dependent positions (Fig. 3.3) with the difference in the colour of organs reflecting how the body was stored [2].

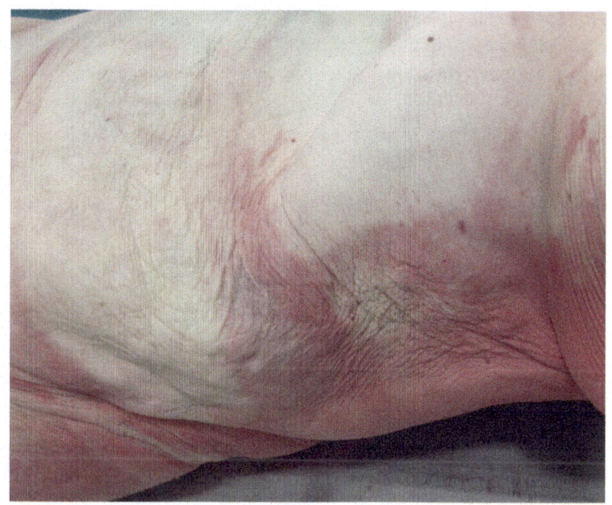

Fig. 3.2 Hypostasis is seen externally with blood settling to dependent parts of the body

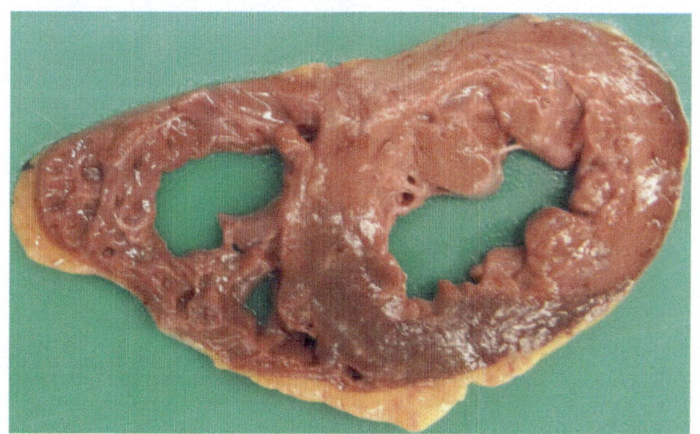

Fig. 3.3 Hypostasis (congestion) is seen internally with blood pooling to the lower side of the heart

On PMCT, hypostasis can also be readily appreciated. Assuming a supine position for the body after death, this is seen as a dependent gradient of increasing attenuation of tissues and organs from anterior to posterior and is usually well demonstrated in the lungs (Fig. 3.4). When death has occurred and the body remains in a lateral position, the gradient will also be lateral (Fig. 3.5).

The skin of dependent regions can display appreciable thickening and subcutaneous fluid accumulation (Figs. 3.6, 3.7, and 3.8). In larger, blood filled structures such as the major vessels and cardiac chambers, there is separation of the blood components (Figs. 3.9 and 3.10) resulting in 'fluid–fluid' levels on imaging [15]. Hypostasis within the vessels should not be mistaken for vascular wall dissection, pathological thrombus or emboli.

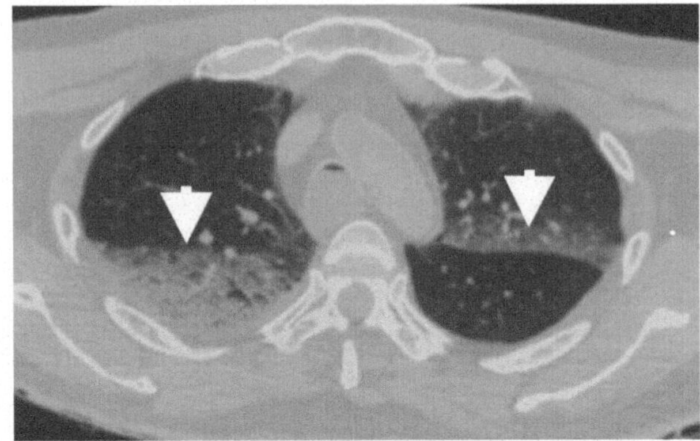

Fig. 3.4 Axial view of the chest on lung windows shows normal hypostasis of fluid (arrows) in the lungs with horizontal demarcation against aerated lung

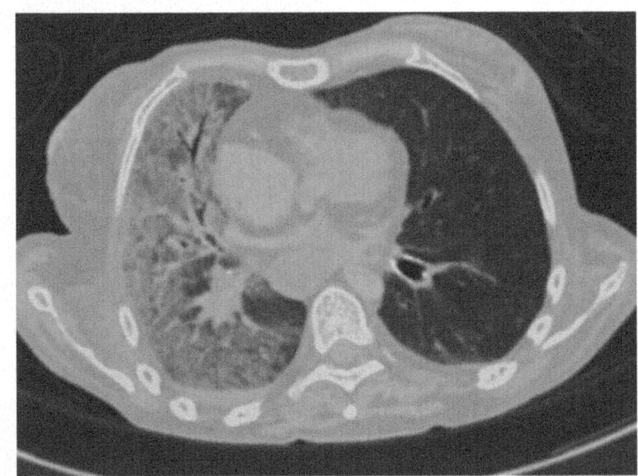

Fig. 3.5 Axial view of the chest on lung windows shows hypostasis of fluid in the right lung, the body was found lying in a right lateral position

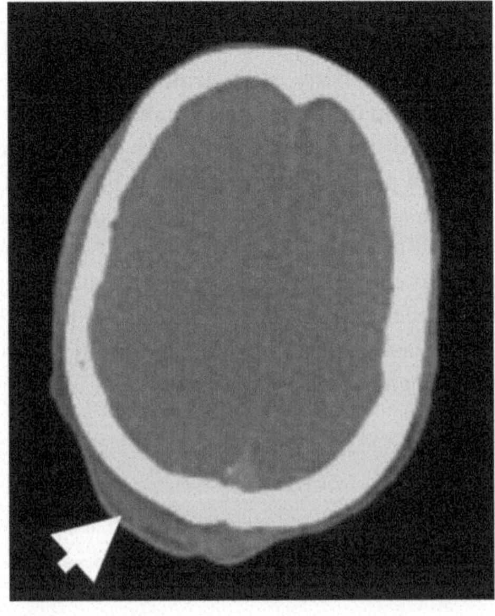

Fig. 3.6 Axial view of the head on soft tissue windows shows fluid collecting in the posterior scalp (arrow) with skin thickening due to hypostasis in the supine position

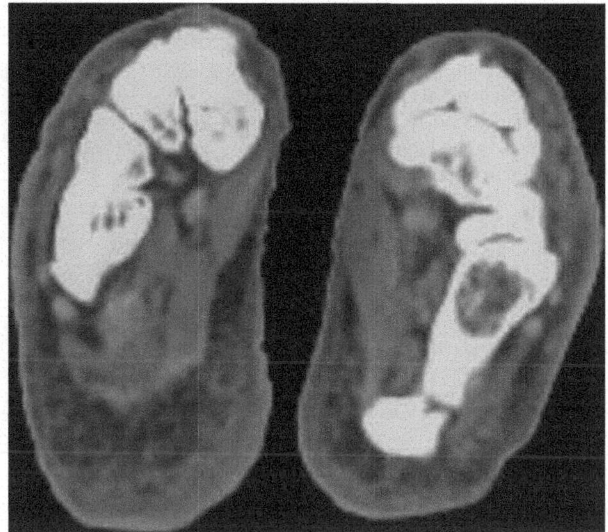

Fig. 3.7 Axial view of both feet on soft tissue windows shows skin thickening and dependent subcutaneous fluid accumulation in both heels due to hypostasis in the supine position

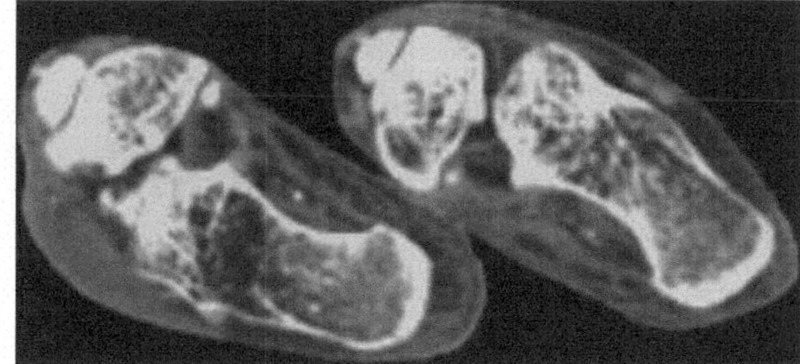

Fig. 3.8 Axial view of both feet on soft tissue windows shows dependent hypostatic fluid in the right lateral foot as the body was found lying on the right side

Rigor Mortis

In basic terms, rigor mortis is stiffening of muscle. The process involves the muscles becoming fixed in position, due to calcium leakage from intracellular muscle cell stores, causing fixed actin–myosin filament cross bridging. This stiffness remains, as there is no oxidative metabolism to create adenosine triphosphate (ATP), which is normally required for muscle relaxation. Yet the muscles do not remain permanently fixed, as later decomposition enzymatic activity degrades the muscle filament binding complexes in the cells and eventually allows release.

Initially, however, in a body seen immediately after death, there is actually a general muscle flaccidity, which may last for a few hours. One might broadly summarise the process as taking around 12 h for general rigor mortis to establish, 12 h to remain, and 12 h to disappear [13], although this timescale is subject to variation due to environmental factors such as temperature [2]. In warm environments, the onset of rigor mortis is earlier than for bodies in cold settings.

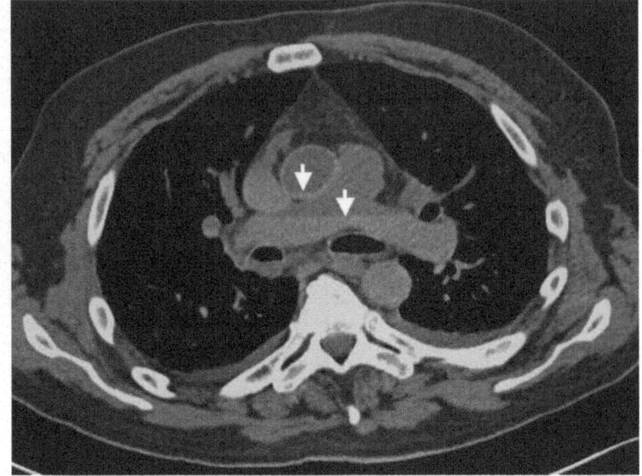

Fig. 3.9 Axial view of the chest on soft tissue windows showing normal post mortem layered separation of blood components in the large vessels due to hypostasis (arrows)

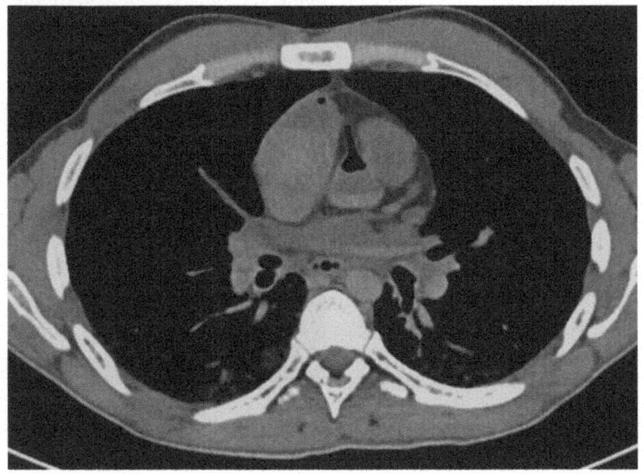

Fig. 3.10 Axial view of the chest on soft tissue windows showing separation of blood products in the great vessels and right atrium with small volume of normal post mortem air rising to outline the right coronary artery origin

It should also be understood that rigor mortis starts in different parts of the body at different times such that the face and neck muscles are earliest affected, with the torso and limbs following later. This same pattern is also seen with the release of the rigor.

Rigor mortis can also be 'broken'. This manipulation is commonly performed by mortuary staff and undertakers [2] usually to aid body transport and storage if the body has become rigid in an awkward position. This process involves firm stretching of the muscle, thereby achieving a normal joint alignment. It must be remembered that excessive force may cause physical rupture of muscles or detachment from their insertions and hence should not be performed by any person without appropriate training. Apart from the obvious physical challenge of scanning a body held in various irregular fixed positions, and the subsequent image reconstructions required to interpret the study, the rigor itself does not affect PMCT appearances.

Later Changes in the Body After Death

Decomposition is progressive, reflecting a combination of processes including autolysis, putrefaction and occasionally animal predation. It is specific to the post mortem state and is unlikely to have been encountered by a clinical radiologist who normally deals with scans of the living.

Post mortem changes on PMCT seem to increase in a regular pattern over time [16], although the timeframe itself and degree of change is highly variable. Influencing factors may be external, such as the environment in which the deceased expired (temperature, humidity, animal predation, trauma), and internal (body habitus, microbial environment and sepsis).

Most bodies in the community will be discovered within a short time after death, others will have death confirmed literally within a few moments of life having ceased (e.g. hospital environments, palliative care settings). Decomposition may have started, without there being significant anatomical change. Even for bodies discovered after several days, significant tissue degradation may not always be evident, unless there is heat in the environment or where the body is exposed to nature.

Bodies that have been discovered after a significant period of time following death may show more structural changes of a potentially confusing nature. The changes involve the progressive tissue lysis that widely affects the body, often driven by the body's own bacterial components. These changes are broadly described as decomposition, although significant tissue destruction, breakdown and loss are commonly referred to as putrefaction. Putrefaction is a process of decomposition caused by microbial activity and fermentation, resulting in gas and fluid production. It is usually seen earliest in the right iliac fossa/lower abdomen (Fig. 3.1) and is accompanied by gaseous tissue/organ distension. It eventually spreads throughout the body, often via blood vessels in a process described as 'marbling' (Fig. 3.11).

A green/grey discolouration of skin can develop as decomposition progresses through putrefaction (Fig. 3.12). There may be blistering with serous fluid (Fig. 3.13) and then loosening of the skin and 'slippage', where skin comes away from the body (Fig. 3.14).

Fluids may leak from any orifice ('purging') that can result in misleading histories of apparent vomiting or haemorrhage at the scene of discovery [2]. To reduce purging, mortuary staff may insert gauze material into the upper aerodigestive tract (Fig. 3.15). This could be a source of misinterpretation if not recognised.

Internal organs decompose naturally at different rates. The pancreas and adrenals undergo relatively early autolysis (Fig. 3.16), and brain changes are also rapid in onset. The heart, prostate and uterus are comparatively resistant to decomposition [14]. The urinary bladder also may appear 'normal' for a considerable period of time (Fig. 3.17).

With time, in cases with unimpeded decomposition, all the soft tissues will be progressively degraded. This is particularly so if the body is in an open environment, where insects and indeed other animals may interact with, or remove body tissues. This tissue loss will be a confounding issue for PMCT but does not automatically imply that a cause of death cannot be defined. Ultimately, if left unchecked,

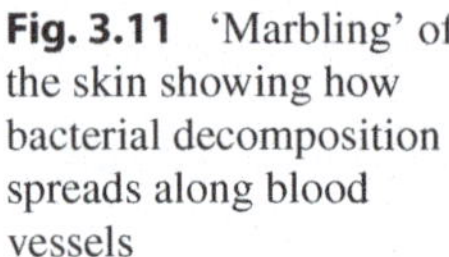

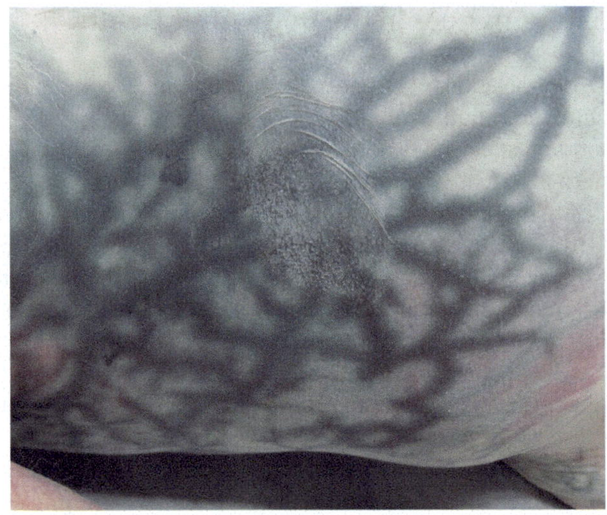

Fig. 3.11 'Marbling' of the skin showing how bacterial decomposition spreads along blood vessels

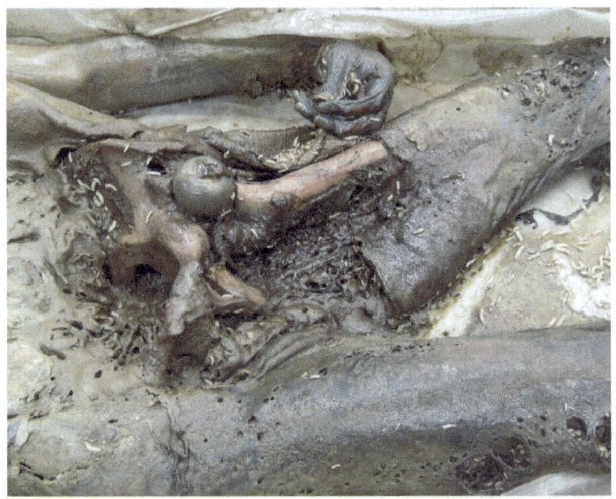

Fig. 3.12 Advanced putrefaction showing pronounced tissue loss and skeletonisation. Numerous small holes are present on the residual tissues reflecting maggot damage

the consequence of autolytic and decomposition phenomena is that one may be left with some skin, thick ligaments and skeleton only, even if the PMI is only a few weeks (Fig. 3.12). Skeletonised bodies will be a particular problem for any PMCT assessment, although the exclusion or discovery of non-accidental osseous injuries may occasionally be valuable.

In some cases, decomposition may occur in a cool and dry environment. Here the tissues may desiccate and become shrivelled, yet structurally may be preserved for many years. These changes are often referred to as 'mummification' but are not akin to the ancient Egyptian practice. Mummified cases are rarely seen in PMCT units.

Clearly, knowledge of extreme ambient temperatures at the scene of death is important, as cases of hypothermia, with freezing of body parts, can result in areas

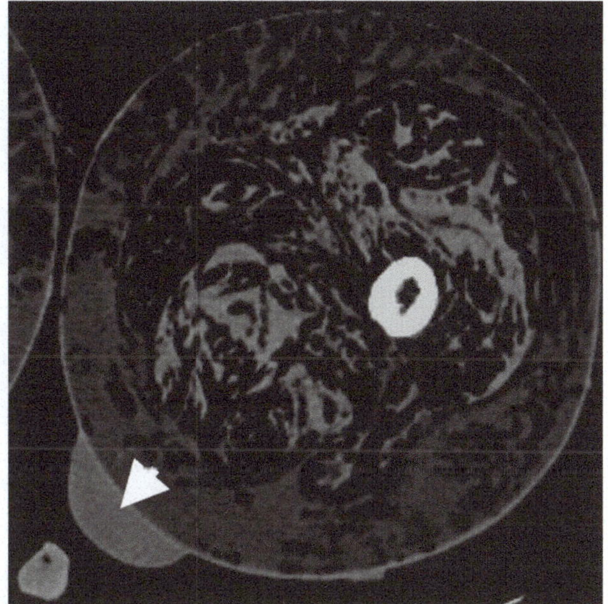

Fig. 3.13 Axial view of the left thigh in soft tissue windows shows extensive soft tissue decomposition gas (hence the general 'blackness' of the image), dependent skin thickening and skin blistering with fluid (arrow)

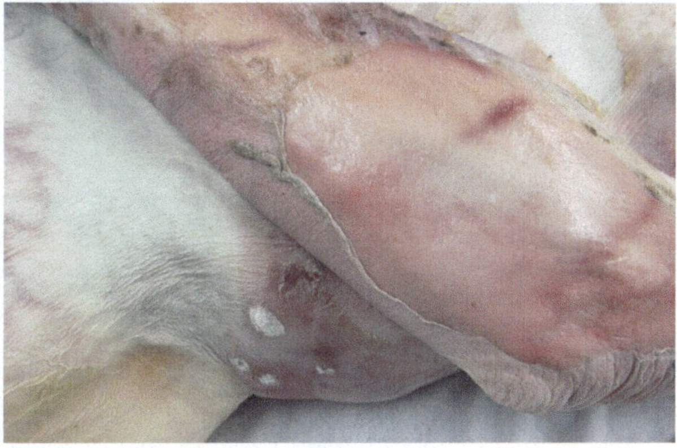

Fig. 3.14 Skin slippage, seen here on the forearm, is commonly seen as decomposition progresses

of low attenuation change on PMCT. In the brain, for example, this may appear similar to infarction but is seen in a non-vascular territory and may be accompanied by preservation of cerebral structure [17].

Refrigeration is thought to have little effect on PMCT, as the density of water remains almost constant when it is between 0 °C and normal body temperature. In contrast, freezing temperatures do affect CT attenuation values. It has been shown ex vivo that the attenuation of frozen water reduces to around −70 to −80 HU [18]. The importance of this in PMCT has not been well researched, but general knowledge of this effect should result in caution when interpreting radiological findings in this unusual setting.

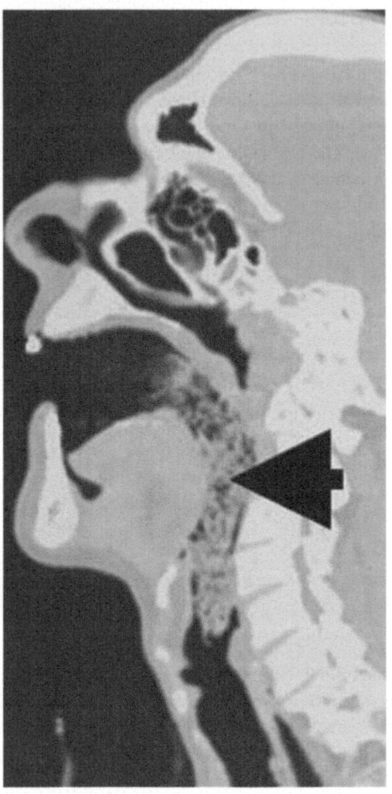

Fig. 3.15 Sagittal view of the face and neck on lung windows showing gauze material in the upper aerodigestive tract (arrow)

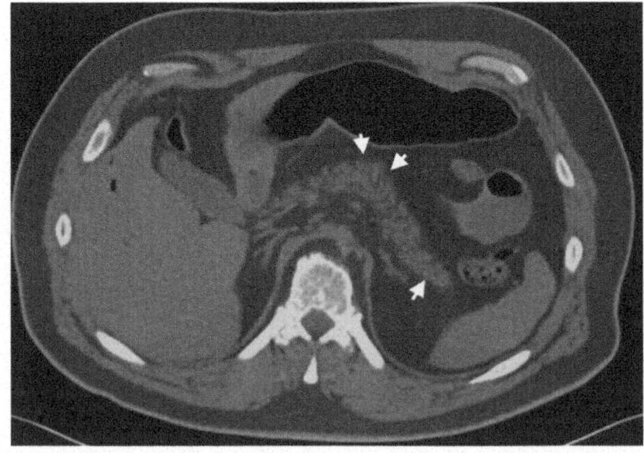

Fig. 3.16 Axial view of the upper abdomen on soft tissue windows shows peri-pancreatic haziness (arrows) in keeping with autolysis, in a patient who died from a myocardial infarct

Finally, one should be aware that whilst whole-body or targeted angiography (PMCTA) may generally be considered a viable and worthwhile technique, if applied early after death [19, 20], its use will be less helpful with advancing decomposition and precluded when vessels eventually lose their integrity.

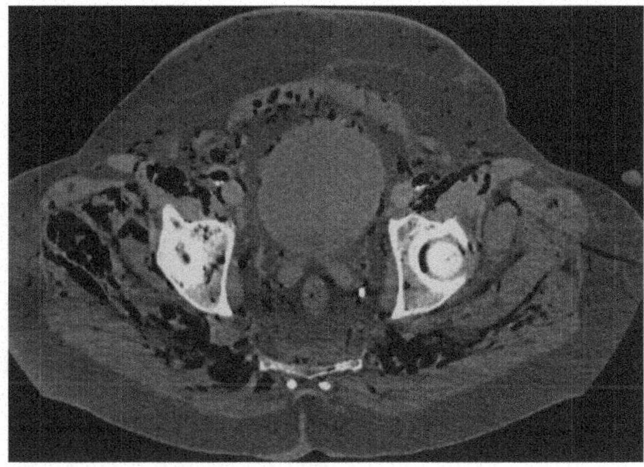

Fig. 3.17 Axial view of the pelvis on soft tissue windows shows a relatively preserved urinary bladder centrally among surrounding tissues with decomposition gas

Decomposition from the Radiology Perspective

The radiologist is not normally required to examine the body directly. This means that the initial external clues of post mortem change and decomposition may be difficult to appreciate, since the body is normally contained within an opaque, sealed body bag. Nevertheless, the presence of gas within the body tissues, dissolution of brain parenchyma and other post mortem degradation effects may indicate that the body is not one that has been secured shortly after death, or one that has not been stored appropriately.

Specific radiological findings that can be attributed to decomposition are also discussed in the subsequent relevant chapters, but broadly include accumulation of intravascular gas (Figs. 3.18, 3.19, and 3.20) and extravascular gas (Figs. 3.21, 3.22, 3.23, and 3.24), fluid settling or 'hypostasis' (Figs. 3.4, 3.25, 3.26), gas and fluid accumulation in cavities (Fig. 3.27), soft tissue collapse (Fig. 3.28) and eventually liquefaction of organs. Teeth may come loose if unsupported by soft tissue (Fig. 3.29), and eventually either mummification or skeletonisation occurs (Figs. 3.30, 3.31, and 3.32).

It is generally appreciated that tissue degradation may proceed variably, with factors as discussed earlier but also relating to natural disease processes (e.g. sepsis) and other metabolic realities (e.g. deaths after a pyrexial illness). Furthermore, aspects of medical intervention, such as invasive or surgical interactions, cancer treatments and immunosuppression, may alter the patterns of sepsis and cause bodily changes. These are potential traps for the unwary radiologist and potentially hinder diagnostic endeavour.

Any signs of decomposition should be described at PMCT. Decomposition can significantly affect the sensitivity of the scan in demonstrating pathology and the degree of certainty with which findings can be reported. Allowing for the general degree of decomposition is of particular value in some circumstances, such as when trying to differentiate air embolism or pneumothorax from decomposition-related gas accumulation.

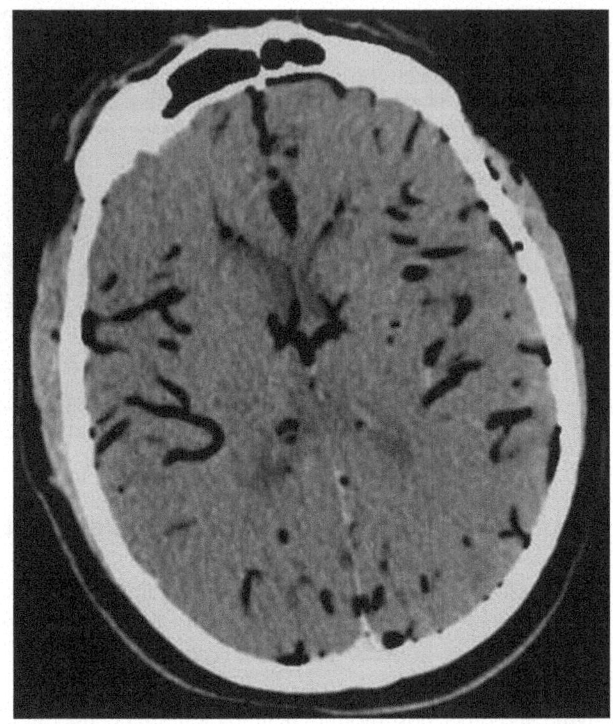

Fig. 3.18 Axial view of the brain on brain windows shows intracranial, intravascular gas (black) due to normal decomposition

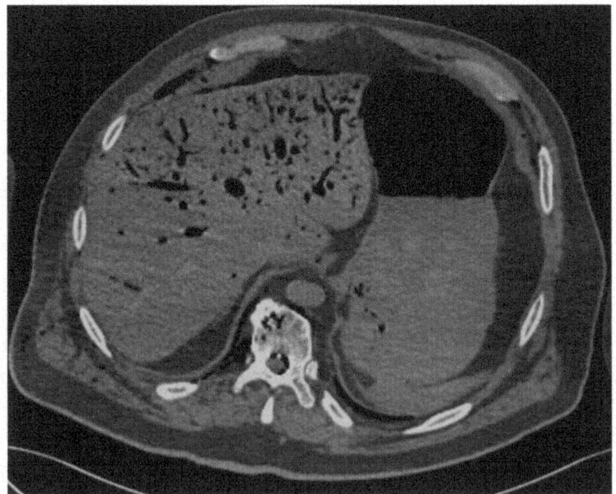

Fig. 3.19 Axial view of the upper abdomen on soft tissue windows shows decomposition gas in the hepatic and portal veins in the liver, mostly in the anterior segments

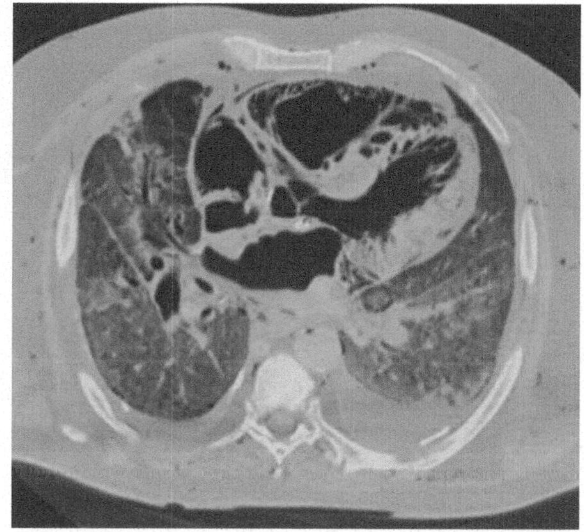

Fig. 3.20 Axial view of the chest on lung windows (accentuating the visibility of gas) shows decomposition gas in the heart chambers, great and superficial vessels

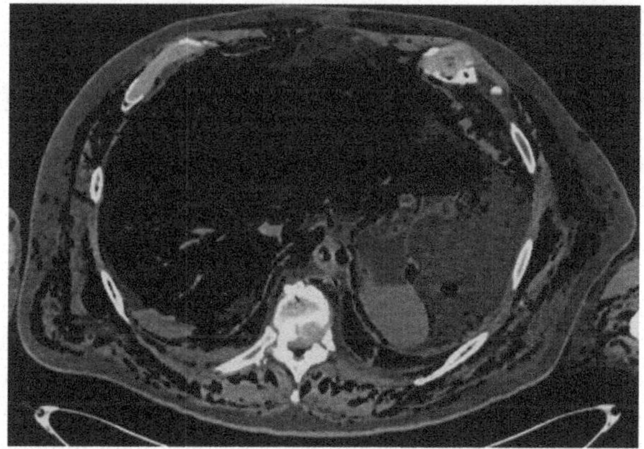

Fig. 3.21 Axial view of the upper abdomen on soft tissue windows shows extensive decomposition gas in the liver and soft tissues, note the liver is barely perceptible

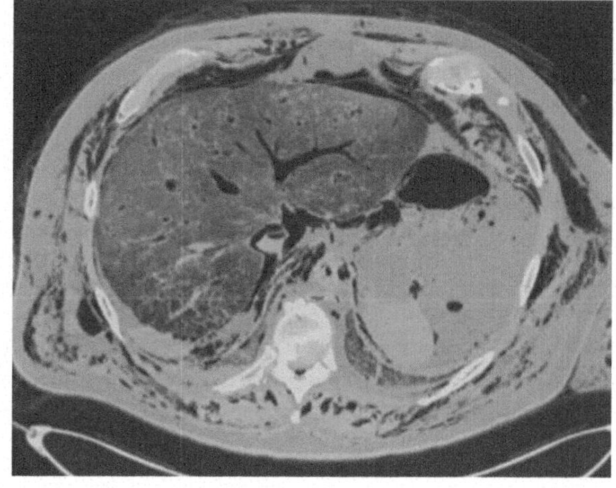

Fig. 3.22 Same case as Fig. 3.21, lung windows better demonstrate the decomposition gas allowing the liver to be visualised

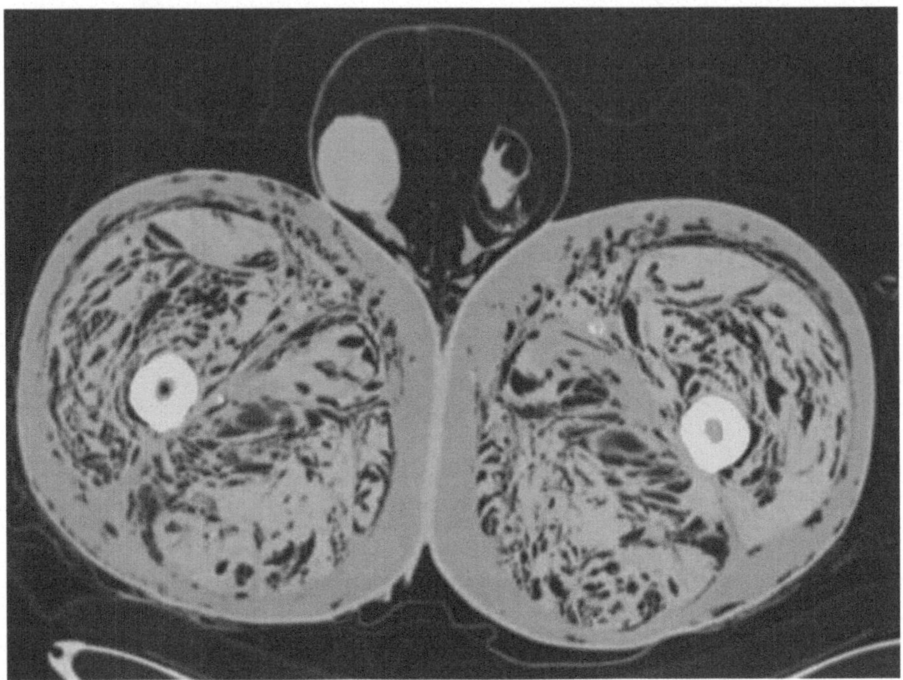

Fig. 3.23 Axial view of the upper thighs on lung windows shows normal decomposition gas in the soft tissues and distending the scrotum

The radiologist may broadly consider whether the degree of decomposition is appropriate for the PMI and given circumstances. The use of the terms such as 'early' or 'late' decomposition is rather subjective and may be misleading if not clarified (does 'early' mean 'minimal' or 'earlier than expected'?). For a non-forensic study, it is more helpful to specifically describe the changes that are believed to be attributable to decomposition and then indicate to what degree, if any, they limit the examination. As expected, with minimal decomposition changes, positive findings on the scan are usually trustworthy. When there are moderate changes, more care should be taken in interpretation. Cases with advanced decomposition changes may have very limited reliability in terms of diagnosing soft tissue pathology (Figs. 3.33, 3.34, and 3.35).

Post Mortem Gas

As gas patterns are well demonstrated at PMCT, it is important to understand their nature in the post mortem setting in order to use them as a diagnostic feature. There is debate about the exact origin and cause of gas in the body of the deceased, although gas production generally relates to putrefaction of tissues and starts to develop in the first few days. During this process, gas in the vessels (Figs. 3.18,

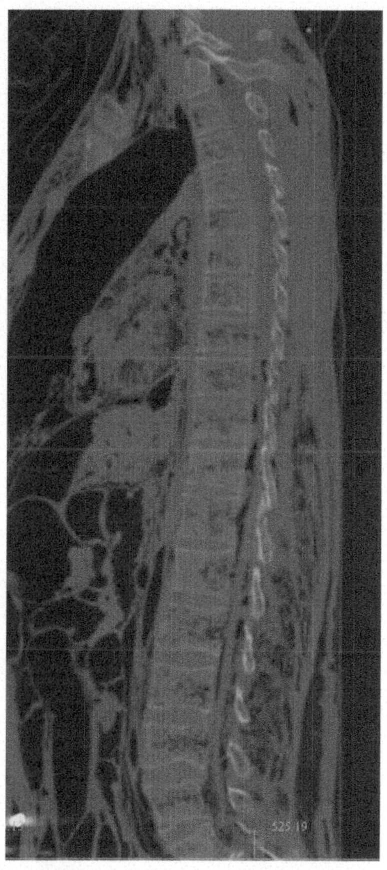

Fig. 3.24 Sagittal view of the thoracolumbar spine on bone windows shows normal decomposition gas (black) in the soft tissues, vertebral canal and marrow

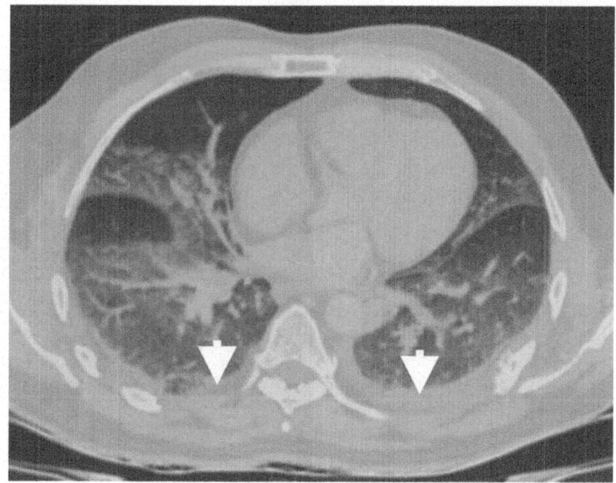

Fig. 3.25 Axial view of the chest on lung windows showing the typical post mortem appearance of fluid hypostasis in the lungs and tiny bilateral pleural effusions (arrows)

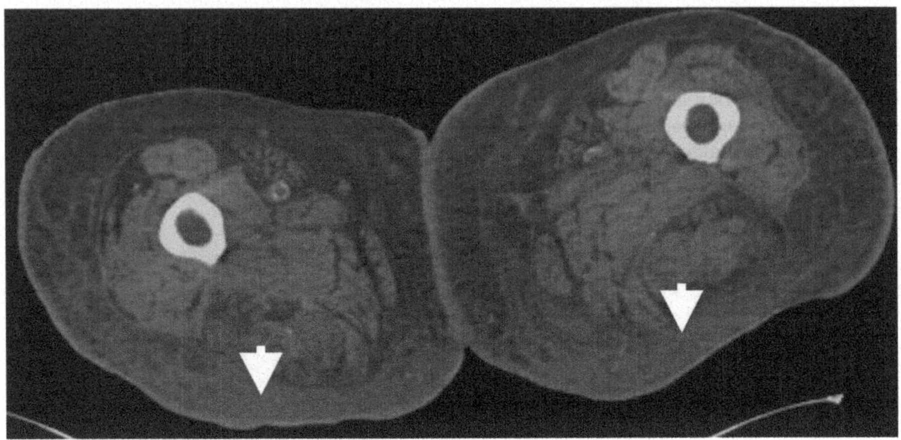

Fig. 3.26 Axial view of both thighs on soft tissue windows demonstrates prominent dependent subcutaneous oedema (arrows) in an obese hospital patient with poor mobility

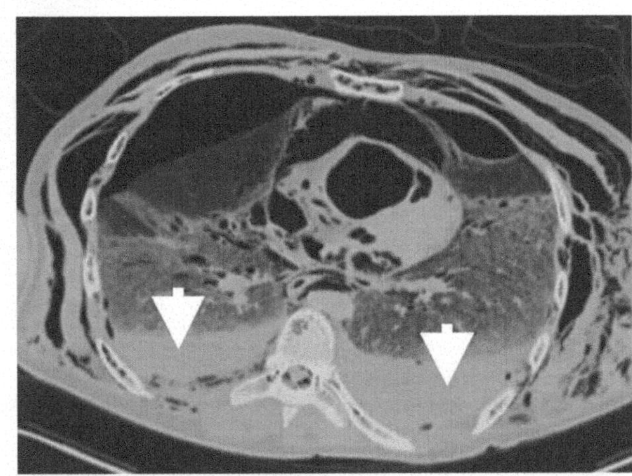

Fig. 3.27 Axial view of the chest on lung windows shows extensive soft tissue gas, free gas and free fluid (arrows) in the pleural spaces due to progressive decomposition

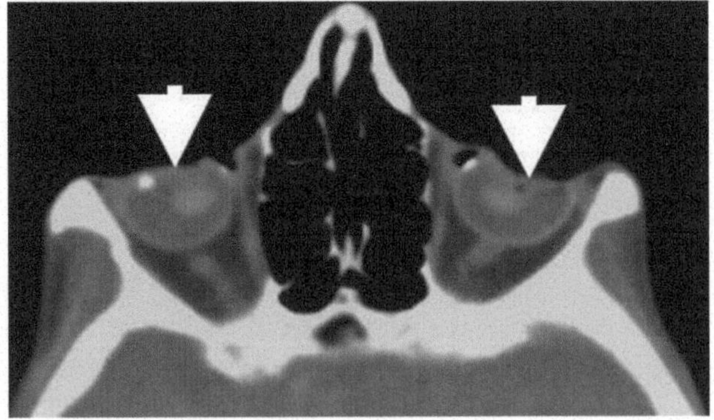

Fig. 3.28 Axial view of the orbits on soft tissue windows shows flattened globes (arrows)

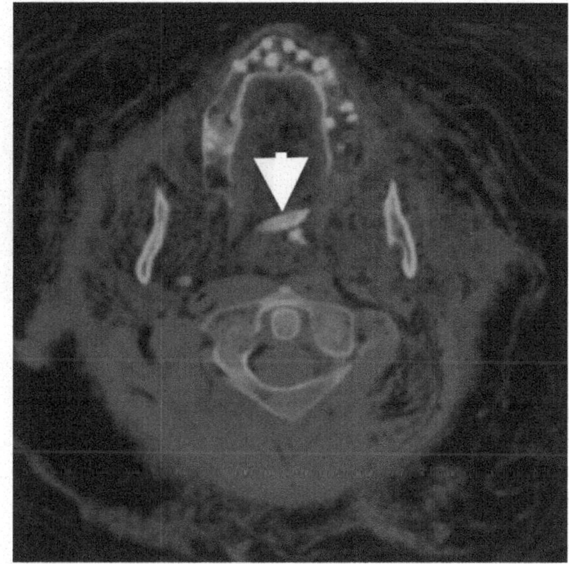

Fig. 3.29 Axial view at the level of the oropharynx shows displaced teeth (arrow) in the setting of extensive surrounding soft tissue decomposition

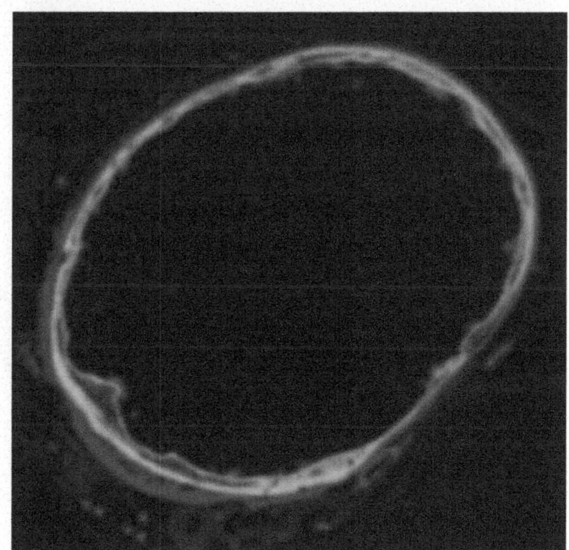

Fig. 3.30 Axial view of the head on bone windows shows near-skeletonisation of the cranium with minimal scalp soft tissue remaining

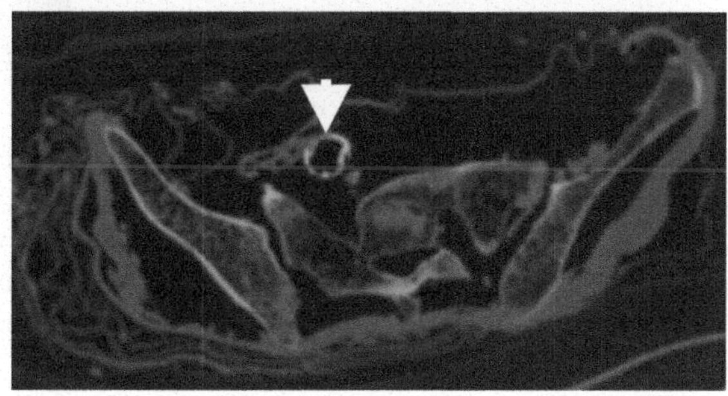

Fig. 3.31 Axial view of the pelvis on bone windows shows a persistent heavily calcified aorta (arrow) in a near-skeletonised pelvis

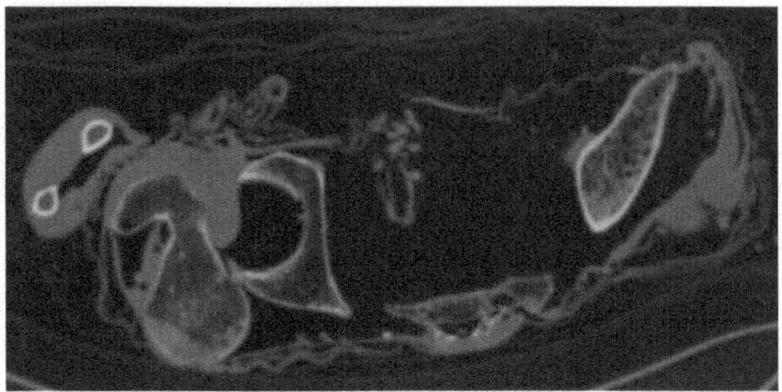

Fig. 3.32 Axial view of the pelvis on bone windows shows a dislocated right hip joint due to loss of soft tissue structural support in a near-skeletonised body

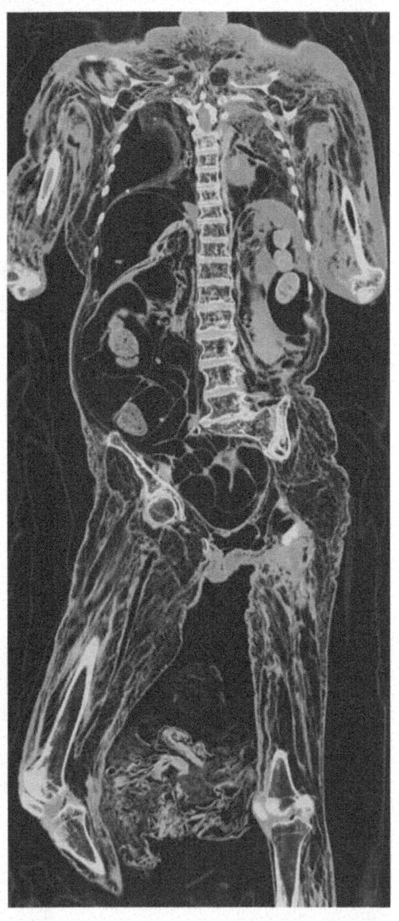

Fig. 3.33 Coronal view of the torso and upper legs on lung windows shows advanced decomposition with extensive soft tissue and free gas, the diagnostic ability of this study is very limited

3.19, and 3.20) is expected before free cavity gas such as pneumothorax (Fig. 3.36) and pneumoperitoneum (Fig. 3.37). With advancing decomposition, gas tends to appear at about the same time in the peritoneal and pleural cavities [21]. When free cavity gas is seen independent of vascular gas (or judged to be out of proportion), careful thought must be given as to whether this signifies a primary pathology.

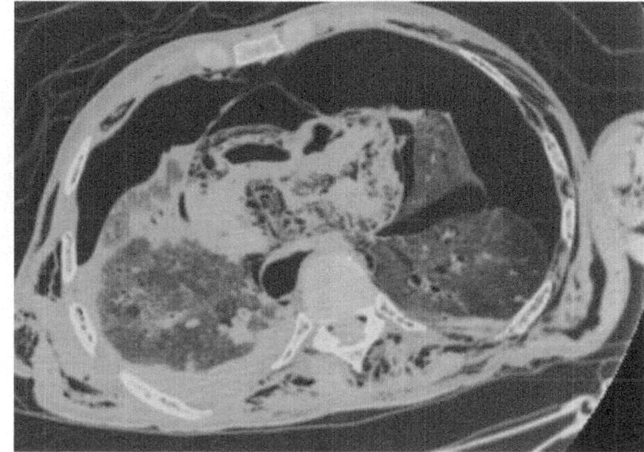

Fig. 3.34 Axial view of the chest on lung windows shows advanced decomposition with soft tissue gas and pneumothoraces, the diagnostic ability of this study is very limited

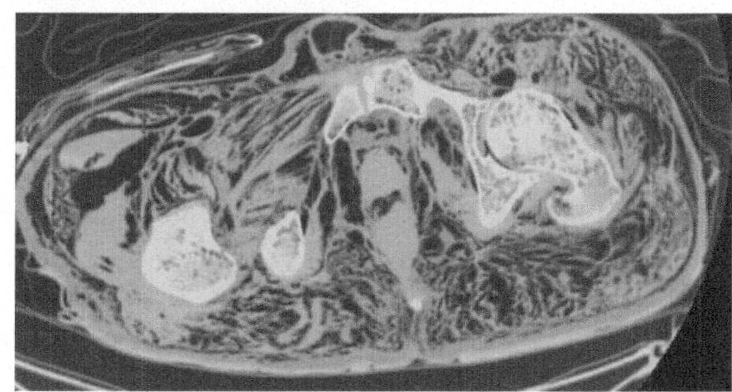

Fig. 3.35 Axial view of the lower pelvis on lung windows shows advanced decomposition with extensive soft tissue and bone marrow gas, soft tissue assessment would be very limited

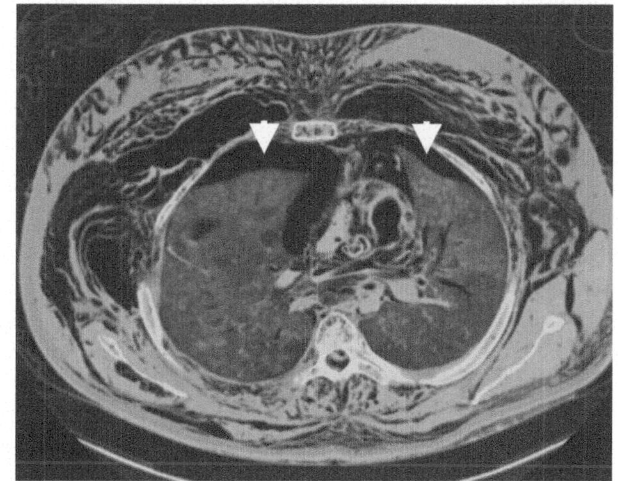

Fig. 3.36 Axial view of the chest on lung windows shows bilateral anterior pneumothoraces (arrows) judged to be due to decomposition as they are in keeping with the degree of vascular and soft tissue gas seen elsewhere

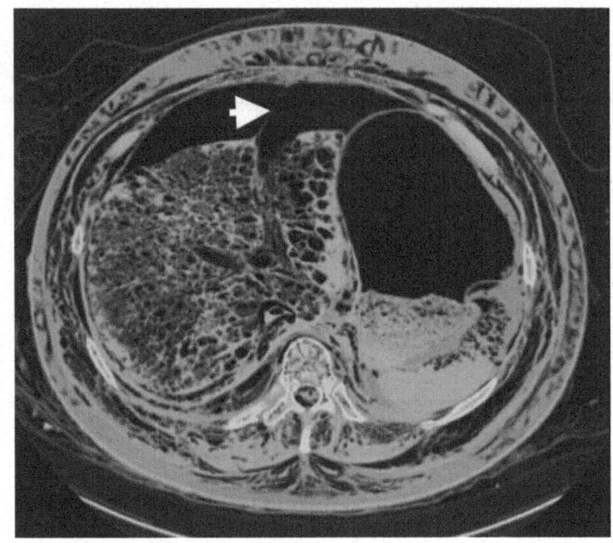

Fig. 3.37 Axial view of the upper abdomen on lung windows shows a pneumoperitoneum and falciform ligament sign (arrow) judged to be due to decomposition rather than primary pathology, given the degree of decomposition gas seen in the soft tissues

It should also be appreciated that the volume of decomposition gas can be generally, or focally, increased in the setting of sepsis, trauma, when lines have been introduced into the body for medical purposes and/or when resuscitation attempts have been made (see Chap. 11).

One method devised to quantify bodily decomposition changes is the 'radiological alteration index' [21]. This objective process, considering the volume of gas at different anatomic locations, is used to derive a numerical score. Cases with a high score (more decomposition) need more questioning of the nature of the findings. The use of such scoring lies outside our routine PMCT practice, and we tend to use a descriptive assessment of any decomposition, with relevance given to the particular case being assessed.

Post Mortem Clot

Post mortem 'clotting' is also highly variable and may be linked to the length of the dying process as well as the underlying pathologies that surround death. Longer deaths tend to exhibit more intravascular clot than rapid deaths. Post mortem clotting may appear prominent in the right heart, pulmonary trunk and great vessels [22], and the large capacity veins may often have coagulum in the post mortem state. It is difficult to reliably distinguish this normal post mortem clot from acute pulmonary embolism (PE), which remains one of the limitations of PMCT (see Chap. 7).

The post mortem separation of blood components can generally result in either this heterogeneous appearance of clots in the great vessels or a simple physical layering of low upon high-density products (hypostasis, Figs. 3.9 and 3.10). When separation of blood products has occurred note that the whole volume is blood and not just the dependent, more dense component.

Animal Predation and Post Mortem Changes

If death occurs outdoors or in an uncontrolled environment, particularly in warmer months, there is a likelihood of animal predation. Examples in the United Kingdom commonly reflect fly maggots, rats and foxes. This predation results in faster tissue loss, and opening the body may accelerate decomposition [2]. This is seen especially in parts of the body that may be exposed, such as the face and hands, and in open wounds or moist areas, such as the eyes, lips and nostrils (Figs. 3.12, 3.38, 3.39, 3.40, 3.41, and 3.42).

Maggot colonies can occasionally present as internal soft tissue masses [23], and this should be considered a differential within the decomposed body. They appear on the scan as discrete soft tissue opacities much the same size and shape as grains of rice. They can add significant bulk to some tissues seen on PMCT and may even appear to fill the upper respiratory tract and/or oral tissue cavities.

Embalmed and Previously Autopsied Bodies

Coronial PMCT will normally be undertaken prior to embalming, and therefore this is not normally an issue to consider. However, occasionally, a body will be repatriated after death has occurred abroad. When transporting a body for repatriation, it is normal practice for the body to be embalmed. Whilst a primary death investigation

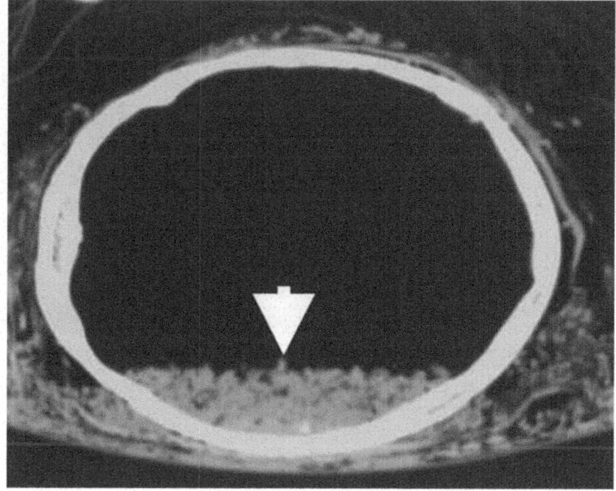

Fig. 3.38 Axial view of the skull (which is turned 90° to the right due to patient positioning) on lung windows shows multiple maggots as small discrete densities (example at tip of arrow) both external and internal to an otherwise empty cranial cavity

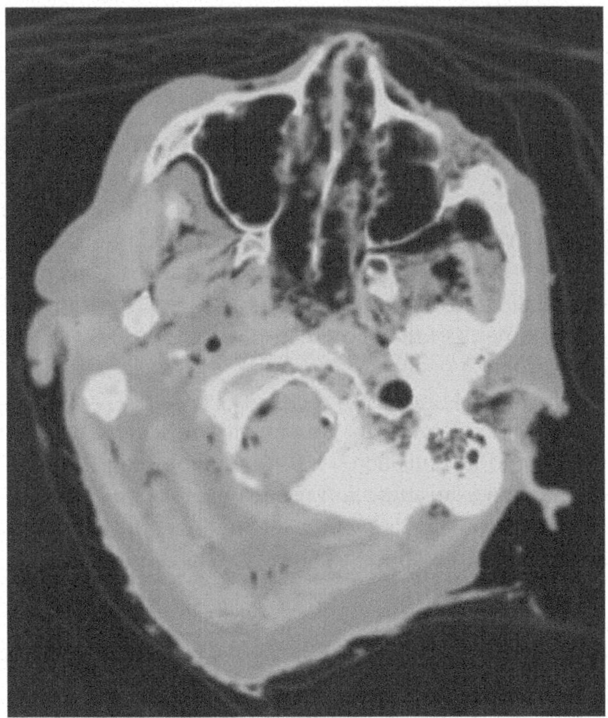

Fig. 3.39 Axial view at the level of the nasal cavity on lung windows shows multiple maggots in the nasal cavities, maxillary sinuses and deeper soft tissues

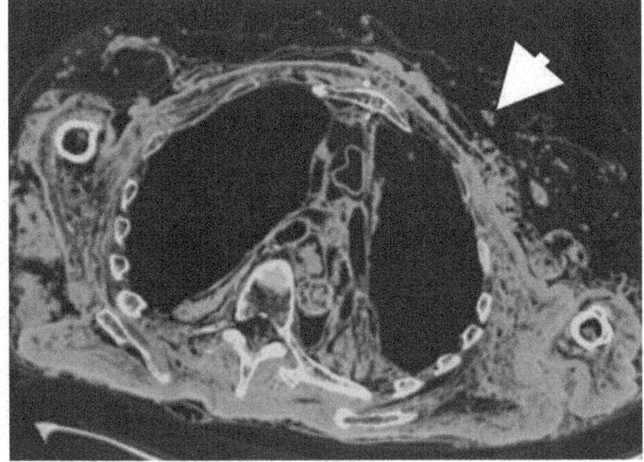

Fig. 3.40 Axial view of the chest on lung windows in the setting of marked decomposition shows extensive soft tissue loss due to maggot activity; multiple maggots are seen in the soft tissues and externally within the body bag (arrow)

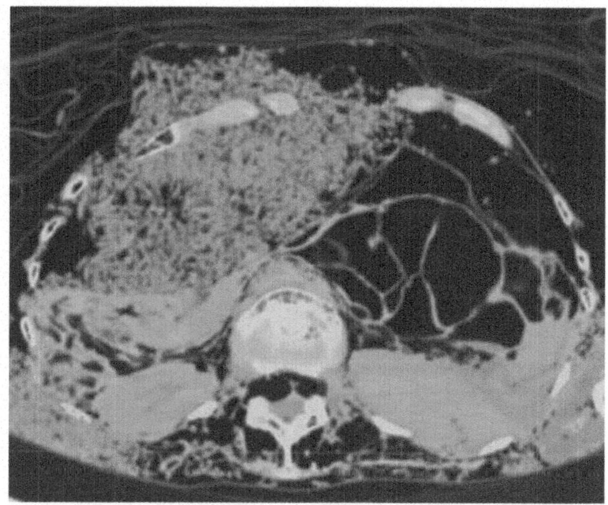

Fig. 3.41 Axial view of the upper abdomen on lung windows shows a mass-like maggot infestation of the abdominal soft tissues through the chest wall anteriorly

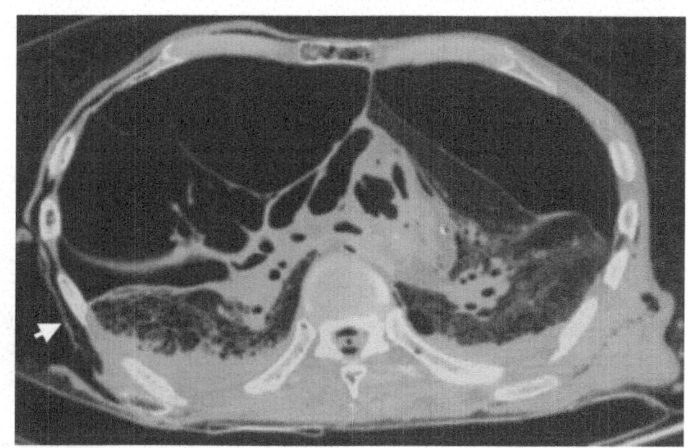

Fig. 3.42 Axial view of the chest on lung windows shows marked decomposition and evidence of predation by the house cat leading to focal right posterior chest wall tissue loss (arrow)

is often conducted by the authorities in that country, a further investigation may be instructed when the body is returned to the United Kingdom.

Embalming is a process of body preservation generally done through chemical agents. This can reduce health (infection) hazards associated with moving the body. Embalming is usually performed by the infusion of fluids through large cannulae in the neck or groin, where gas tracks may then later be seen on PMCT (Fig. 3.43). It has been suggested that the process itself may have a detrimental effect on the quality of subsequent PMCT images [24], although this is not always the case and an individual case assessment will need to be made. If the embalming is suboptimal, there may be further confusion with partially preserved and partially decomposed tissues [25].

Some bodies are returned after an initial autopsy performed abroad (Figs. 3.44 and 3.45). These autopsies are of variable quality, may be partial or complete

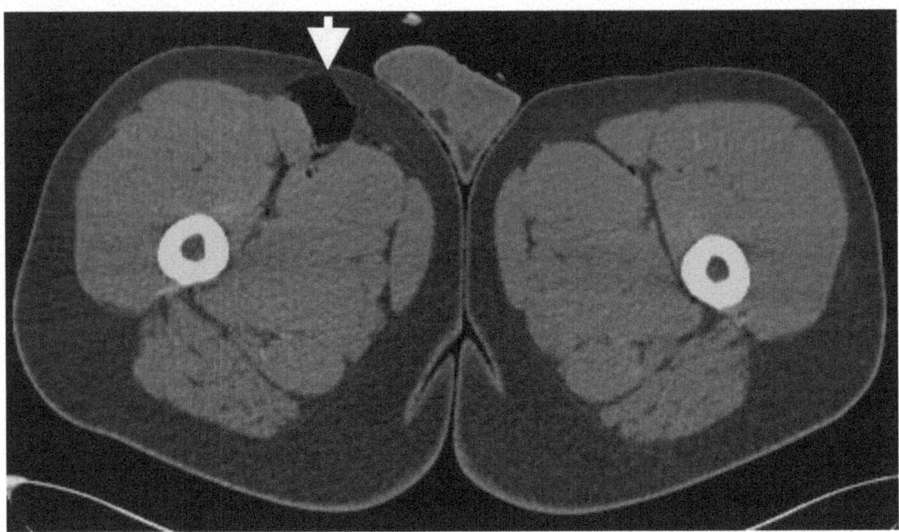

Fig. 3.43 Axial view of the upper thighs on soft tissue windows shows focal gas in the anterior superficial right groin (arrow) due to cannulation for embalming, with little evidence of decomposition elsewhere. Note also the subtle dependent thickening of the skin due to hypostasis

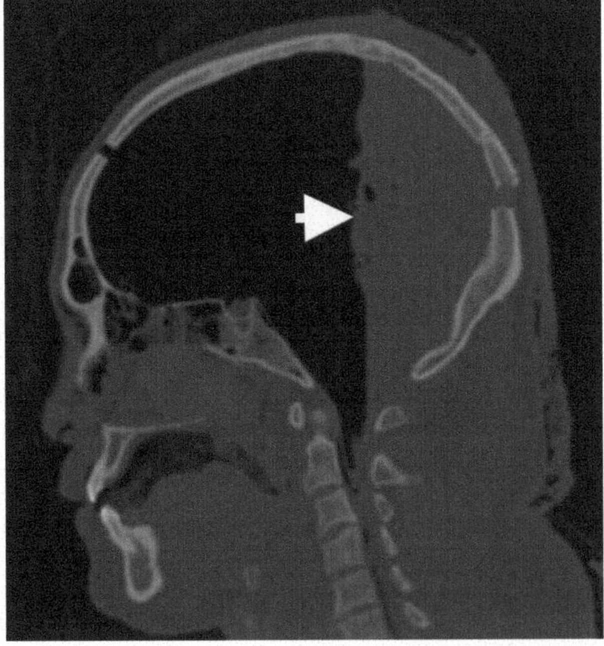

Fig. 3.44 Sagittal view of the head and neck on bone windows showing skull cap fractures from autopsy craniotomy, gauze in oral cavity, absent brain and an intracranial fluid level (arrow—this appears vertical as the study has been reconstructed)

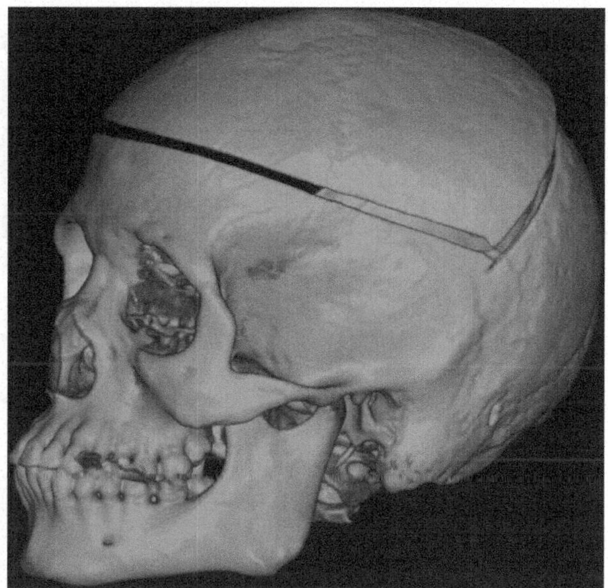

Fig. 3.45 Volume rendered three-dimensional PMCT image showing craniotomy fractures performed during open autopsy

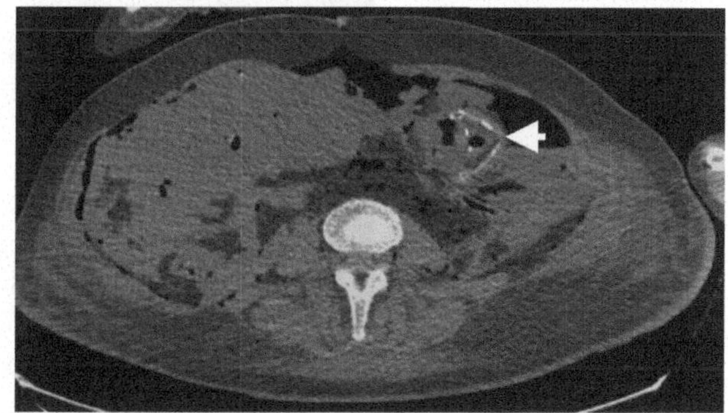

Fig. 3.46 Axial view of the abdomen on soft tissue windows following open autopsy shows mal-positioning of a calcified larynx in the abdomen (arrow) and no discernible normal abdominal viscera

invasive examinations, often with no accompanying information given back to the UK authorities. Furthermore, the prior autopsy practitioners may have placed any or all the tissues in a variably dissected fashion into a sealed bag placed into the abdomen (Fig. 3.46), and it is common to see gauze used to pack any resultant cavities (Figs. 3.47, 3.48, and 3.49). Organs placed in a bag are not accessed by embalming fluids, with resultant pronounced tissue degradation/autolysis. It is further recognised that major organs of importance may be retained in the original mortuary. Indeed, many pathologists would have seen cases where there are few or no internal organs within the returned body!

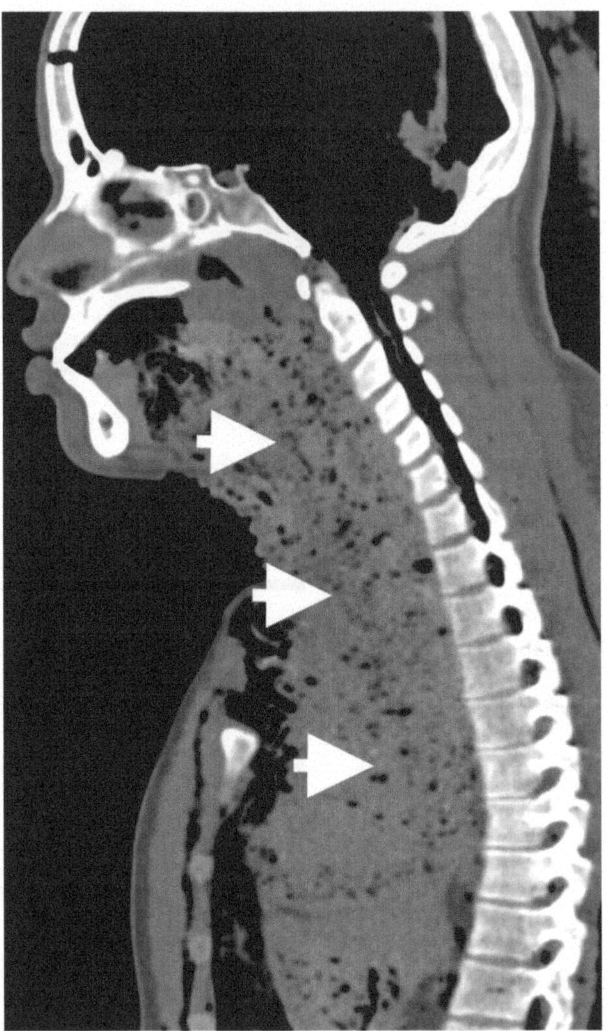

Fig. 3.47 Sagittal view of the upper body windowed to show absent cranial, neck and thoracic structures following autopsy and the resultant contiguous cavity packed with extensive gauze material (arrows)

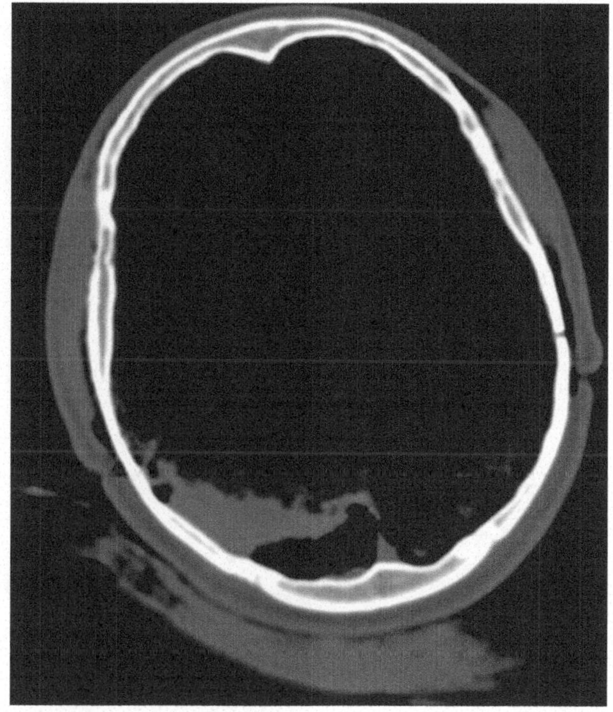

Fig. 3.48 Axial view of the head on soft tissue windows shows an apparently 'empty' cranial cavity following an open autopsy

PMCT interpretation of such previously autopsied cases is often futile if one wants to establish a medical cause of death. The role of PMCT is therefore different here. First, it can be used to exclude that a fraudulent autopsy has taken place—a finding of only a stitched incision without underlying dissection of organs [2]. Second, it can reveal the extent of the performed invasive autopsy, for example, some parts of the body may not have been examined. Limb and bony pathology should still be apparent, and the scan can be used to reveal any retained implants or potentially dangerous foreign bodies (Figs. 3.50 and 3.51). In such situations, PMCT is usually considered an adjunct to further autopsy investigation.

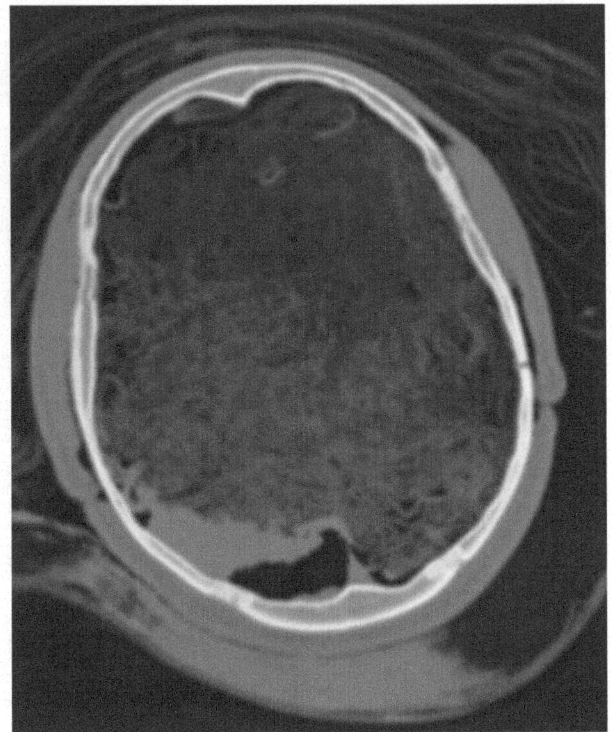

Fig. 3.49 Same case as Fig. 3.48, lung windows readily reveal the intracranial gauze packing highlighting the need to assess the body with multiple window settings

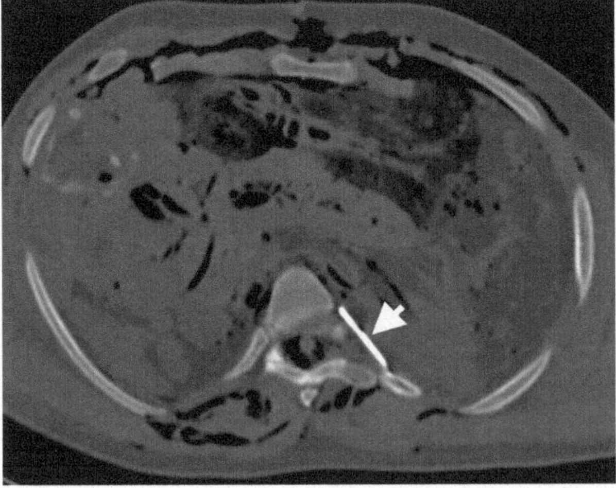

Fig. 3.50 Axial view of the chest following autopsy (note discontinuous anterior thoracic wall and midline incision) windowed to highlight linear radio-dense foreign body in the left paraspinal thoracic cavity (arrow)

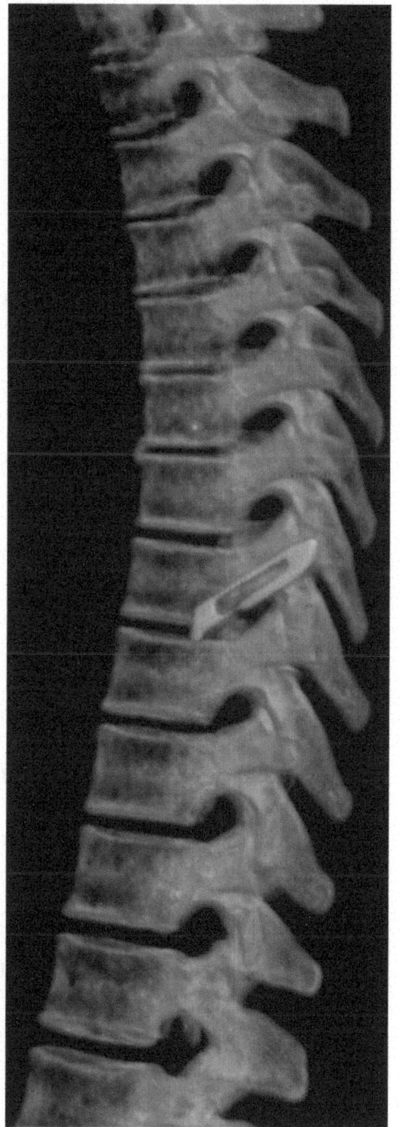

Fig. 3.51 Same case as Fig. 3.50, volume rendered PMCT image demonstrates the foreign body to be a retained scalpel blade therefore requiring a cautious approach to any subsequent open examination

Reporting Post Mortem Change and Decomposition: Pearls and Pitfalls

There is almost always evidence of post mortem change on routine PMCT, and therefore common findings should be considered to be 'normal for the nature of the study'. Certainly, hypostasis, putrefactive gas and fluids should not be mistaken for pathology.

As a general rule, the degree of decomposition should be similar throughout the body. Asymmetrical or peripheral putrefactive changes (perhaps due to body position near a heat source or partial exposure) can be normal, but the reporter should assess this on an individual basis, correlating with the environment in which the body was found if necessary.

When reporting the scan of a heavily decomposed body, there are limitations as to the detail that can be given regarding the soft tissues, and this should be clearly conveyed in the report.

Implanted medical devices can still easily be seen, and a quantification of coronary artery calcification remains possible, even in cases of advanced decomposition (see Chap. 8).

Bony findings such as fractures can be defined giving value to the study, despite soft tissue limitations.

Example PMCT report phrases:

- The post mortem interval at time of scan is (if known).
- Appearances are consistent with normal post mortem change.
- Appearances are consistent with minimal/moderate/advanced decomposition.
- Extensive vascular gas and a small pneumoperitoneum secondary to decomposition.
- The presence of decomposition change severely limits the diagnostic capability of this study.

References

1. Schofield GM, Urch CE, Stebbing J, Giamas G. When does a human being die? QJM [Internet]. 2015;108(8):605–9. https://academic.oup.com/qjmed/article-lookup/doi/10.1093/qjmed/hcu239.
2. Saukko P, Knight B. Knight's forensic pathology [Internet]. 4th ed. Boca Raton: CRC Press; 2015. https://www.routledge.com/Knights-Forensic-Pathology/Saukko-Knight/p/book/9780340972533.
3. Kastenbaum R. Death, society, and human experience. 11th ed. Abingdon: Routledge; 2011.
4. Benbow E. Ageing and death. In: Cross S, editor. Underwood's pathology: a clinical approach [Internet]. 7th ed. Elsevier; 2019. p. 219–28. https://www.elsevier.com/books/underwoods-pathology-a-clinical-approach/cross/978-0-7020-7212-3.

5. Offiah CE, Dean J. Post-mortem CT and MRI: appropriate post-mortem imaging appearances and changes related to cardiopulmonary resuscitation. Br J Radiol [Internet]. 2016;89(1058):20150851. http://www.birpublications.org/doi/10.1259/bjr.20150851.
6. Takahashi Y, Sano R, Kominato Y, Takei H, Kobayashi S, Shimada T, et al. Usefulness of postmortem computed tomography for demonstrating cerebral hemorrhage in a brain too fragile for macroscopic examination. J Forensic Radiol Imaging [Internet]. 2013;1(4):212–4. https://linkinghub.elsevier.com/retrieve/pii/S221247801300083X.
7. Ruder TD, Zech W-D, Hatch GM, Ross S, Ampanozi G, Thali MJ, et al. Still frame from the hour of death: acute intracerebral hemorrhage on post-mortem computed tomography in a decomposed corpse. J Forensic Radiol Imaging [Internet]. 2013;1(2):73–6. https://linkinghub.elsevier.com/retrieve/pii/S2212478013000440.
8. Hatch GM, Dedouit F, Christensen AM, Thali MJ, Ruder TD. RADid: a pictorial review of radiologic identification using postmortem CT. J Forensic Radiol Imaging [Internet]. 2014;2(2):52–9. https://linkinghub.elsevier.com/retrieve/pii/S2212478014000501.
9. Takahashi N, Satou C, Higuchi T, Shiotani M, Maeda H, Hirose Y. Quantitative analysis of intracranial hypostasis: comparison of early postmortem and antemortem CT findings. AJR Am J Roentgenol [Internet]. 2010;195(6):W388–93. http://www.ncbi.nlm.nih.gov/pubmed/21098169.
10. Jackowski C, Thali M, Aghayev E, Yen K, Sonnenschein M, Zwygart K, et al. Postmortem imaging of blood and its characteristics using MSCT and MRI. Int J Legal Med [Internet]. 2006;120(4):233–40. http://link.springer.com/10.1007/s00414-005-0023-4.
11. Ishida M, Gonoi W, Hagiwara K, Takazawa Y, Akahane M, Fukayama M, et al. Hypostasis in the heart and great vessels of non-traumatic in-hospital death cases on postmortem computed tomography: relationship to antemortem blood tests. Leg Med [Internet]. 2011;13(6):280–5. https://linkinghub.elsevier.com/retrieve/pii/S134462231100112X.
12. Ishikawa N, Nishida A, Miyamori D, Kubo T, Ikegaya H. Estimation of postmortem time based on aorta narrowing in CT imaging. J Forensic Leg Med [Internet]. 2013;20(8):1075–7. https://linkinghub.elsevier.com/retrieve/pii/S1752928X13002655.
13. Kori S. Time since death from rigor mortis: forensic prospective. J Forensic Sci Crim Investig [Internet]. 2018;9(5). https://juniperpublishers.com/jfsci/JFSCI.MS.ID.555771.php.
14. Levy AD, Harcke HT. Essentials of forensic imaging [Internet]. Boca Raton: CRC Press; 2010. https://www.taylorfrancis.com/books/9781420091120.
15. Ishida M, Gonoi W, Okuma H, Shirota G, Shintani Y, Abe H, et al. Common postmortem computed tomography findings following atraumatic death: differentiation between normal postmortem changes and pathologic lesions. Korean J Radiol [Internet]. 2015;16(4):798. https://www.kjronline.org/DOIx.php?id=10.3348/kjr.2015.16.4.798.
16. Klein WM, Kunz T, Hermans K, Bayat AR, Koopmanschap DHJLM. The common pattern of postmortem changes on whole body CT scans. J Forensic Radiol Imaging [Internet]. 2016;4:47–52. https://linkinghub.elsevier.com/retrieve/pii/S2212478015300289.
17. Kawasumi Y, Usui A, Ikeda T, Ishibashi T, Funayama M. Post-mortem computed tomography findings of the frozen brain. J Forensic Radiol Imaging [Internet]. 2017;10:37–40. https://linkinghub.elsevier.com/retrieve/pii/S2212478016300284.
18. Hyodoh H, Ogura K, Sugimoto M, Suzuki Y, Kanazawa A, Murakami R, et al. Frozen (iced) effect on postmortem CT—experimental evaluation. J Forensic Radiol Imaging [Internet]. 2015;3(4):210–3. https://linkinghub.elsevier.com/retrieve/pii/S2212478015300186.
19. Franckenberg S, Flach PM, Gascho D, Thali MJ, Ross SG. Postmortem computed tomography-angiography (PMCTA) in decomposed bodies—a feasibility study. J Forensic Radiol Imaging [Internet]. 2015;3(4):226–34. https://linkinghub.elsevier.com/retrieve/pii/S2212478015300265.
20. Ruder TD, Schulze K, Ross S, Ampanozi G, Gascho D, Laberke P, et al. Into the decomposed body—feasibility of post-mortem CT angiography in a decomposed cadaver. J Forensic Radiol Imaging [Internet]. 2014;2(3):149–52. https://linkinghub.elsevier.com/retrieve/pii/S2212478014000793.

21. Egger C, Vaucher P, Doenz F, Palmiere C, Mangin P, Grabherr S. Development and validation of a postmortem radiological alteration index: the RA-index. Int J Legal Med [Internet]. 2012;126(4):559–66. http://link.springer.com/10.1007/s00414-012-0686-6.
22. Ross SG, Bolliger SA, Ampanozi G, Oesterhelweg L, Thali MJ, Flach PM. Postmortem CT angiography: capabilities and limitations in traumatic and natural causes of death. Radiographics [Internet]. 2014;34(3):830–46. http://pubs.rsna.org/doi/10.1148/rg.343115169.
23. Roberts I, Traill Z. The radiological autopsy. In: Suvarna SK, editor. Atlas of adult autopsy [Internet]. Cham: Springer International Publishing; 2016. p. 362. http://link.springer.com/10.1007/978-3-319-27022-7_13.
24. Balta JY, Twomey M, Moloney F, O'Connor OJ, Murphy KP, Cronin M, et al. Assessing radiological images of human cadavers: is there an effect of different embalming solutions? J Forensic Radiol Imaging [Internet]. 2017;11:40–6. https://linkinghub.elsevier.com/retrieve/pii/S2212478017300564.
25. Williams EJ, Davison A. Autopsy findings in bodies repatriated to the UK. Med Sci Law [Internet]. 2014;54(3):139–50. http://journals.sagepub.com/doi/10.1177/0025802413499325.

External Findings, Tubes and Devices on Post Mortem Computed Tomography

4

Introduction

The external examination of a body forms an essential part of the overall post mortem investigation. It provides the opportunity to spot features that point to underlying pathology, alongside allowing one to consider the possibilities of unnatural death. The latter could stop any routine open autopsy and prompt further specialist investigation or forensic involvement.

Standard diagnostic imaging has a limited role in the examination of the external surface of a body. Indeed, post mortem CT (PMCT) cannot depict skin colour, superficial bruising, tattoos, scars or abrasions to name but a few findings. Yet, these could be potentially significant. Therefore, both a review of external findings on the PMCT scan/report and a visual external inspection are necessary tasks for the pathologist.

In addition, usually following deaths in hospital or where cardiopulmonary resuscitation has been attempted, various tubes and devices may be encountered on post mortem scans. Examples are given and their importance in relation to the cause of death is discussed. Some devices also have relevance to handling of the body, along with issues in relation to cremation.

The External Examination: The Pathologist's Perspective

An external examination occurs prior to evisceration for open autopsies and is also required in those cases that will be certified without invasive studies. For routine coronial cases, this is usually performed by a pathologist. A radiologist would not usually externally examine the physical body.

The external examination provides the pathologist with information about likely internal disease. It should also be remembered that personal adornments such as piercings and rings may be part of case identification. The presence of jaundice, petechial haemorrhages or peripheral oedema may indicate liver failure, infections/

A. Shenton et al., *Post Mortem CT for Non-Suspicious Adult Deaths*,
https://doi.org/10.1007/978-3-030-70829-0_4

terminal hypoxia and cardiac dysfunction. Natural disease can also be indicated by clubbing, tobacco tar staining, joint deformities and drug patches. Accelerated marbling of the skin (whereby the pattern of underlying vessels is clearly visible, see Chap. 3) may suggest sepsis as would also be supported by diffuse petechial haemorrhages.

Vascular lines, drainage tubes, airways, feeding tubes and other devices can indicate medical intervention alongside review of medical tattoos. The position of these items should be confirmed as correct and should also be mapped against the background history. Furthermore, the identification of scars (fresh/healed) should support the medical history provided.

Livor mortis will point to the position of the body after death. Non-natural pathology may be indicated by superficial self-inflicted injuries, crease marks around the neck from ligatures, superficial skin ulcers and sinuses reflecting intravenous drug use and unusual bruises in cases of abuse. The degree of body nutrition (undernourished/emaciated, through to obesity) may be relevant in terms of assessment, particularly in terms of evaluation of care before death.

Criminal act pathology may be indicated by incised wounds, abrasions and penetrating injuries along with the pattern of bruising around vital structures, such as the neck. Rarely, skin colour can be a clue as to the pathology—such as pink discolouration in carbon monoxide poisoning, grey discolouration in methemoglobinemia and general pallor in association with pronounced blood loss. Examples and full discussion on the value of the external examination can be found in autopsy pathology texts [1].

External Findings on PMCT

Ideally, visual external examination should be performed in advance of PMCT in order to better inform the imaging interpretation. This is not always practical, due to mortuary workflow realities, and will need to be locally negotiated.

When performed prior to the scan, the results of the external examination, tubes removed and sites of any toxicological sampling (Figs. 4.1 and 4.2 and see Chap. 2) should be indicated to the radiologist. Any/all remaining devices should be noted in the PMCT report such that the information can be correlated at a later date if necessary.

To review the external body on PMCT, the scout views may be reviewed, standard axial images can be 'windowed' to better demonstrate external items (Figs. 4.3 and 4.4) or volume-rendered surface reformats can be produced (Figs. 4.5 and 4.6). Some forensic centres use three-dimensional surface scanning or photogrammetry to obtain a detailed picture of the body surface to aid forensic reconstructions, for example to correlate injury with a suspected instrument [2]. These data may also be of value in public court settings, rather than using actual photographs of the body.

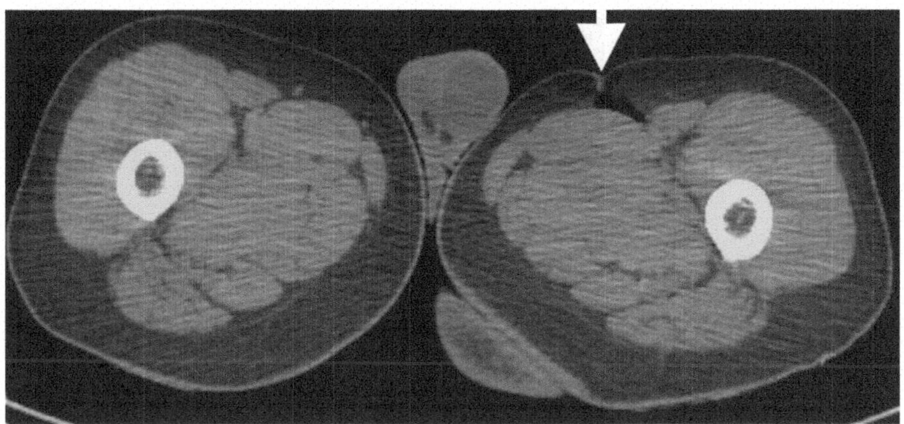

Fig. 4.1 Axial view of the upper thighs on soft tissue windows shows left groin soft tissue gas track (arrow) following toxicological blood sampling from the femoral vessels

Fig. 4.2 Sagittal view of the pelvis on lung windows to highlight suprapubic gas track (arrow) from urine sampling

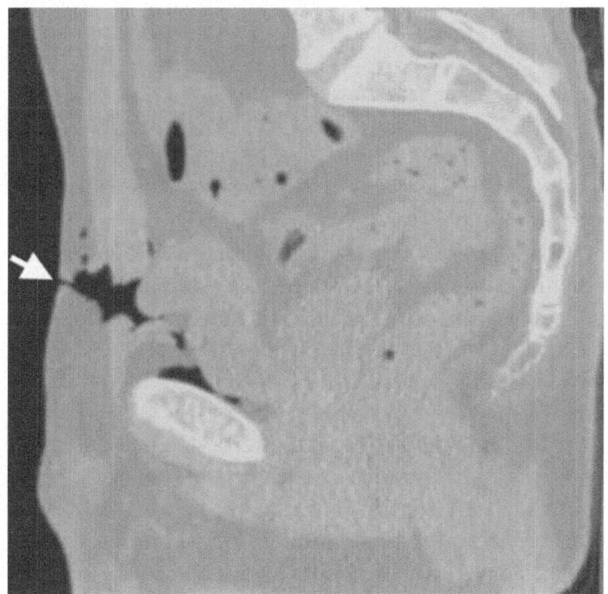

In the non-forensic setting, common external findings of note on PMCT include the presence of medical equipment from attempted cardiopulmonary resuscitation (Figs. 4.5, 4.7, 4.8, 4.9, and 4.10, see also later in this chapter and Chap. 11), nutritional support (Fig. 4.11), traumatic injuries (Figs. 4.12 and 4.13) or, in cases of suicidal hanging, the ligatures (Fig. 4.14, see also Chap. 6).

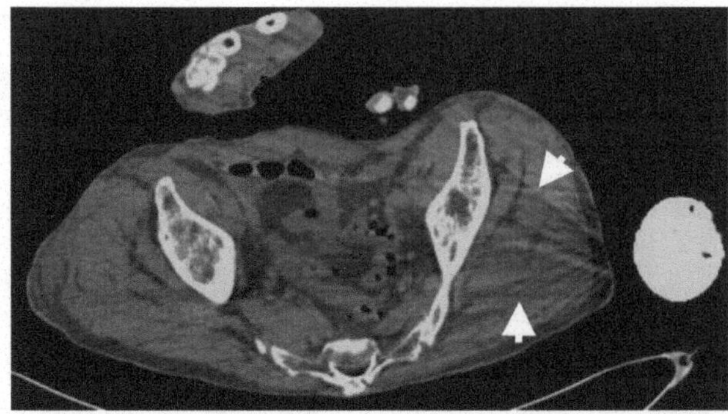

Fig. 4.3 Axial view of the pelvis on soft tissue windows shows streak artefact (arrows) from a dense metallic object on the left forearm

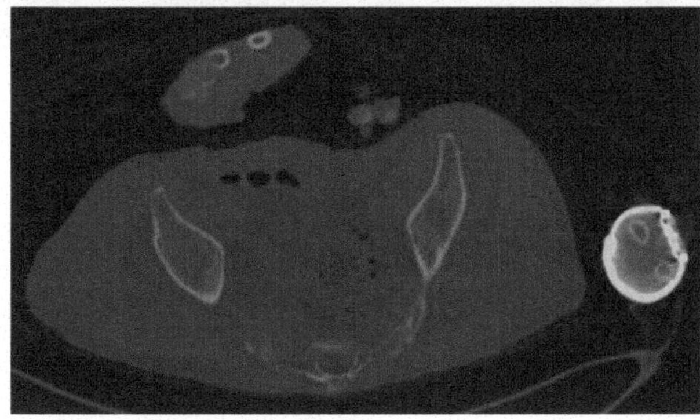

Fig. 4.4 Same image as Fig. 4.3 on bone windows reveals the object to be a wristwatch

Particularly in community sudden death cases, items of clothing, jewellery or other objects can be seen to remain with the body (Figs. 4.15, 4.16, 4.17, 4.18, and 4.19). They may occasionally be valuable in terms of patient identification but may cause artefacts that merit consideration. With agreement from the Coroner's office, these items may need to be removed for the scan if they render aspects of the study non-diagnostic.

It has been suggested that after a detailed external examination of the physical body, the PMCT can be used to 'triage' the need to proceed to open autopsy. If the circumstances, clinical information, findings on visual inspection and PMCT provide enough information to establish a cause of death on the 'balance of probabilities', then one should be able to derive a cause of death formulation and release the body without further investigation [3].

Tubes Seen on PMCT

General Comments

After deaths in hospital, medical care or following resuscitation attempts, various 'tubes' may be left in place. These include airway adjuncts, central venous or arterial lines, urinary catheters, nasogastric tubes and cavity drains (Figs. 4.20 and 4.21).

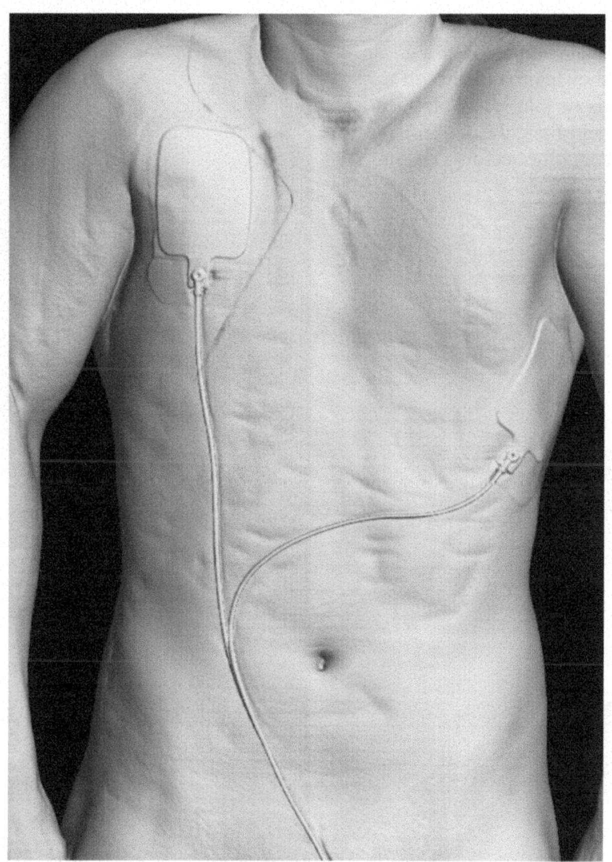

Fig. 4.5 Volume-rendered PMCT image showing defibrillator pads in place on the anterior chest wall

One benefit of PMCT is the ability to assess the body 'as it is' and observe potential complications such as tube misplacement (Fig. 4.22), underlying tissue trauma, pneumothorax or air embolism [4] prior to destructive dissection. PMCT in polytrauma patients can identify a badly positioned tube or line to provide the medical team with feedback and improve training [5]. Such poor placements may also be debated as pertinent to the cause of death, for example an airway incorrectly positioned in the oesophagus.

The radiologist should however keep in mind that tube positions may have altered after death, such as during body handling or transport. Whilst it is important to correctly identify any malposition of a tube or other device, it should not be assumed that this is relevant to the cause of death without other supportive data [4].

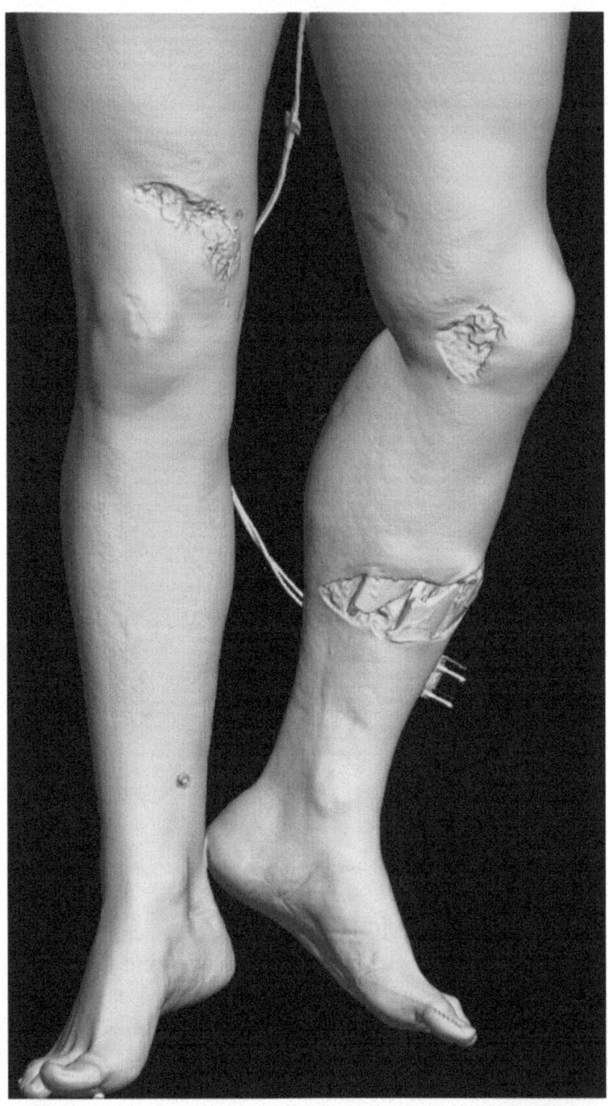

Fig. 4.6 Volume-rendered image of the lower legs showing traumatic soft tissue injuries and left leg deformity, the defibrillator pad wires are also visible

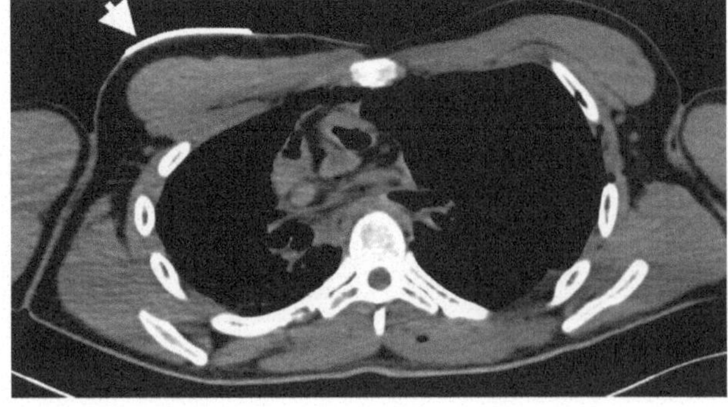

Fig. 4.7 Axial view of the chest on soft tissue windows shows a hyperdense right anterior chest wall defibrillator pad (arrow)

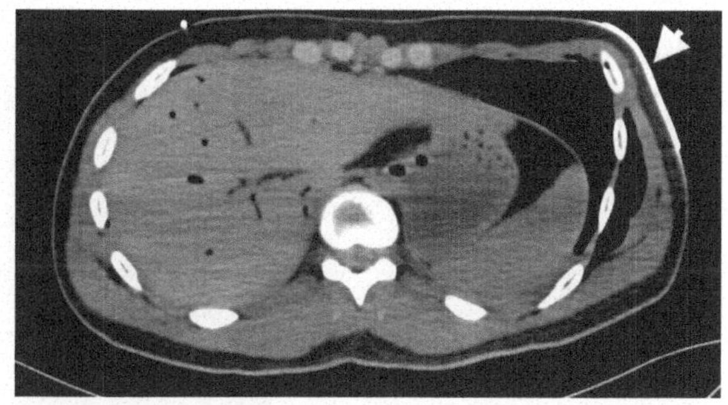

Fig. 4.8 Same case as Fig. 4.6, axial view of the upper abdomen shows hyperdense left lateral chest wall defibrillator pad (arrow), note the underlying traumatic soft tissue and rib cage shape deformity

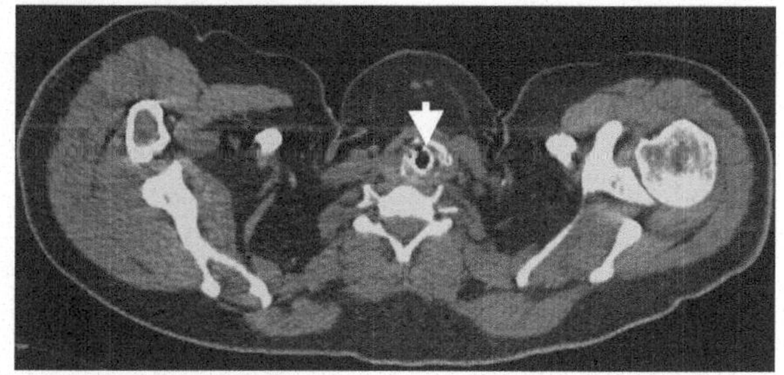

Fig. 4.9 Axial view of the lower neck on soft tissue windows shows an endotracheal tube (arrow) traversing the larynx

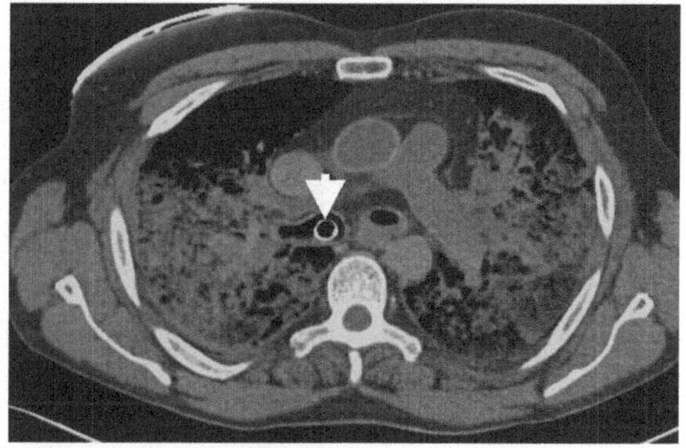

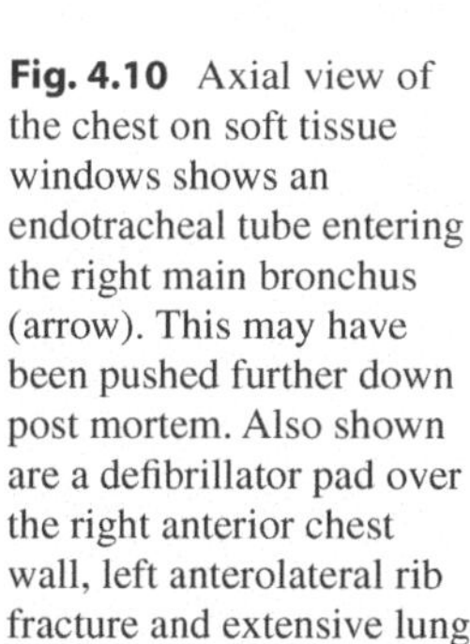

Fig. 4.10 Axial view of the chest on soft tissue windows shows an endotracheal tube entering the right main bronchus (arrow). This may have been pushed further down post mortem. Also shown are a defibrillator pad over the right anterior chest wall, left anterolateral rib fracture and extensive lung changes

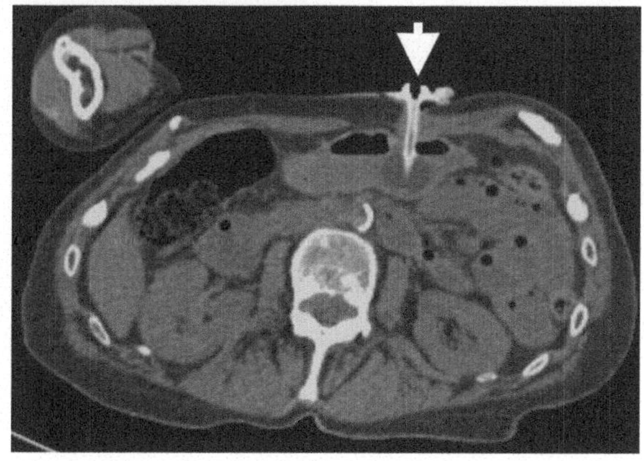

Fig. 4.11 Axial view of the abdomen on soft tissue windows shows an anterior abdominal wall percutaneous gastrostomy (arrow) with external flange and balloon correctly inflated in the stomach lumen

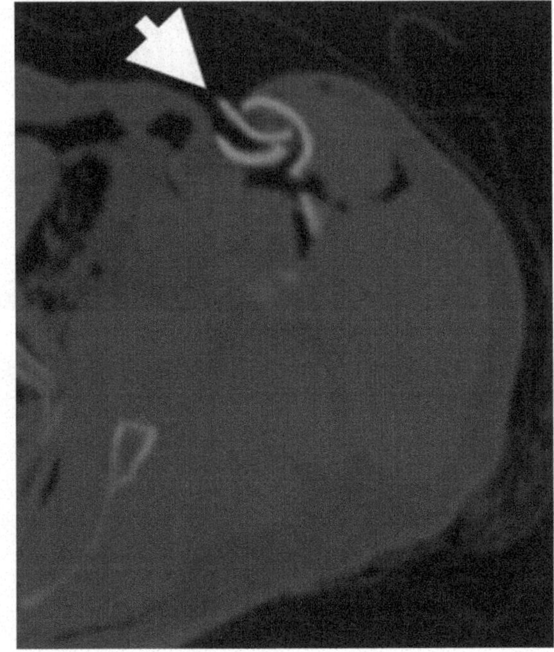

Fig. 4.12 Axial view of the left shoulder on bone windows showing a comminuted open fracture of the left humerus with skin and soft tissue disruption (arrow) following a road traffic collision suicide

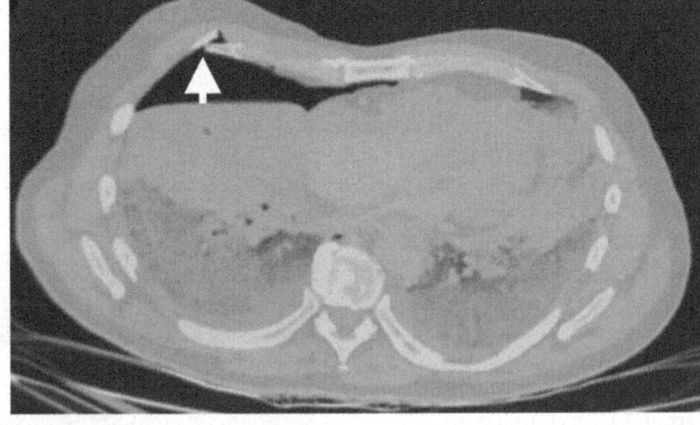

Fig. 4.13 Axial view through the chest on lung windows shows rib fractures causing thoracic wall distortion (arrow) and a pneumothorax, judged to be due to CPR chest compressions

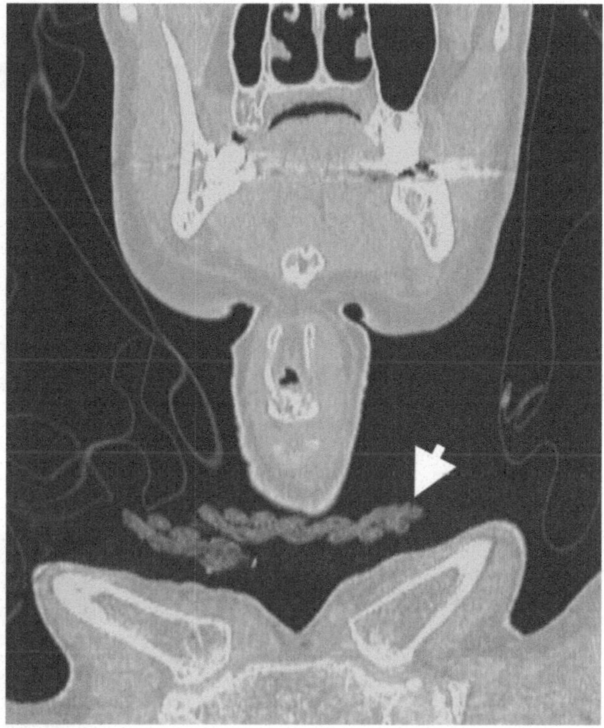

Fig. 4.14 Coronal view of the neck on lung windows shows a rope ligature (arrow) and thin folds of the body bag in a case of suicide by hanging

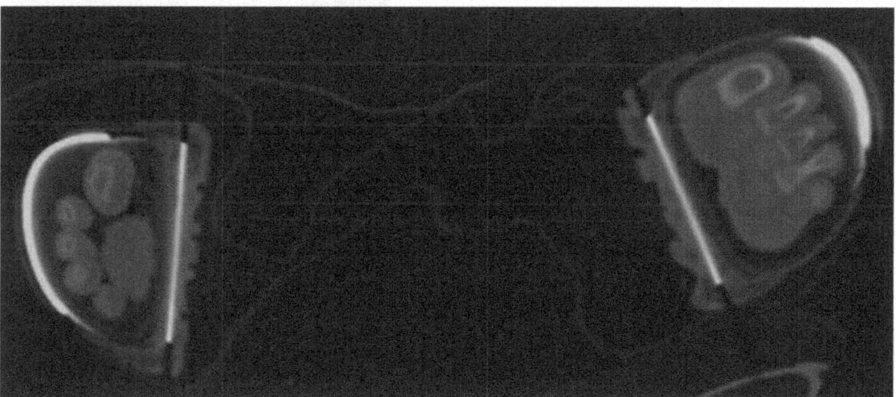

Fig. 4.15 Axial view of both feet on bone windows shows that the body has been imaged wearing clothes and steel toe cap shoes following death at the workplace

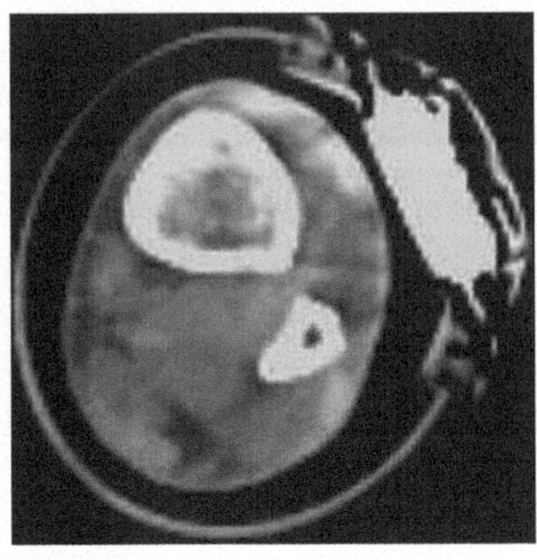

Fig. 4.16 Axial view of the left lower leg on soft tissue windows showing an electronic monitoring tag which is causing some artefact at this level

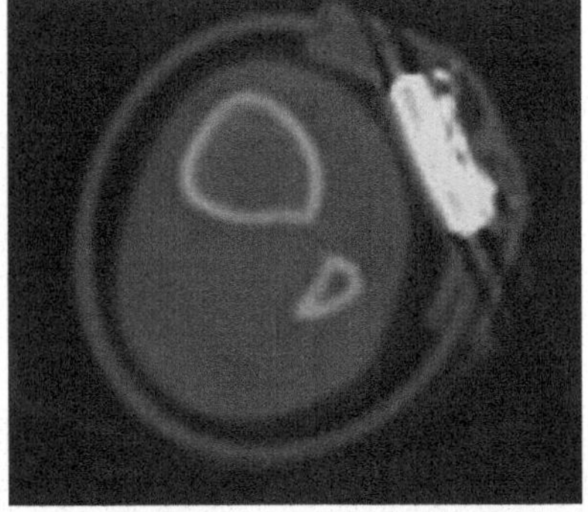

Fig. 4.17 Same case as Fig. 4.16, the electronic monitoring tag itself is better visualised on bone windows and the underlying bones can be assessed

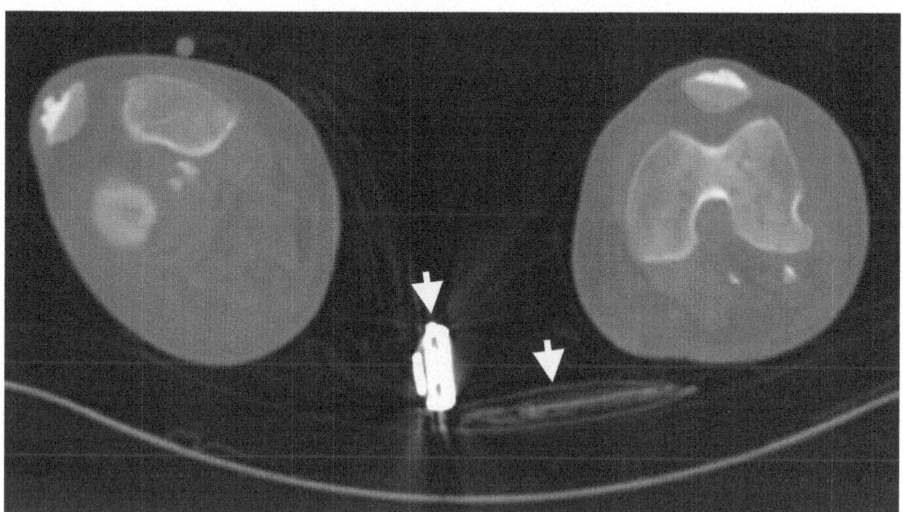

Fig. 4.18 Axial view at the level of the knees on bone windows shows that the body has been scanned with wallet and watch (arrows) between the legs in the body bag

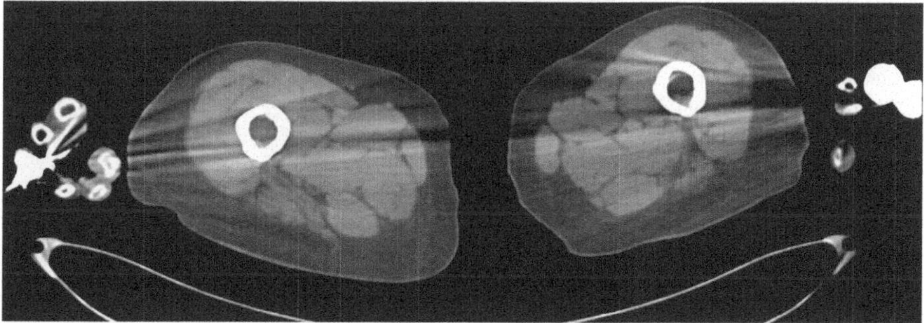

Fig. 4.19 Axial view at the level of the upper thighs on soft tissue windows, scanned with 'arms by the sides' shows streak artefact from multiple metallic rings on the fingers of both hands

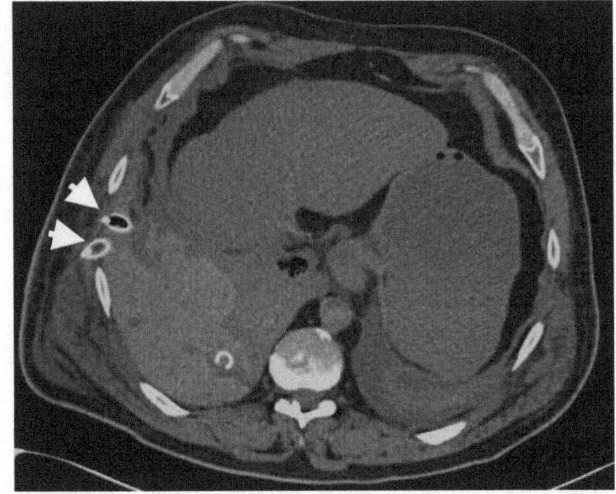

Fig. 4.20 Axial view of the lower chest/upper abdomen on soft tissue windows shows two large right-sided intercostal chest drains (arrows) inserted to treat a known empyema. In addition, there is a hyperdense irregular clot in keeping with haemothorax

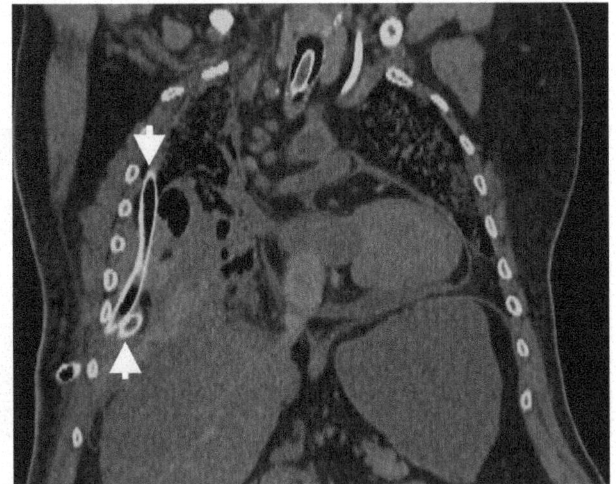

Fig. 4.21 Coronal view of same patient in Fig. 4.20 demonstrates apical (down arrow) and basal (up arrow) placements of the chest drains. There is also an endotracheal tube and left internal jugular vein catheter, as death occurred in hospital

Airway Adjuncts

A wide variety of airway adjuncts exist, including oropharyngeal and nasopharyngeal airways, supraglottic airways, tracheostomies and endotracheal (ET) tubes (Figs. 4.23, 4.24, 4.25, 4.26, and 4.27). The type and position of the airway adjunct *at the time of scanning* should be factually documented. The reporter should be aware of spurious foreign bodies such as dentures dislodged during resuscitation attempts (Fig. 4.28).

ET tubes enter the trachea via the mouth and larynx. After death, they are commonly pushed further inwards by nursing or mortuary staff, so that the face of the deceased can be viewed with the mouth closed. This procedure causes the tube to

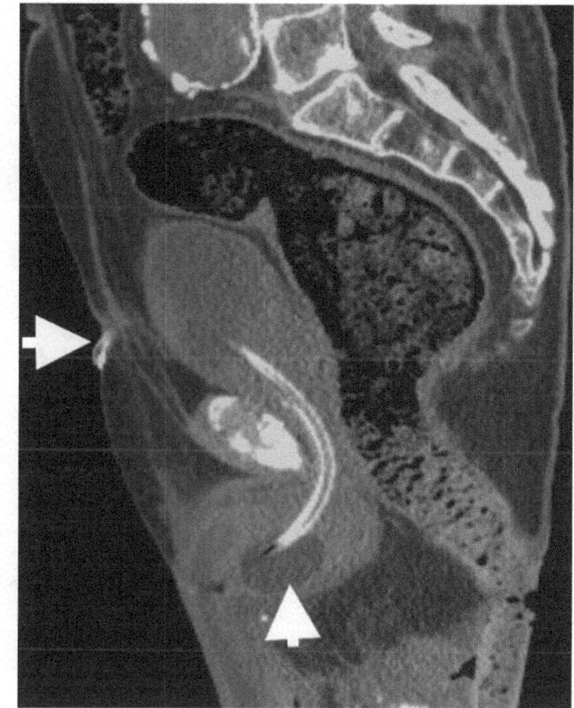

Fig. 4.22 Sagittal view of the pelvis on soft tissue windows showing a suprapubic catheter entering the lower anterior abdominal wall (horizontal arrow) but which has been misplaced with the balloon (vertical arrow) inflated in the urethra. Note extensive faecal loading and partly visualised peripherally calcified abdominal aortic aneurysm

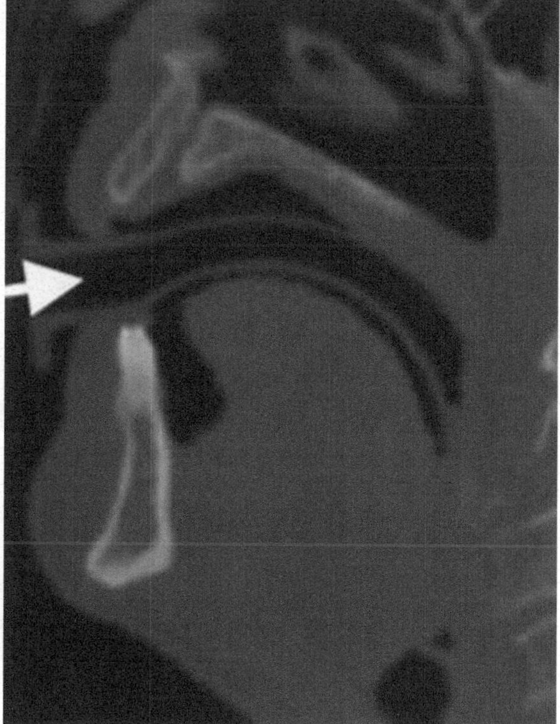

Fig. 4.23 Sagittal view of the oral cavity on bone windows showing an oropharyngeal airway (arrow) and also a partially visualised C2 anteroinferior corner fracture

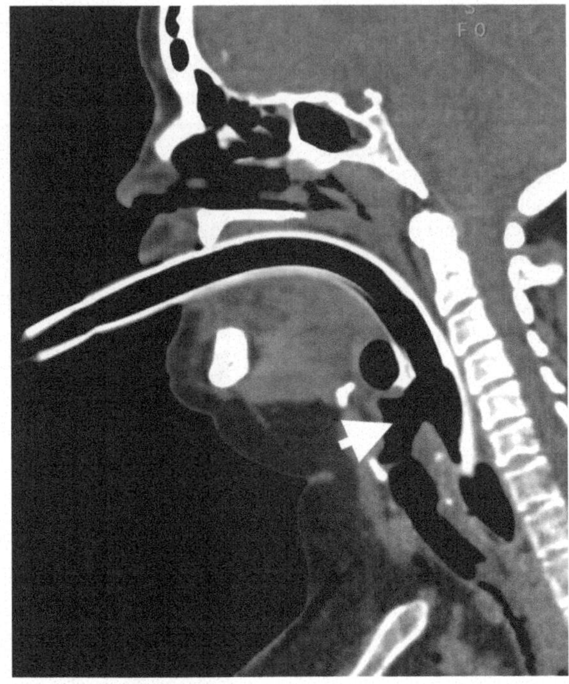

Fig. 4.24 Sagittal view of the neck on soft tissue windows showing a supraglottic laryngeal airway device and widely patent laryngeal inlet (arrow)

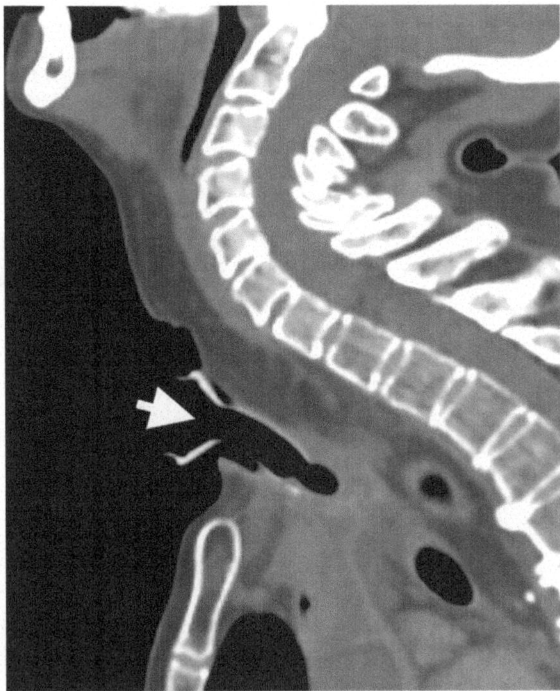

Fig. 4.25 Sagittal view of the neck windowed to show laryngectomy and tracheostomy (arrow)

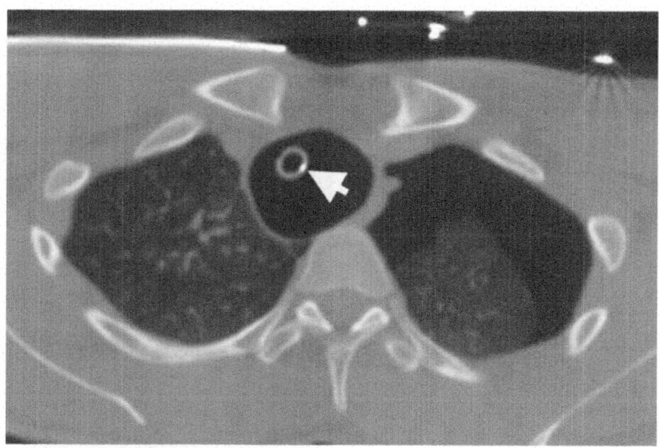

Fig. 4.26 Axial view at the level of the lung apices windowed to show an endotracheal tube (arrow pointing to the radiographic marker) with inflated cuff distending the tracheal wall. In addition, there is a left pneumothorax and a right chest wall defibrillator pad

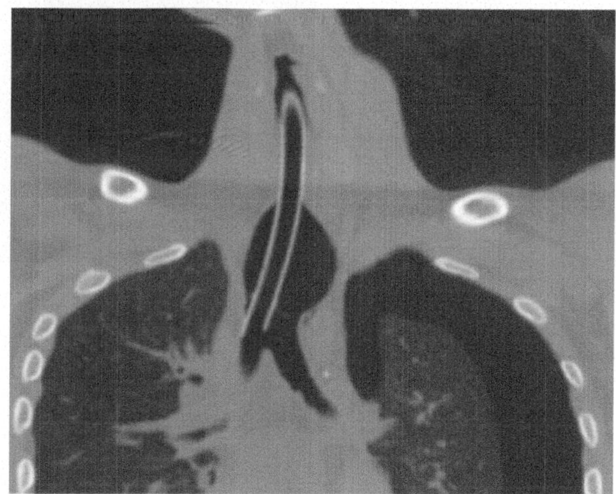

Fig. 4.27 Same case as Fig. 4.26, coronal view again shows endotracheal tube with inflated cuff and the left pneumothorax

move distally into the central airways, usually with the tip in the right main bronchus (Fig. 4.29). This should therefore not be automatically assumed as misplacement. If, however, the ET tube is seen in the oesophagus, it is unlikely to have been the result of any post mortem movement. Failure of correct endobronchial intubation may go unnoticed in the pre-hospital setting with oesophageal intubation being unrecognised [4].

Supraglottic airways are increasingly used in emergency settings owing to their relatively quick and easy placement. This type of airway also enters the mouth and usually has an elliptical, inflatable, or malleable plastic cuff that should sit in the hypopharynx (Figs. 4.30 and 4.31).

Vascular Access

Peripheral vascular cannulae can be difficult to identify on PMCT due to their small calibre but are unlikely to be of any significance. Potential local complications

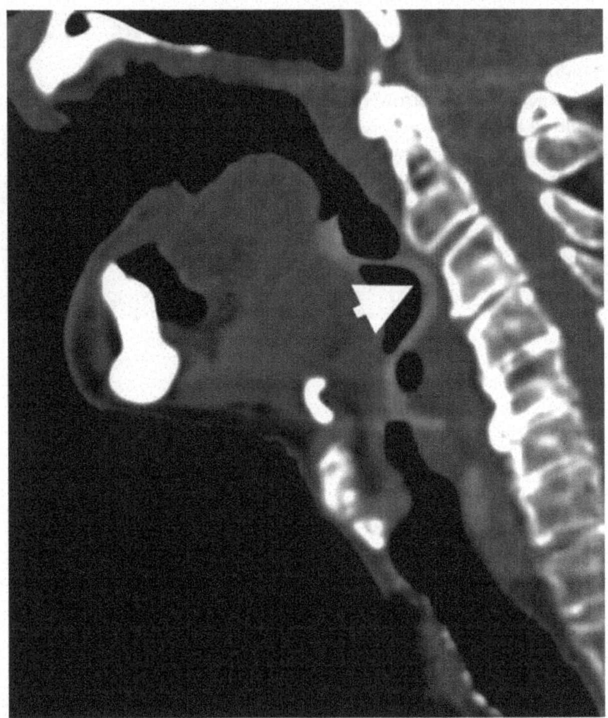

Fig. 4.28 Sagittal view of the upper aerodigestive tract on soft tissue windows shows an 'omega' shaped foreign body (arrow) consistent with dislodged dentures

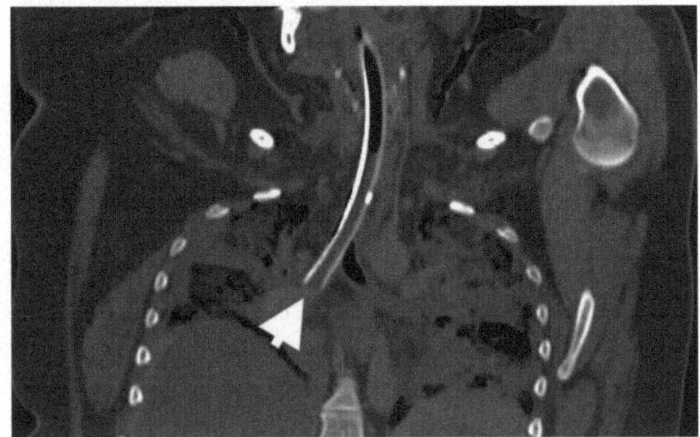

Fig. 4.29 Coronal view of the chest on soft tissue windows showing misplaced endotracheal tube tip in the right main bronchus (arrow), fluid in the tube lumen is a common post mortem finding

include extravasation including that of iodinated contrast, peripherally injected for clinical CT (Fig. 4.32).

Central venous access catheters are more important as they indicate significant medical intervention and are more complex to place. Complications include haematoma around the catheter track (Fig. 4.33) although some blood is often seen around central lines. The tip of a central venous catheter should lie centrally in the lumen of the vessel, usually the superior vena cava. It can unfortunately be difficult to precisely assess the position of catheter (or wire) tips with respect to lumen or wall as post mortem vessels are often collapsed, but a lack of perivascular stranding or haematoma argues against vessel rupture.

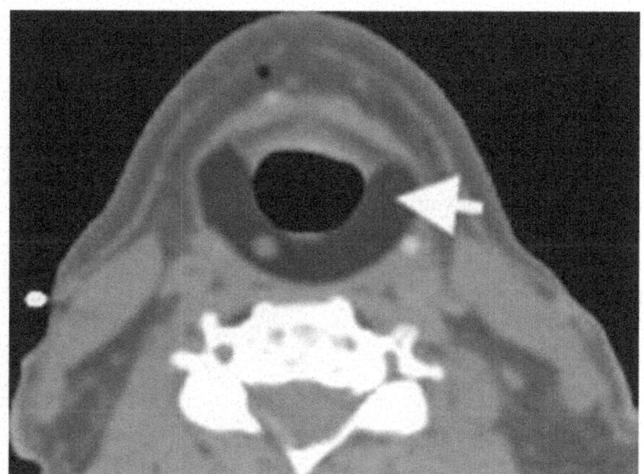

Fig. 4.30 Axial view at the level of the supraglottis, windowed to show a supraglottic airway device cuff (arrow)

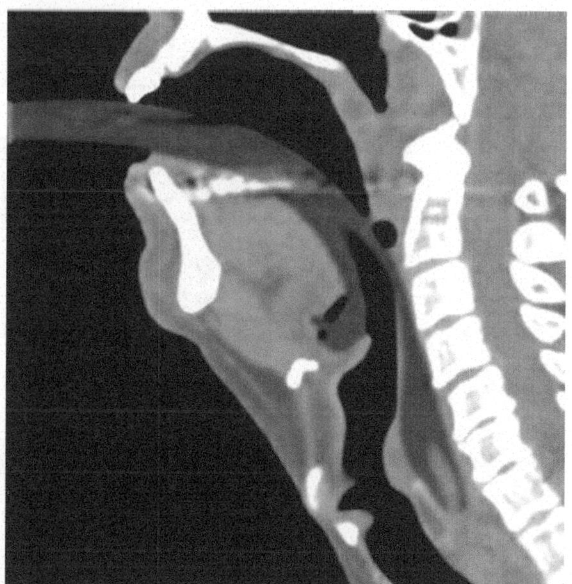

Fig. 4.31 Same case as Fig. 4.30, sagittal view of the neck shows the supraglottic airway device and a patent upper airway

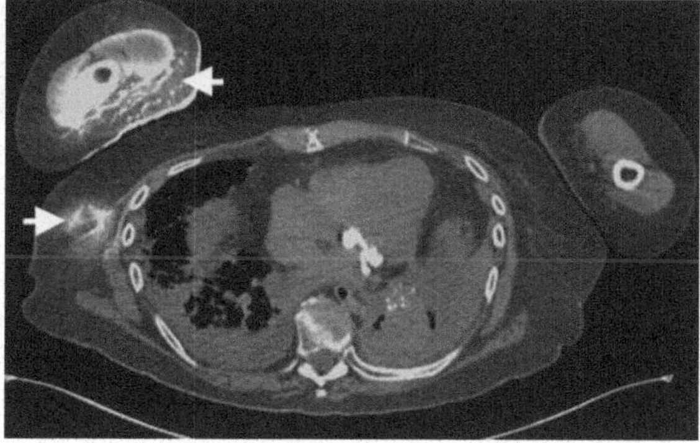

Fig. 4.32 Axial view of the chest and arms at the level of the heart, on soft tissue windows, shows dense, streaky iodinated contrast extravasation in the right upper arm and chest wall (arrows)

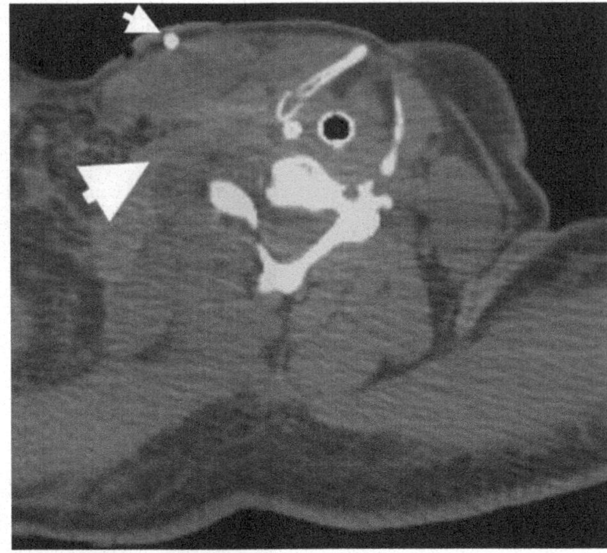

Fig. 4.33 Axial view of the neck on soft tissue windows shows a right internal jugular vein haematoma (large arrow) with loss of clear fat planes and mass effect deviating the larynx away, following vascular catheter placement (small arrow). Note also an endotracheal tube in the upper airway

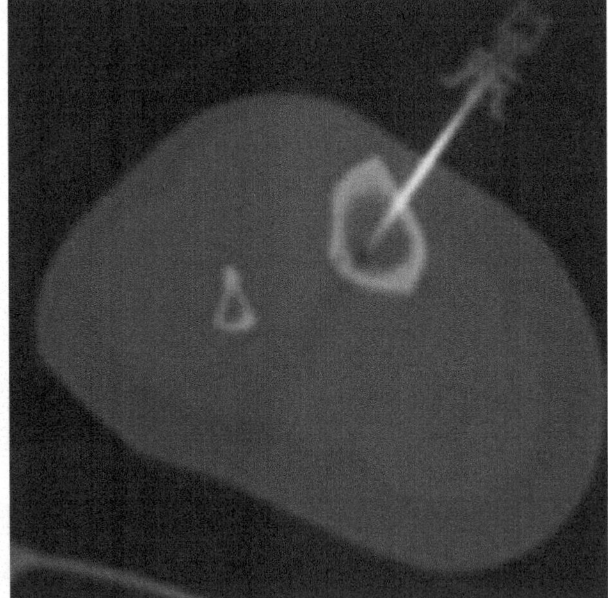

Fig. 4.34 Axial view of the right tibia on bone windows shows an intra-osseous needle with tip correctly positioned in the marrow cavity

Intraosseous Needles

Intraosseous (IO) needles may be used during resuscitation attempts when vascular access is insufficient or has failed. They are commonly inserted into the proximal tibia (Fig. 4.34), as well as the proximal humerus (Fig. 4.35) but also distal femur, distal tibia and sternum. Due to the cross-sectional nature of CT, needle position can be easily assessed. The tip should lie within the medullary cavity of the bone, not in

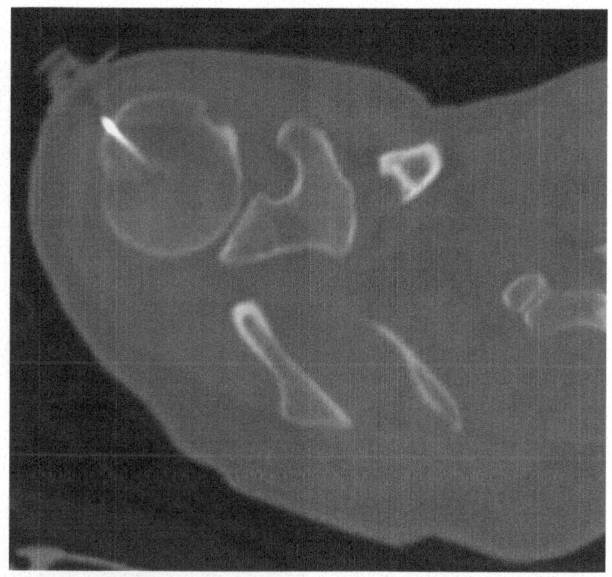

Fig. 4.35 Axial view at the level of the gleno-humeral joints on bone windows showing a right proximal humeral intra-osseous needle with tip in the marrow cavity

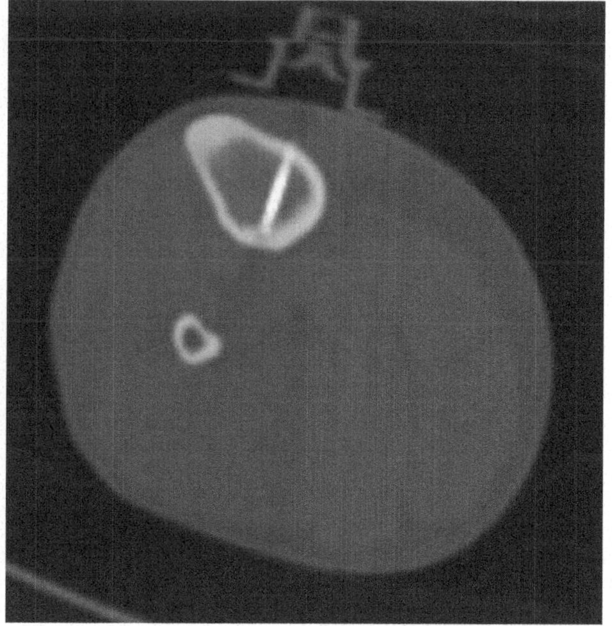

Fig. 4.36 Axial view of the right upper tibia on bone windows shows an intra-osseous needle with tip into the distal cortex; this needle was non-flushing

the cortex (Fig. 4.36), and the shaft should not be bent (Fig. 4.37). When entirely misplaced (Fig. 4.38) there can be extravasation into surrounding tissues and, of course, a limited or non-therapeutic result. Venous air embolism has also been associated although the exact mechanism is undetermined [4]. When removed prior to the scan, these needles can leave an intra-osseous gas track (Fig. 4.39) and should not be mistaken for fractures.

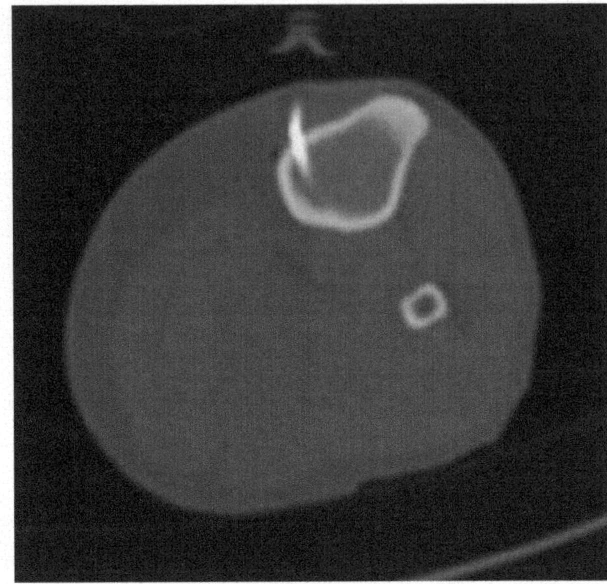

Fig. 4.37 Axial view of the left upper tibia on bone windows shows an intra-osseous needle with bent metal shaft; this needle was non-flushing

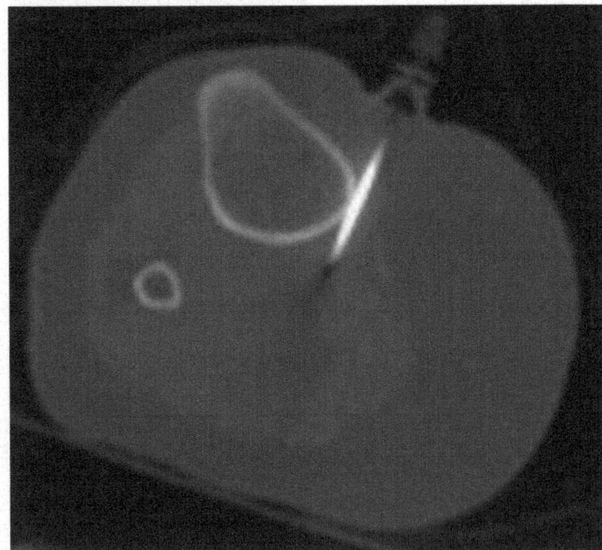

Fig. 4.38 Axial view of the right upper tibia on bone windows shows a misplaced intra-osseous needle which does not penetrate the bone cortex

Devices Seen on PMCT

Implantable Cardiac and Other Electrical Devices

It is important to identify these battery-operated internal devices which include implantable loop recorders, pacemakers, re-synchronisation therapy devices and cardiac defibrillators (Figs. 4.40, 4.41, 4.42, 4.43, and 4.44) as they must be removed prior to cremation, due to their risk of exploding [6].

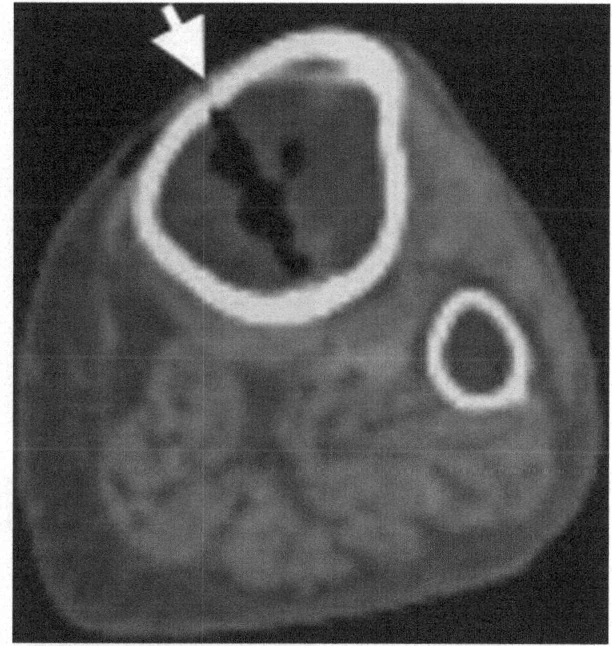

Fig. 4.39 Axial view of the left upper tibia on soft tissue windows shows intra-osseous gas track (arrow) from a removed intra-osseous needle

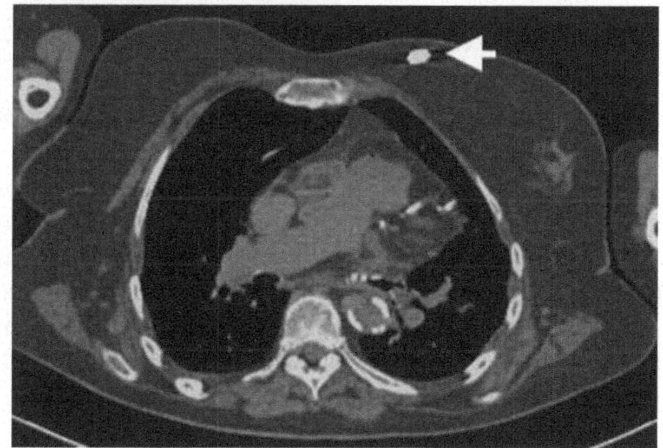

Fig. 4.40 Axial view of the chest on soft tissue windows showing an implantable loop recorder device in the subcutaneous left anterior chest wall (arrow)

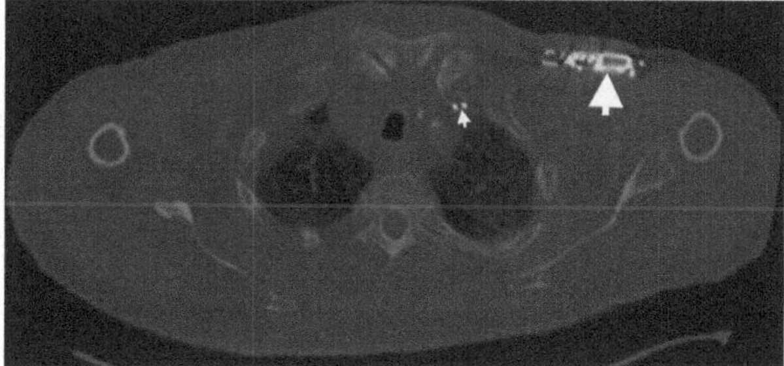

Fig. 4.41 Axial view of the upper chest on bone windows showing a pacemaker unit in the left anterior chest wall (large arrow) and two leads/metallic wires in the left subclavian vein (small arrow)

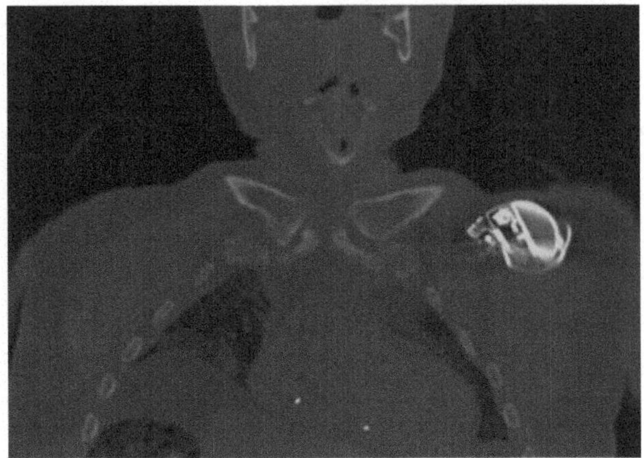

Fig. 4.42 Coronal view of the chest on bone windows showing the conventional position of a pacemaker device in the left anterior chest wall

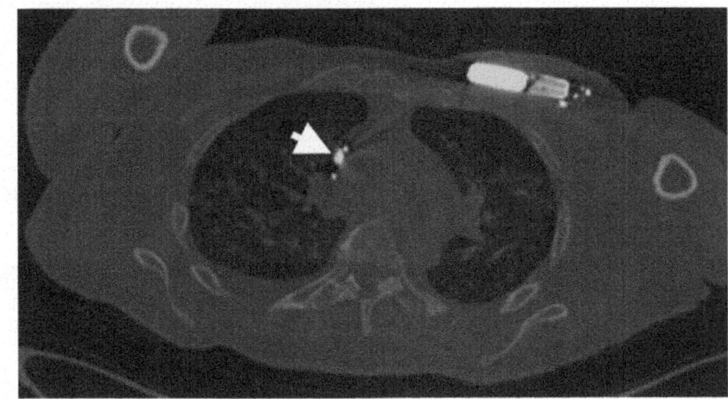

Fig. 4.43 Axial view of the chest on bone windows showing an implantable cardiac defibrillator and pacemaker combination device (larger than pacemaker only) with thicker lead containing the 'shock coil' at the level of the superior vena cava (arrow)

Implantable defibrillators also require deactivation prior to removal in order to avoid risk of injury to anyone handling the body. Such devices are used to prevent and treat cardiac arrhythmias, which might otherwise lead to sudden cardiac death. Conversely, there is a risk of discharge and inducing a fatal arrhythmia to mortuary staff when removing a device after death [7, 8]. Some of these devices record data that may be retrieved for evaluation of potential arrhythmias or even device malfunction, if this is in question.

On PMCT, the wires of such devices may cause localised streak artefact (Fig. 4.45). This can hamper assessment of the heart, in particular accurate coronary calcium scoring and can also make luminal assessment more difficult on a CT coronary angiogram.

Other electrical devices one may encounter include vagal or sacral nerve root stimulators, baclofen or other battery-operated pumps (Figs. 4.46 and 4.47). These should all be mentioned as they mostly require removal prior to cremation.

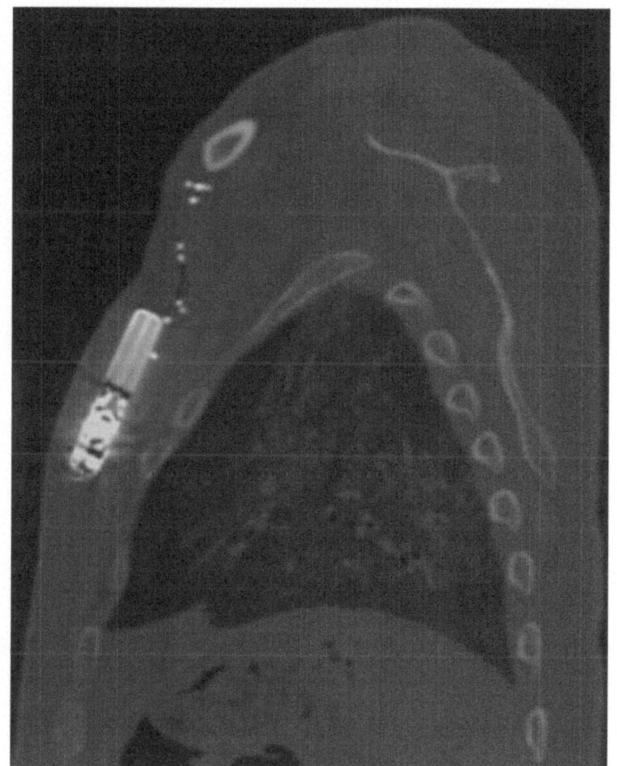

Fig. 4.44 Same case as Fig. 4.43, para-sagittal view of the chest showing the superficial placement of the implantable cardiac defibrillator/pacemaker device and its multiple leads

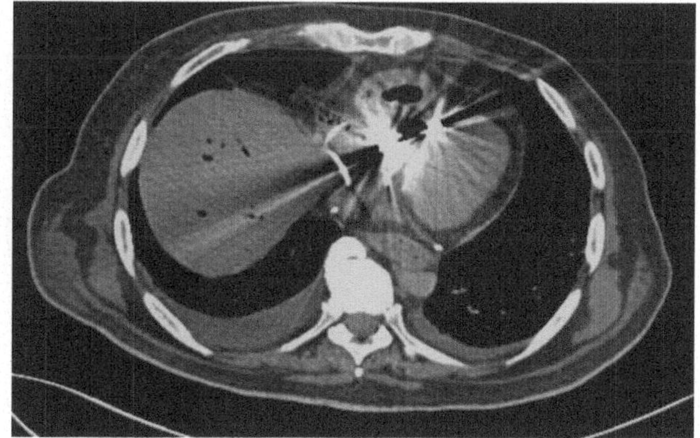

Fig. 4.45 Axial view of the chest on soft tissue windows shows that there is considerable streak artefact from implantable cardiac defibrillator wires. This can make the coronary calcium score difficult to measure

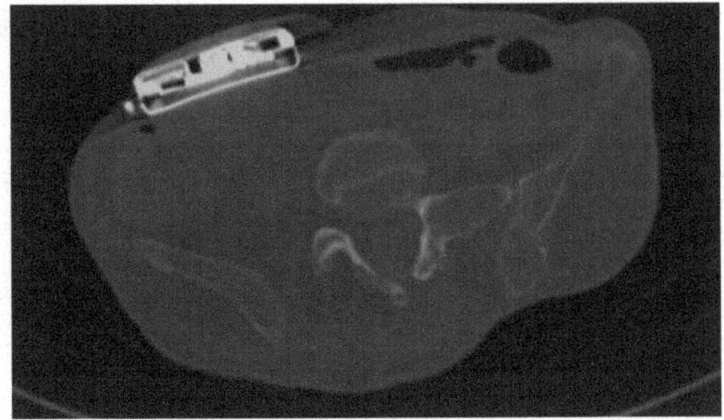

Fig. 4.46 Axial view of the pelvis on bone windows shows a right lower anterior abdominal wall placement of a baclofen pump, the tubing usually exits laterally and traverses the subcutaneous plane before entering the vertebral canal (Fig. 4.47)

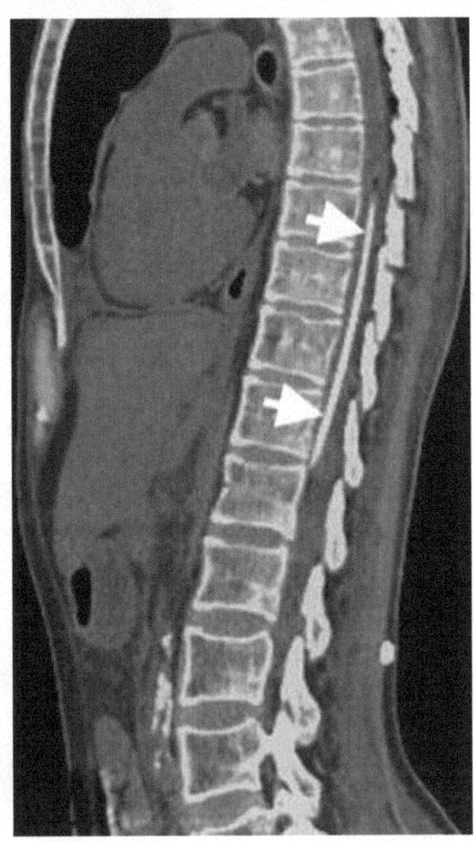

Fig. 4.47 Same case as Fig. 4.46, a sagittal view of the thoracolumbar spine on soft tissue windows shows the baclofen pump tubing ascending the vertebral canal (arrows)

Non-electrical Implants

Beyond those mentioned, there are a myriad of other implanted devices, including stents, grafts and prostheses, some more unusual than others (Fig. 4.48) that should be mentioned in the report. They may be relevant in indicating underlying disease

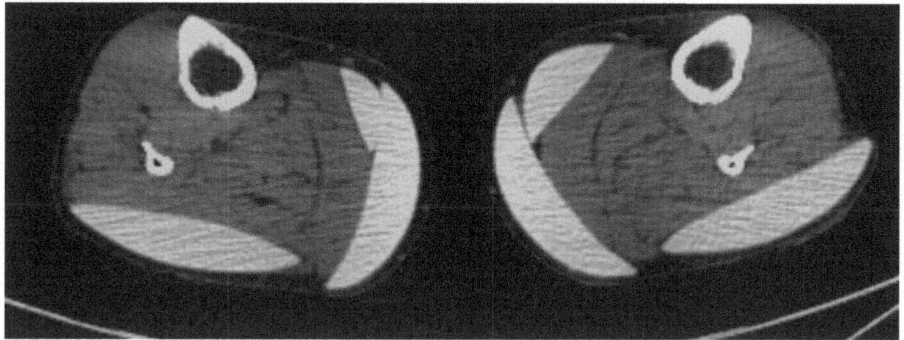

Fig. 4.48 Axial view at the level of the lower legs on soft tissue windows showing bilateral dense surgical calf implants

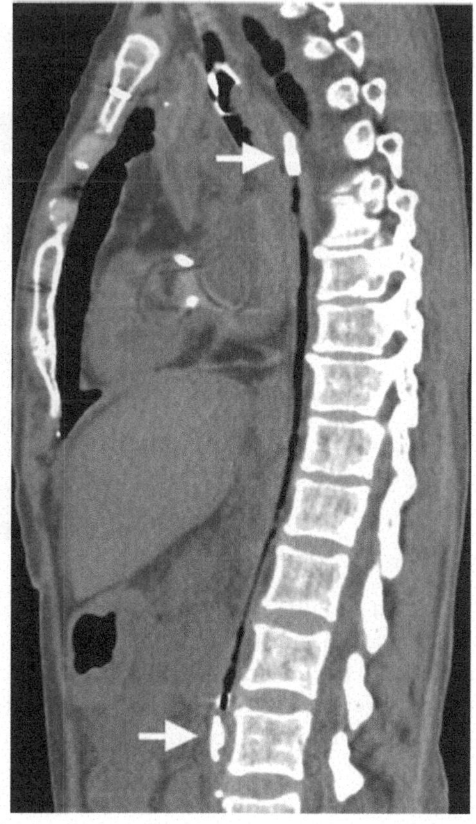

Fig. 4.49 Sagittal view of the chest on soft tissue windows shows the radio-opaque markers (arrows) of a collapsed intra-aortic balloon pump

or recent illness (Figs. 4.49, 4.50, and 4.51). Others require removal or specialist handling. They may have item numbers to permit patient identification—in cases of decomposed bodies.

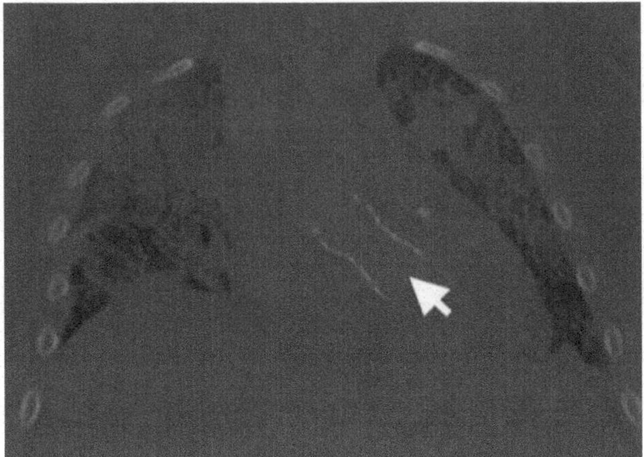

Fig. 4.50 Coronal view of the chest on bone windows showing a transcatheter aortic valve implantation/TAVI (arrow)

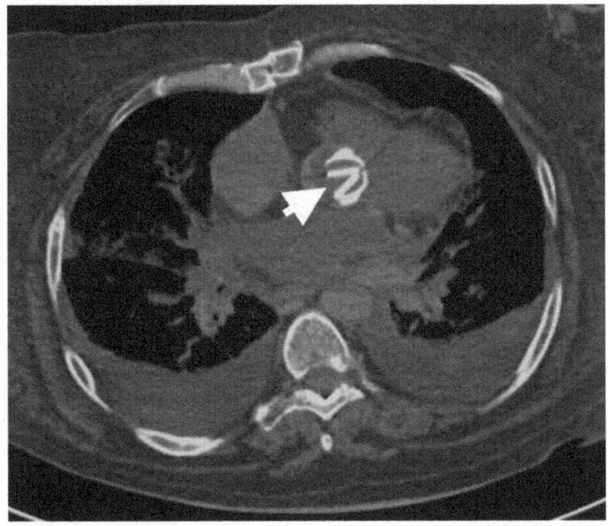

Fig. 4.51 Axial view of the chest on soft tissue windows shows a metallic aortic valve (arrow). Note also a healed surgical sternal fracture and moderate bilateral pleural effusions

Whilst metallic joint prostheses and fracture fixations (Fig. 4.52) are usually of no consequence, an uncommon type of intramedullary nail (Fixion®) has been reported to have a risk of explosion during cremation due to an internal saline component over-expanding [9]; we have not however come across this device. It is expected that not all types of specialised implant will be familiar to every radiologist, but the reporter should mention any and all implanted devices as a matter of routine and seek clarification from medical notes if there are queries or concerns as to the nature or function of the device.

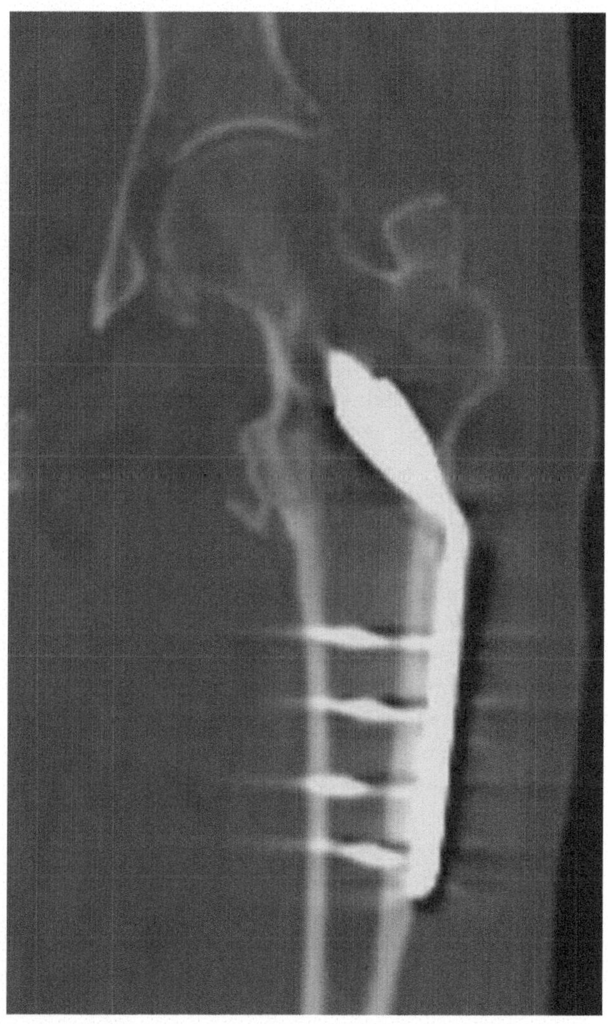

Fig. 4.52 Coronal view of the left proximal femur on bone windows showing a dynamic hip screw and remodelled, healed intertrochanteric fracture

Finally, if there are implanted radioactive seeds (such as used in the prostate or breast for the treatment of cancer), these should also be specifically mentioned. The radiation risk is low to those working in the PMCT suite, owing to the locally acting nature of such implants, however, appropriate radiation protective wear may be advised. For high-radiation devices one may need to delay scanning or open autopsy.

Reporting External Findings and Devices: Pearls and Pitfalls

Make note in the report if you have performed or received details of any external examination including knowledge of sites of toxicological sampling.

Review any scout imaging and window standard images to demonstrate any external or superficial items of interest.

It is suggested that the presence of any/all implanted tubes and devices is mentioned in each report as a matter of routine.

State clearly when there is an absence of such devices, particularly those that may preclude cremation or if they were indicated as present in the clinical record.

Of note, the following list of implants merit consideration before cremation is permitted, as they are considered potentially dangerous [10]:

- Pacemakers
- Implantable Cardioverter Defibrillators (ICDs)
- Cardiac resynchronization therapy devices (CRTDs)
- Implantable loop recorders
- Ventricular assist devices (VADs)
- Implantable drug pumps including intrathecal pumps
- Neurostimulators (including for pain & Functional Electrical Stimulation)
- Bone growth stimulators
- Hydrocephalus programmable shunts
- Fixion® nails
- Any other battery powered or pressurised implant
- Radioactive implants
- Radiopharmaceutical treatment (via injection)

Finally, note any finding that seems out of the ordinary even, if the significance is unknown, as relevance may potentially become apparent later.

Example PMCT report phrases:

- I have not performed an external examination of the body or received details of such an examination.
- An endotracheal tube is present with its tip in the mid oesophagus. This is unlikely to have migrated in the post mortem setting.
- An intra-osseous needle is placed in the proximal right tibia and the tip is correctly sited in the medullary cavity.
- There is a pacemaker/other device in place at the time of PMCT.
- There is no implantable cardiac or other battery-powered device in place.
- A soft tissue gas track in the groin suggests there has been prior aspiration for toxicology, please correlate with mortuary records.

References

1. Lloyd KL, Suvarna SK. External examination. In: Suvarna SK, editor. Atlas of adult autopsy [Internet]. Cham: Springer International Publishing; 2016. p. 13–45. http://link.springer.com/10.1007/978-3-319-27022-7_2.
2. Grabherr S, Egger C, Vilarino R, Campana L, Jotterand M, Dedouit F. Modern post-mortem imaging: an update on recent developments. Forensic Sci Res [Internet]. 2017;2(2):52–64. https://www.tandfonline.com/doi/full/10.1080/20961790.2017.1330738.
3. Chatzaraki V, Heimer J, Thali M, Dally A, Schweitzer W. Role of PMCT as a triage tool between external inspection and full autopsy—case series and review. J Forensic Radiol Imaging [Internet]. 2018;15:26–38. https://linkinghub.elsevier.com/retrieve/pii/S2212478018300601.
4. Bolster F, Ali Z, Fowler D, Daly B. Imaging of resuscitation and emergency resuscitation devices—Lessons learned from post mortem computed tomography. J Forensic Radiol Imaging [Internet]. 2019;17:23–30. https://linkinghub.elsevier.com/retrieve/pii/S2212478019300383.
5. Lotan E, Portnoy O, Konen E, Simon D, Guranda L. The role of early postmortem CT in the evaluation of support-line misplacement in patients with severe trauma. Am J Roentgenol [Internet]. 2015;204(1):3–7. http://www.ajronline.org/doi/10.2214/AJR.14.12796.
6. Johnson C, Lowe J, Osborn M. Guidance for pathologists conducting post-mortem examinations on individuals with implanted electronic medical devices [Internet]. The Royal College of Pathologists, London; 2015. https://www.rcpath.org/uploads/assets/4f04f871-257e-446b-b94f38095defaf0d/guidance-for-pathologists-conducting-post-mortem-examinations-on-individuals-with-implanted-electronic-and-medical-devices.pdf.
7. Ackerman MJ, Giudicessi JR. Post-mortem cardiovascular implantable electronic device interrogation: Clinical indications and potential benefits. J Am Coll Cardiol [Internet]. 2016;68(12):1265–7. https://linkinghub.elsevier.com/retrieve/pii/S0735109716345983.
8. Mitchell LB, Pineda EA, Titus JL, Bartosch PM, Benditt DG. Sudden death in patients with implantable cardioverter defibrillators: The importance of post-shock electromechanical dissociation. J Am Coll Cardiol [Internet]. 2002;39(8):1323–8. https://linkinghub.elsevier.com/retrieve/pii/S0735109702017849.
9. Phillips AW, Patel AD, Donell ST. Explosion of Fixion® humeral nail during cremation: novel "complication" with a novel implant. Inj Extra [Internet]. 2006;37(10):357–8. https://linkinghub.elsevier.com/retrieve/pii/S1572346106000365.
10. Ministry of Justice. The cremation (England and Wales) regulations 2008. Guidance to applicants. [Internet]. 2018. https://www.cremation.org.uk/content/files/2018-guidance-to-applicants.pdf.

Post Mortem Computed Tomography of the Brain and Spinal Cord

5

Introduction

As with cranial computed tomography (CT) in the living, non-contrast–enhanced post mortem computed tomography (PMCT) can readily identify significant haemorrhage, mass effect, hydrocephalus, large vessel territory infarction and, additionally, fatal trauma. Cranial PMCT may therefore permit a cause of death solution without open autopsy being needed.

One should also be mindful of further benefit in cases where (more commonly) no cranial pathology is demonstrated. In these scenarios, opening the head at invasive autopsy can usually be avoided [1]. This advantage focuses the pathologist onto areas likely to be relevant to the cause of death, such as the heart and lungs (see Chaps. 7 and 8).

However, before reporting cranial PMCT, it is imperative to become familiar with normal post mortem findings in order not to mistake decomposition changes for genuine pathology. PMCT of the brain can generally be considered to be reliable, although its value may fall quickly in cases with significant tissue decomposition.

Autopsy of the Brain and Spinal Cord: The Pathologist's Perspective

The post mortem examination of the brain and spinal cord is technically difficult, since these soft structures are very well protected by cranial and vertebral bone [2]. Such examination is potentially disfiguring to the body and thereby often a particular concern for relatives of the deceased. Indeed, many pathologists and Coroners prefer not to engage with head and nervous system tissues unless there is a good reason requiring open access.

A. Shenton et al., *Post Mortem CT for Non-Suspicious Adult Deaths*, https://doi.org/10.1007/978-3-030-70829-0_5

Should the brain need to be removed, then a coronal slice through the scalp tissues down to the skull is accomplished from behind the ear on both sides, with the scalp and deeper soft tissues being reflected anteriorly and posteriorly. The calvarium of the skull is removed using a circumferential saw cut, including a step in the cut, usually made in order to facilitate reassembly of the skull and reconstitution of the head tissues following examination. In this manner, the top of the skull is removed, allowing direct inspection of the dura, leptomeninges and underlying brain with the cranial nerves, tentorium cerebelli and vasculature being transected to facilitate extraction. The pituitary can be accessed at this juncture if desired.

Once the brain has been removed and weighed, there are two possibilities for the examination. First, one could progress through direct inspection of the meninges, removal of the brainstem and cerebellum at the mid-brain level and a section of the cerebellum through the peduncles, thereby exposing the fourth ventricle. Serially slicing through the mid-brain, pons and medulla in transverse fashion allows good inspection of the brainstem tissues. The cerebellum is traditionally cut centrally in a sagittal fashion through the vermis, with oblique sections taken to expose the dentate nucleus and cortical grey ribbon tissues.

The cerebral hemispheres are examined by coronal slices, commencing anteriorly and generally passing progressively backwards in 1 cm steps. This exposes the outer grey cortical ribbon, the inner white matter, the deep nuclei, the ventricles and choroid plexus tissues. It also facilitates identification of the pineal gland.

If one is interested in the arterial vasculature, then this is usually resected in one piece from the under surface of the brain before the brain tissue slicing. This is generally reserved for complex vascular malformations and confirmation of thrombosis.

It has to be recognised that examination of the unfixed brain is complex because the brain parenchyma is so soft. Block sampling is complicated, as some lesions may be difficult to identify in the unfixed state.

The second and alternative solution to brain tissue examination is to suspend the intact brain in a large bucket of formalin for approximately 6 weeks, allowing the tissues to fix and harden. This is particularly useful for complex neuropathology cases, as it allows smaller step sections to be taken through the brain tissues. Clearly, retaining the brain at the end of an autopsy for a period of time may be less acceptable to relatives compared to examination of the fresh tissues, with this having to be balanced against the need to acquire good histology.

The examination of the spinal cord can be accomplished in two ways. The first is to turn the body into a prone position and make a longitudinal slice from the occiput down towards the sacrum with dissection of underlying soft tissue and musculature down to the posterior bony components of the vertebral canal. These need to be sawn in a stepwise fashion on both sides with the ligamentous tissues as well as the vertebral spine/posterior arch elements then being removed. This allows exposure of the spinal cord, which can be removed intact, after transecting the relevant spinal nerves.

Alternatively, the body can be left in its supine position, with the vertebral bony tissues being exposed. The anterior vertebral arch bone is cut sequentially. One then removes the vertebral bodies and anterior arch tissues as well as the intervertebral discs in one piece. This also allows exposure of the spinal cord and its removal.

Both techniques are time-consuming, labour intensive and complicated, requiring good-quality mortuary staff assistance and a good reason to perform these tasks. It has to be remembered that simply fragment autopsy sampling of parts of the brain tissues is often an unrewarding experience unless one knows where lesions reside. Often, it is the totality of the brain tissues and spinal cord examination that allows one to make a value judgement as to any neuropathology. It should also be remembered that brain tissues can be a particular hazard in certain circumstances. The most important of these is that of prion diseases, with the infectious agent being potentially aerosolised during cranial examination. Indeed, there is still deemed to be a hazard for fixed tissue and even slide material according to some sources [3].

As a consequence, many pathologists prefer to start with the thoracic and abdominal tissues in order to try to define a cause of death. If examination has been achieved adequately beforehand, by imaging, then there is often no need to examine the brain or related tissues. It has been shown that there is a very low frequency of positive diagnoses in cases when there is no prompt to open the head—and opening the head should therefore not be an automatic protocol [4].

The advent of PMCT has shown confidence in assessing the brain and to a lesser degree the vertebral tissues, permitting the avoidance of unnecessary head and spinal cord tissue examination in many cases.

Normal PMCT Findings

Brain

Very early post mortem imaging appearances (within approximately 6 h after death) are comparable to those of the living. However, as time progresses, there are normal changes of brain autolysis, characterised by a loss of grey–white matter differentiation, decreased cerebral attenuation and mild diffuse swelling (Figs. 5.1 and 5.2) [5–7]. Whilst perhaps less reliable than in the living for subtle change, a gross estimate of cerebral volume and/or significant atrophy can still be made. If present, significant periventricular ischaemic changes can also remain visible.

The decomposition process results in the study becoming progressively less sensitive for the detection of brain abnormalities, although pathology such as significant haemorrhage can be seen for some time. Subtle brain changes are potentially critical findings in imaging the living, but they are unlikely to be fatal.

As decomposition progresses, gas begins to accumulate in the tissues. Initially this is within the blood vessels, eventually becoming free within the cranium. Over time the brain ‘slumps’ or ‘settles’ in a dependent (gravity-based) position, initially maintaining recognisable architecture. Later it becomes soft and eventually liquefies, resulting in a dependent fluid level with enlarging putrefactive pneumocephalus (Figs. 5.3, 5.4, 5.5, 5.6, and 5.7). At this point, the brain parenchyma can no longer be reliably assessed by imaging.

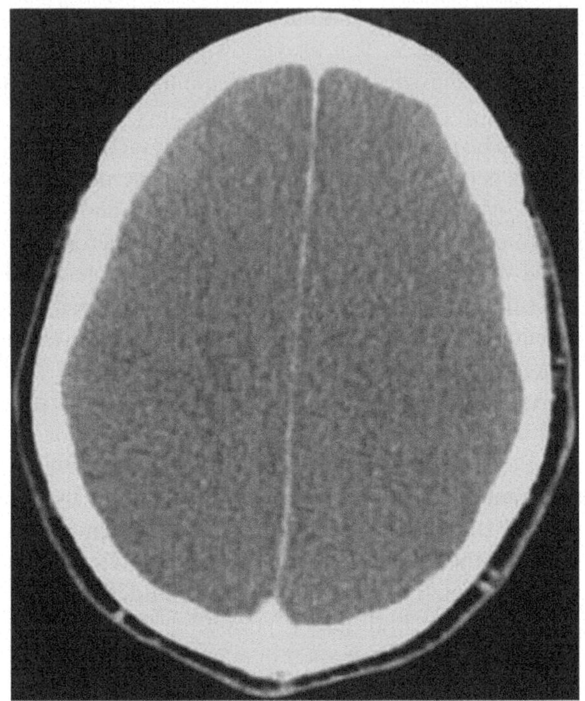

Fig. 5.1 Axial view of the brain cranial to the ventricles, on brain windows, shows the early normal post mortem changes of brain autolysis. There is loss of grey–white matter differentiation, diffuse swelling and loss of sulcal visualisation

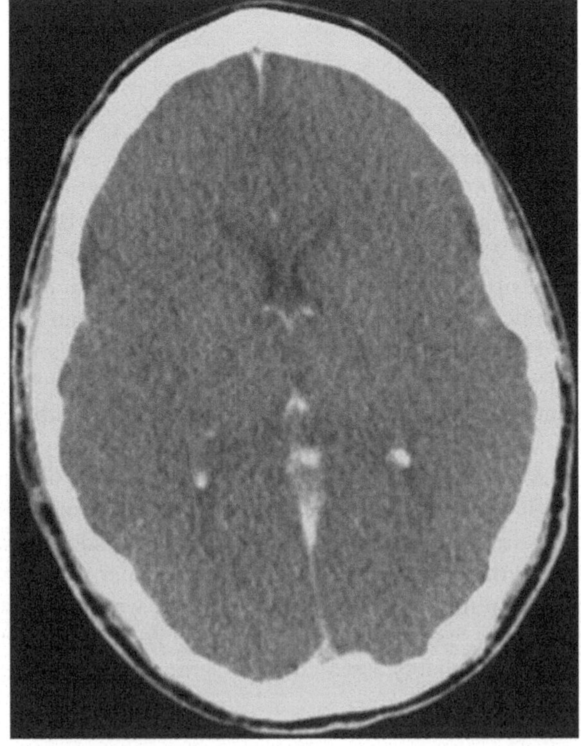

Fig. 5.2 Axial view of the brain at the level of the lateral ventricles shows normal post mortem changes. There is loss of grey–white matter differentiation, generally decreased cerebral attenuation and mild diffuse swelling

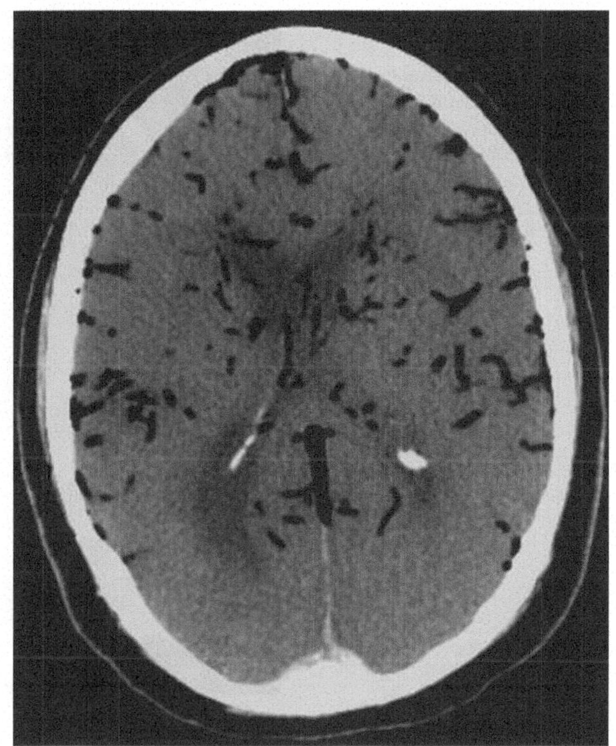

Fig. 5.3 Axial view of the brain, on brain windows, shows early intracranial decomposition evidenced by vascular gas (black in the image) and a very tiny pneumocephalus anteriorly

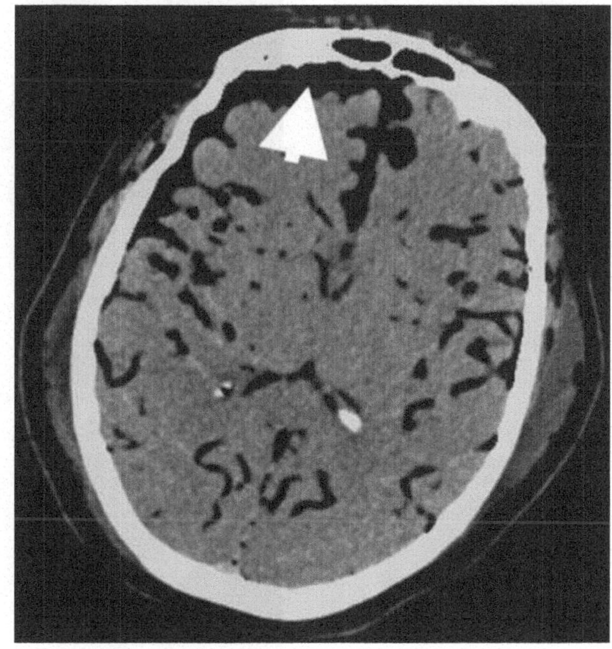

Fig. 5.4 Axial view of the brain shows an increasing pneumocephalus anteriorly (arrow) compared to Fig. 5.3 and more extensive vascular gas

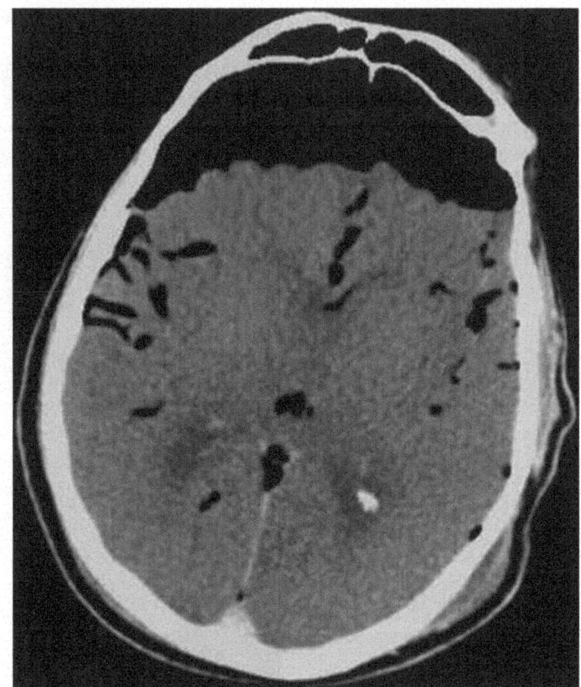

Fig. 5.5 Axial view of the brain shows further evolution of intracranial decomposition with enlarging pneumocephalus and dependent brain settling. Some of the gyral outlines and the ventricles can still be appreciated

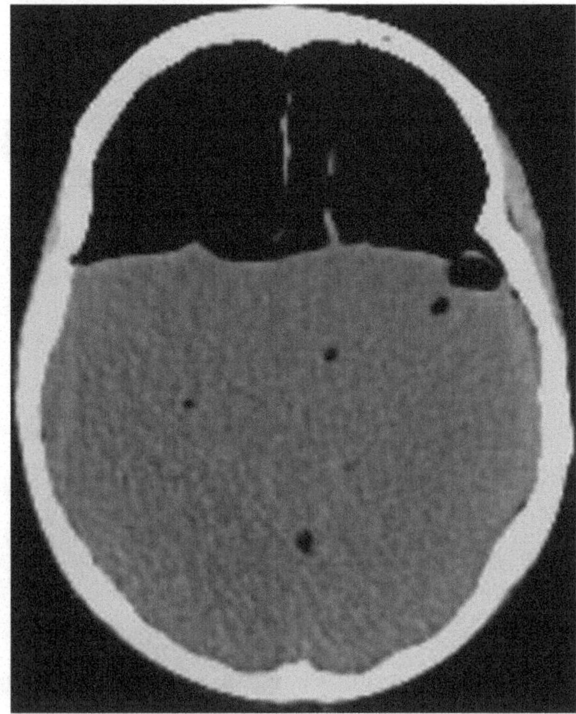

Fig. 5.6 Axial view of the brain shows a large decomposition pneumocephalus and loss of normal brain features in keeping with liquefaction. The parenchyma is unrecognisable

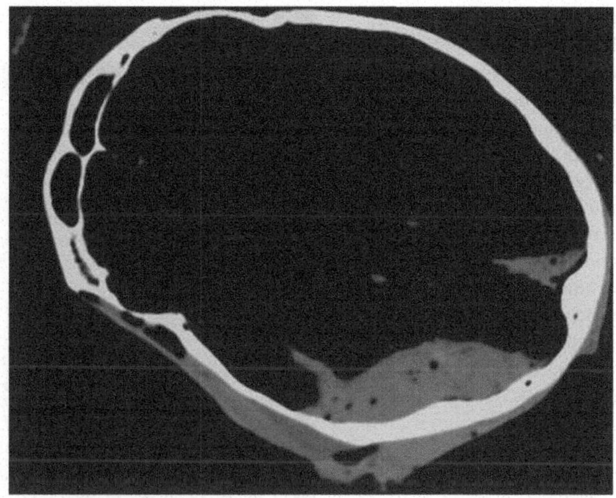

Fig. 5.7 Axial view of the brain (cranium rotated towards the right due to positioning), on soft tissue windows shows a near-empty cranial vault with small volume of residual brain tissue dependently, bounded by meninges

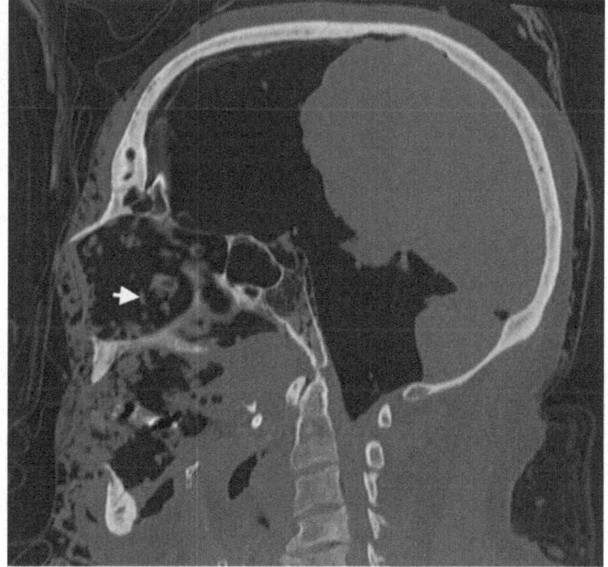

Fig. 5.8 Sagittal view of the head on bone windows shows multiple discrete densities in the nasal and oral cavities (example at tip of arrow), some within the cranial cavity, and a large decomposition pneumocephalus. Note the folds of multiple body bags external to the body

Occasionally, as the face is usually exposed, localised decomposition can be further accelerated by maggot activity (Fig. 5.8, see also Chap. 3) or another animal predation.

Intracranial Vessels

The cerebral venous sinuses, cortical veins and intracranial arteries are often hyperdense at PMCT due to post mortem clotting (Fig. 5.9). If there is generalised and

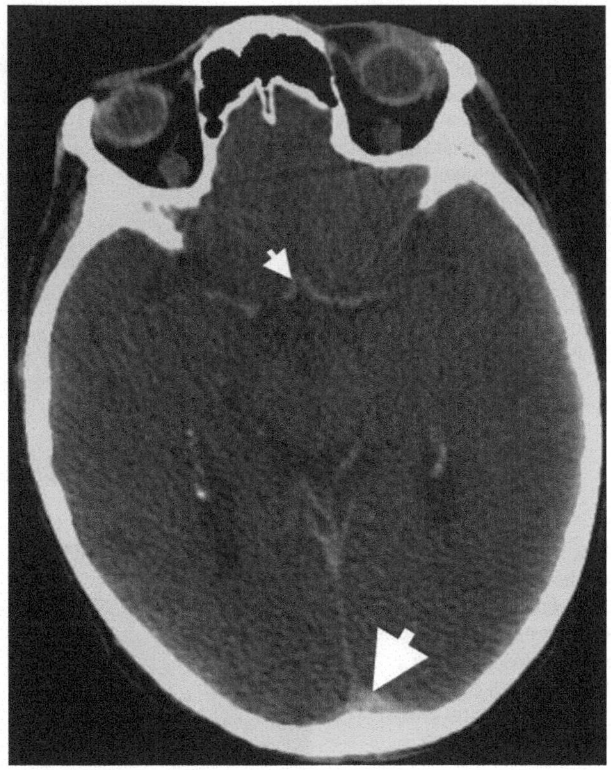

Fig. 5.9 Axial view of the brain, windowed to demonstrate normal post mortem vessel hyperdensity of the cerebral venous sinuses (large arrow) and intracranial arteries (small arrow). This can mimic a contrast-enhanced examination or thrombus, especially when compounded by the normal decreased cerebral attenuation

symmetrical vascular density, this finding can be disregarded as a normal post mortem change [5, 8] although it is noted that if the body has been in a lateral position for some time there may be asymmetry in the density—perhaps mimicking pathology. The cerebral venous sinuses (in particular the large superior sagittal sinus) may also show a 'fluid–fluid level' or an apparent 'filling defect' due to separation of blood products and hypostasis (Fig. 5.10). This should not be interpreted as pathological venous sinus thrombosis.

Owing to this normal post mortem vessel hyperdensity, the post mortem falx has been described as having a 'nodular' appearance [8] due to visualisation of adjacent venous structures. With knowledge of these normal post mortem appearances, such a finding should not be mistaken for an abnormal falx or parafalcine subarachnoid haemorrhage.

Decomposition results in the gradual accumulation of intravascular gas (Figs. 5.3 and 5.4) and is the usual explanation for gas presence. In other appropriate circumstances, this should not be confused with the sequela of infection, trauma or air embolus. Arterial and venous air emboli may occur in the setting of penetrating trauma, attempted cardiopulmonary resuscitation and iatrogenic interventions. PMCT is superior to open autopsy in identifying both normal and pathological gas collections [9]. For the pathologist to demonstrate intracranial gas emboli, they

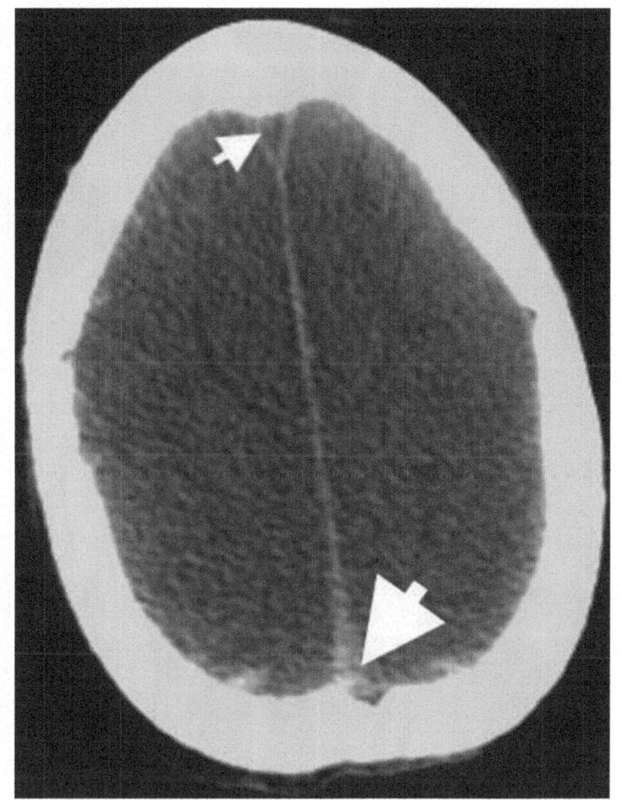

Fig. 5.10 Axial view of the brain windowed to demonstrate the normal post mortem separation of blood products in a larger vessel. This can result in low density of the anterior superior sagittal sinus (small arrow) and high-density posteriorly (large arrow)

would have to undertake complicated/specialised autopsy techniques, such as opening the head under water [7]. It is important not to overcall this common finding on imaging.

Spinal Cord

As with clinical CT, PMCT is not generally suitable or reliable to detect intrinsic changes in the spinal cord, although fortunately such pathology is not often in question. This is therefore a potential 'blind spot' of PMCT, much like routine open autopsy.

Gas or blood collecting in the vertebral canal may occasionally be seen to outline the cord and allow a gross assessment of cord integrity, most relevant when there is a history of trauma (see also Chaps. 6 and 10). When gas collects in the vertebral canal it is referred to as pneumorachis. Whilst this can reflect trauma, in the post mortem setting, this is more commonly caused by advancing decomposition (Figs. 5.11, 5.12, and 5.13).

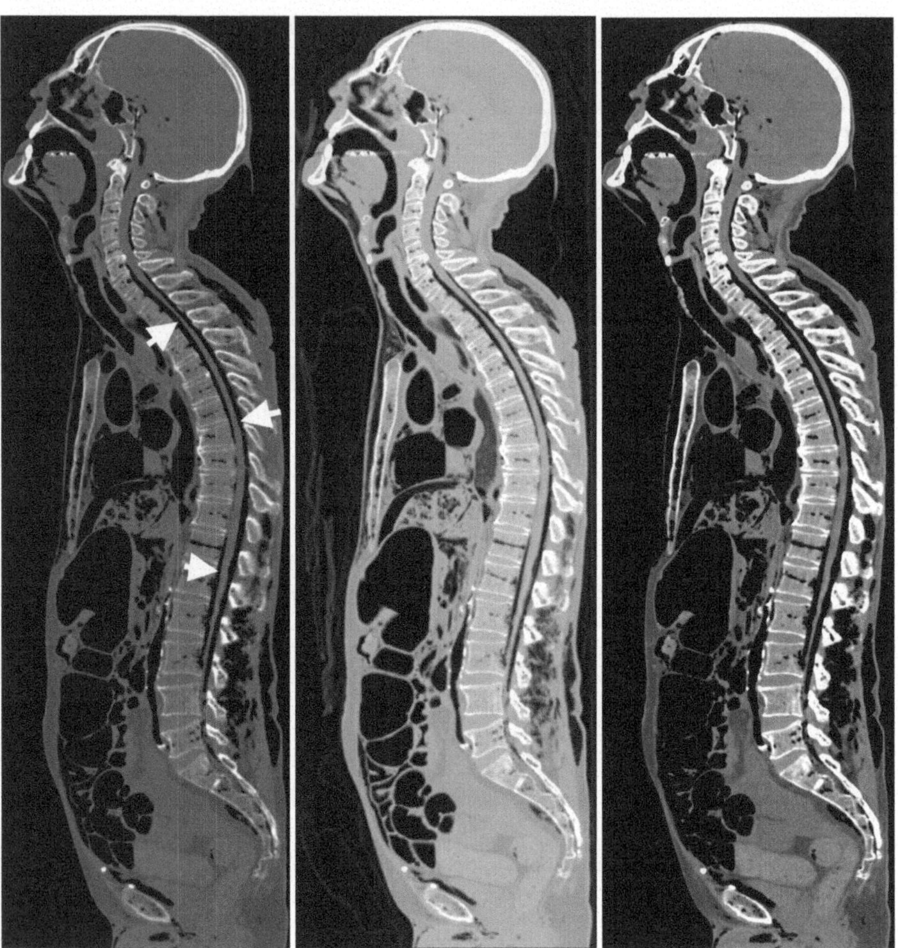

Fig. 5.11, 5.12 and 5.13 Sagittal view of the whole spine presented on bone, lung and soft tissue windows respectively showing pneumorachis—air in the vertebral canal which outlines the spinal cord (arrows). At PMCT this is usually seen secondary to decomposition (in this example there is vertebral body and soft tissue gas also due to decomposition)

Abnormal PMCT Findings

Cranial and Cervical Traumatic Injury

Fatal traumatic injuries are usually accompanied by relevant history, often with police reports and prior exclusion of a suspicious nature. In such circumstances, a reasonably detailed PMCT report should allow the cause of death to be formulated without further invasive investigation, aside perhaps from toxicology studies.

PMCT will easily demonstrate traumatic cranial and intracranial injuries sufficient to have caused death. Indeed, findings include extensive haemorrhage, crush fractures, brain herniation, pneumocephalus and vascular gas emboli (Figs. 5.14, 5.15, 5.16, 5.17, 5.18, and 5.19). Some appearances may seem more challenging, such as a significant burn injury that results in destruction of brain tissues (Fig. 5.20), although correlation with the history and external features will normally resolve this matter quickly.

Occasionally, gunshot injury may be encountered in non-suspicious circumstances, following accidental or suicidal deaths (Figs. 5.21 and 5.22). Determination of the injuries sustained (for example damage to vital structures or overwhelming haemorrhage) will inform the cause of death, although there may be devastating injury and no defined *singular* cause. In such cases, the cause of death may be recorded as 'multiple injuries' secondary to gunshot, 'or gunshot injuries to head'. For such non-forensic cases, the information regarding the weapon and events surrounding the gunshot should be known and available. For interest, and for informing correct terminology, the reader may refer to further texts, usually of a forensic nature [10–13].

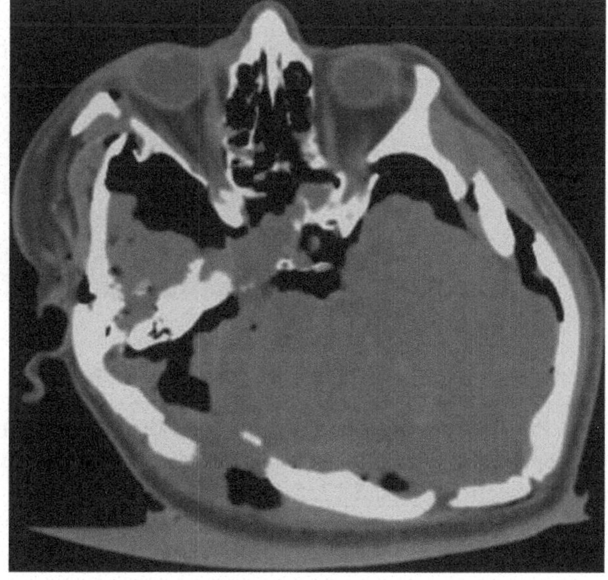

Fig. 5.14 Axial view of the head on soft tissue windows showing multiple displaced fractures, resulting in cranial deformity. There is a traumatic pneumocephalus, brain parenchymal injury and external haemorrhage, overall totalling a fatal cranial injury

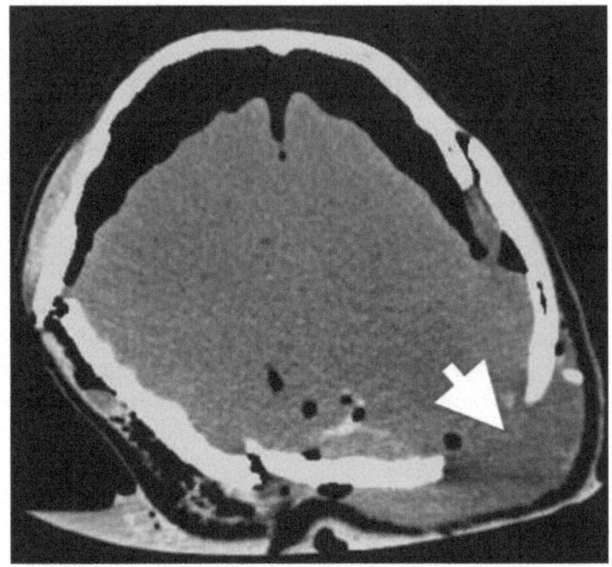

Fig. 5.15 Axial view of the head on brain windows following crush injury shows a traumatic pneumocephalus, external brain herniation (arrow) and high-density haemorrhagic fluid in the body bag beneath the head

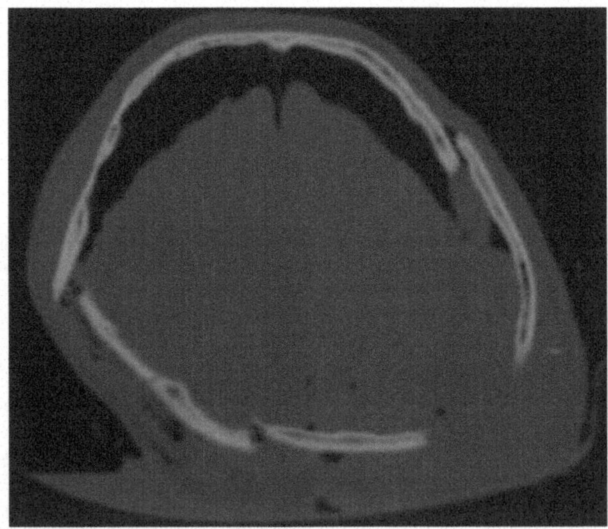

Fig. 5.16 Same case as Fig. 5.15, axial view of the head on bone windows shows multiple, severely displaced cranial fractures

Catastrophic skull vault fractures, especially those resulting from crush injury (Figs. 5.14, 5.15, and 5.16), will be clearly evident on the visual external examination. PMCT however has the additional distinct advantage of also easily demonstrating additional skull base and cervical spine injury without the need for extensive open dissection (Figs. 5.17, 5.18, and 5.19).

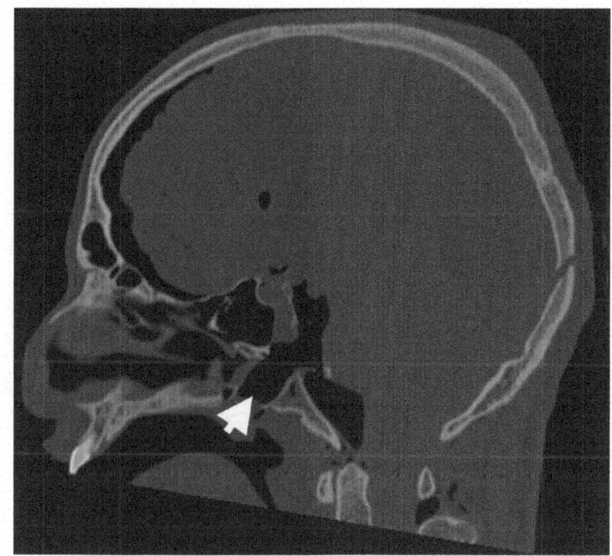

Fig. 5.17 Sagittal view of the skull on bone windows following a road traffic accident shows significantly displaced basal skull fractures which involve the clivus (arrow) and occiput, with a traumatic pneumocephalus

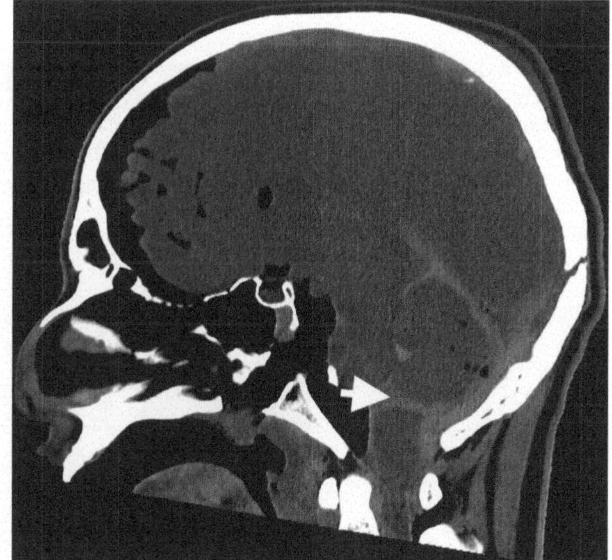

Fig. 5.18 Same case as Fig. 5.17, soft tissue windows demonstrate extensive hyperdense subarachnoid haemorrhage in the posterior fossa, outlining the cerebellum and revealing traumatic pontomedullary transection (arrow)

Intracranial Infection and Masses

Findings relating to intracranial infection and mass lesions are more difficult to confidently diagnose on PMCT without a known history or previous imaging to correlate. As found in the clinical setting, PMCT would also usually be normal in cases

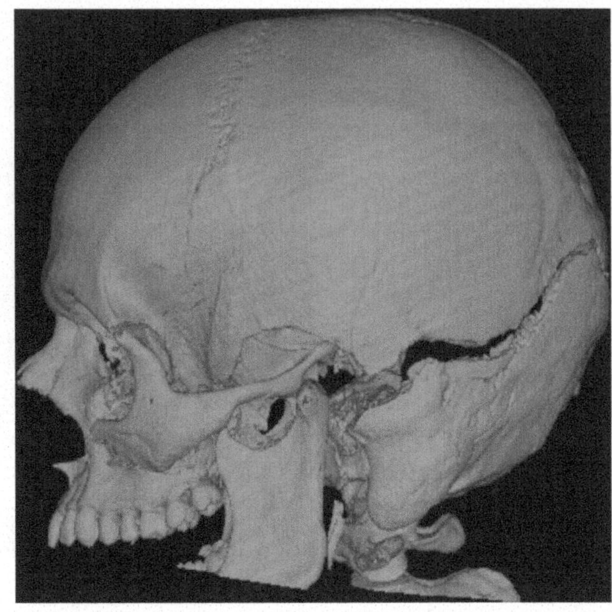

Fig. 5.19 Same case as Fig. 5.17, volume-rendered image of the skull demonstrating the contiguous skull base and occipital fractures

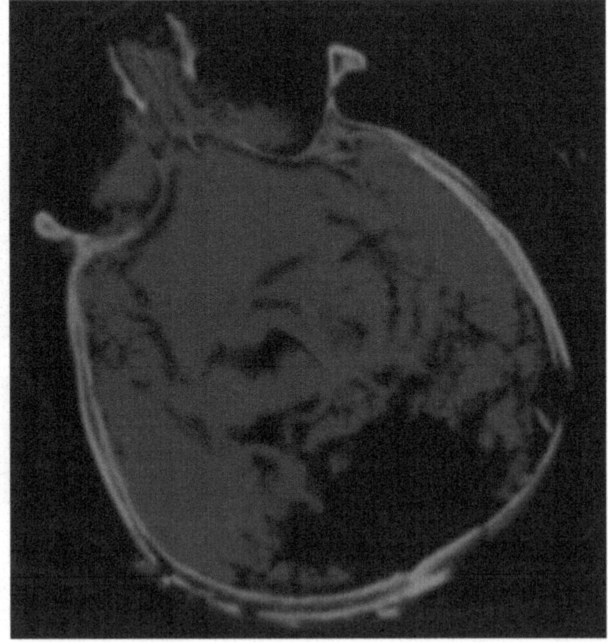

Fig. 5.20 Axial view of the head on bone windows shows extensive intracranial and extracranial irregular tissue destruction resulting from a fatal burn injury (accidental house fire)

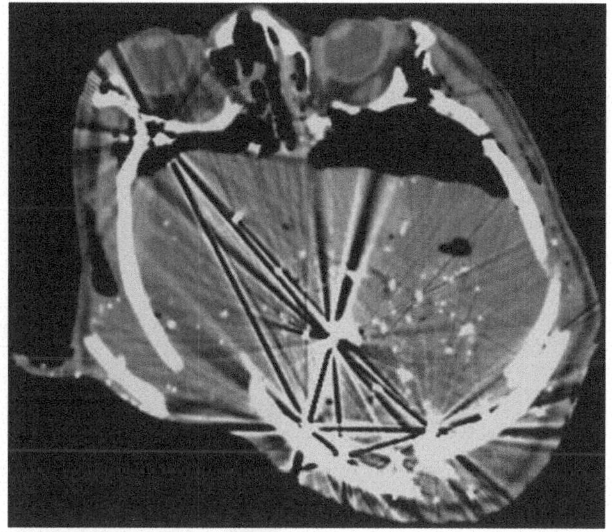

Fig. 5.21 Axial view of the head on soft tissue windows shows multiple displaced skull fractures, intracranial metallic shot particles (with linear beam hardening artefact) and debris from an intra-oral shotgun suicide

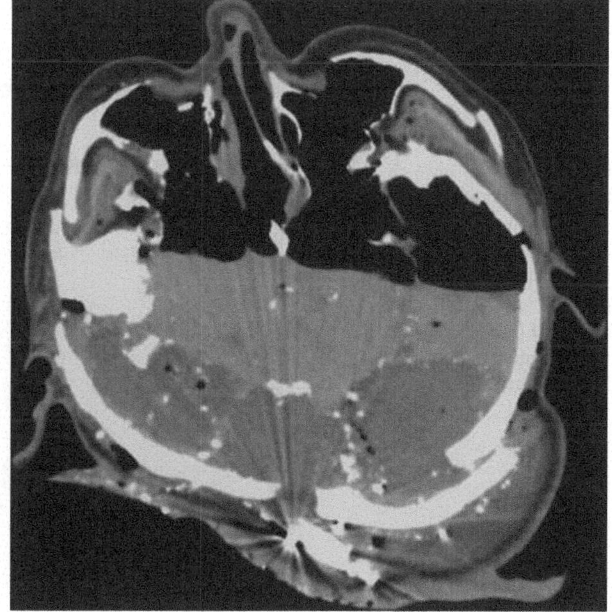

Fig. 5.22 Same case as Fig. 5.21, at a different level, showing the unsurvivable brain tissue injury with multiple projectile tracks, fractures, layered haemorrhage and pneumocephalus

of meningitis or early cerebritis. Such potential infection will often be missed as a PMCT diagnosis [14], even in the setting of sepsis/cranial symptoms [15].

An intracranial abscess, however, may be seen as a mass lesion (Fig. 5.23), often accompanied by peri-lesional oedema, although it cannot reliably be distinguished from an intracranial tumour or metastasis (Fig. 5.24) on imaging alone. Careful

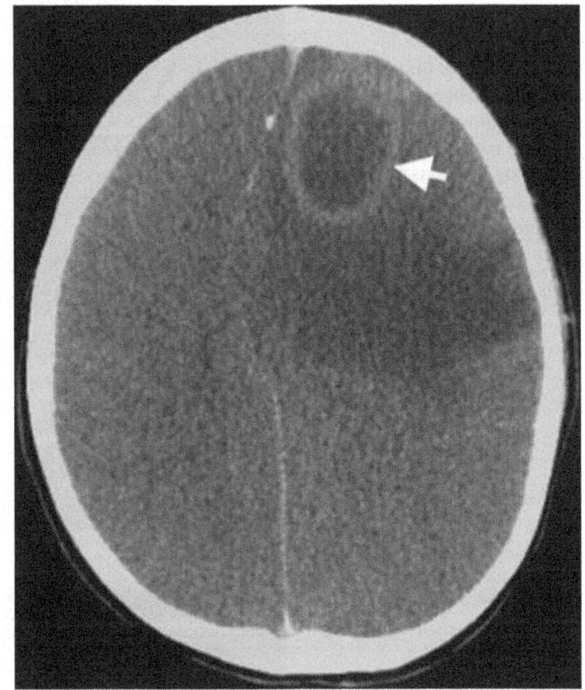

Fig. 5.23 Axial view of the brain on brain windows shows an autopsy-confirmed left frontal brain abscess with ring-like appearance (arrow). There is hypoattenuating perilesional oedema and positive mass effect with midline shift toward the right

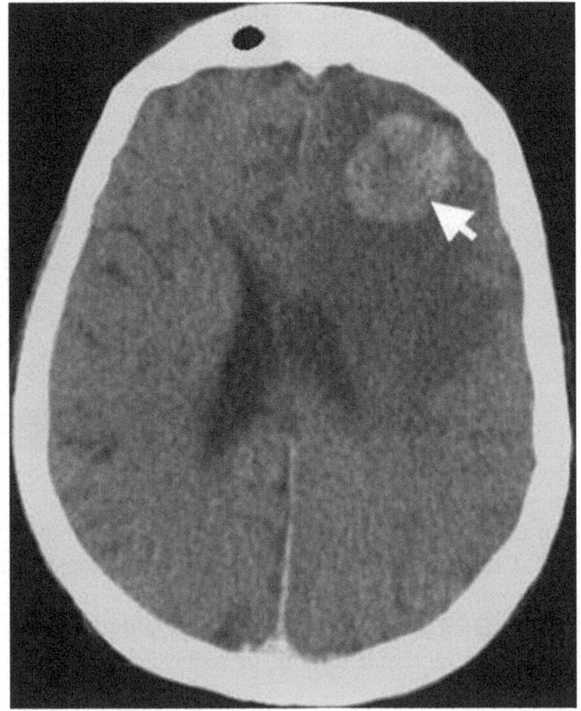

Fig. 5.24 Axial view of the brain on brain windows shows an autopsy-confirmed left frontal metastasis (arrow) with perilesional oedema and localised mass effect; this was secondary to known lung malignancy

correlation with the supporting information/clinical data and a thorough assessment of the remaining body should be undertaken to seek out other signs of infection or malignancy.

Intracranial Haemorrhage

As for clinical imaging, intracranial haemorrhage appears hyperdense on PMCT (Fig. 5.18). Blood collections may visibly persist even in cases of advanced decomposition and brain liquefaction [16–18]. Indeed, it has been described that PMCT demonstrates a 'still frame' regarding haemorrhage, as it must have been at or around the time of death [19].

PMCT is particularly valuable at demonstrating bleeding within the brain substance (Figs. 5.25 and 5.26), although a potential underlying pathology (such as tumour or vascular malformation) may remain obscure [18]. Occasionally, as with clinical imaging, the location or morphology of the haemorrhage may suggest the underlying cause, such as hypertension or amyloid angiopathy (Fig. 5.27). Mass effect, midline shift and asymmetric sulcal effacement should all be visible with such large bleeds, until decomposition obscures these secondary effects.

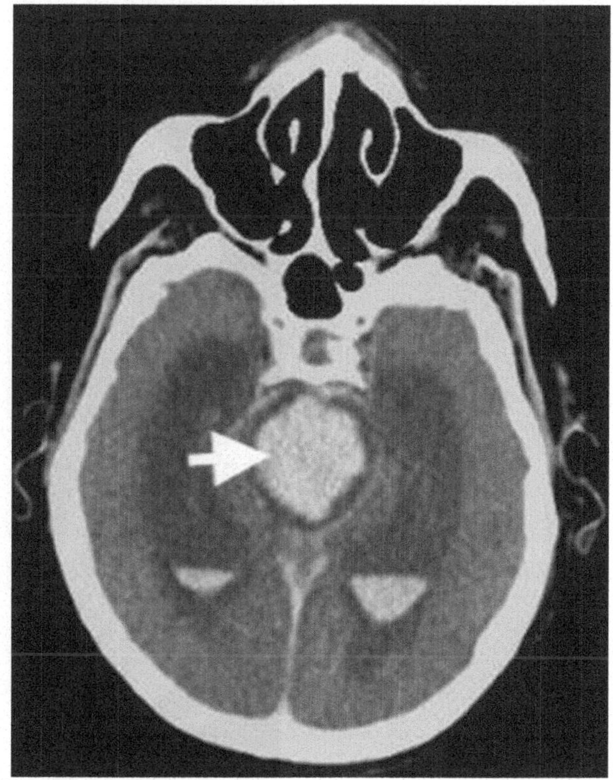

Fig. 5.25 Axial view of the brain on brain windows shows a fatal extensive brainstem haemorrhage (arrow) with layered intraventricular extension and enlarged lateral ventricles in keeping with obstructive hydrocephalus

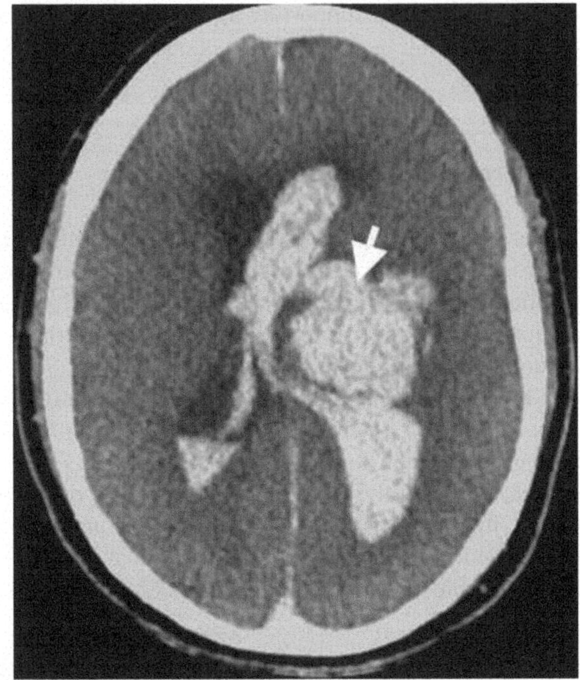

Fig. 5.26 Axial view of the brain on brain windows shows an acute left parenchymal haemorrhage (arrow) with mass effect, midline shift toward the right and intraventricular extension, in a patient with known hypertension. Post mortem brain swelling and loss of grey–white matter differentiation are compounded by the additional mass effect

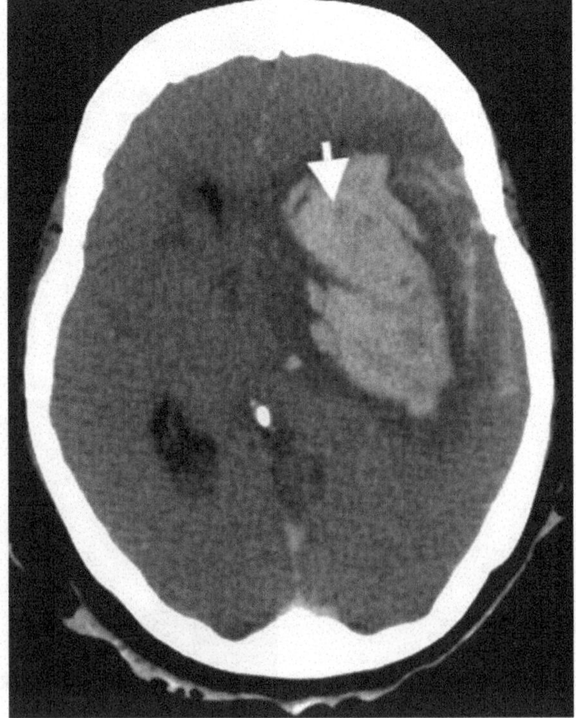

Fig. 5.27 Axial view of the brain on brain windows shows an acute left frontal intracranial haematoma (arrow) with finger-like projections, in keeping with cerebral amyloid angiopathy associated haematoma. Note also superficial subarachnoid extension of the haemorrhage

In terms of sensitivity, PMCT has been shown to identify small areas of intracranial haemorrhage, over a size of about 5 mm [18], which would be potentially missed at open autopsy [15]. Conversely, it is also possible to miss small haemorrhages [7, 8], which may be overlooked amongst the normal post mortem hyperdensity of small cortical vessels. Such small haemorrhages, without secondary effects, are however often judged unlikely to have been fatal in isolation (but might be present as part of a constellation of other findings).

It is important to be aware that a true subarachnoid haemorrhage can occasionally be difficult to distinguish from the misleading, relatively hyperdense basal cisterns and cortical sulci due to the decreased attenuation of the normal post mortem, ischaemic or oedematous brain. This misleading appearance is termed 'pseudo-subarachnoid haemorrhage' and is also seen in clinical imaging.

A true subarachnoid haemorrhage tends to be of striking higher attenuation [20] (Figs. 5.28 and 5.29) and, in the absence of trauma, can be associated with underlying pathology such as aneurysms (Figs. 5.30 and 5.31). Of note, normal decomposition will never lead to true subarachnoid haemorrhage [8]. Occasionally, when extensive, the haemorrhage can track caudally into the spinal subarachnoid space and outline the cord (Fig. 5.32).

In cases of true pathological cerebral oedema, with or without suspected 'pseudo subarachnoid haemorrhage', one may see supporting signs of narrowed temporal horns and herniation of the cerebral tonsils [21], but distinguishing such findings from normal post mortem swelling and decreased attenuation can be extremely challenging.

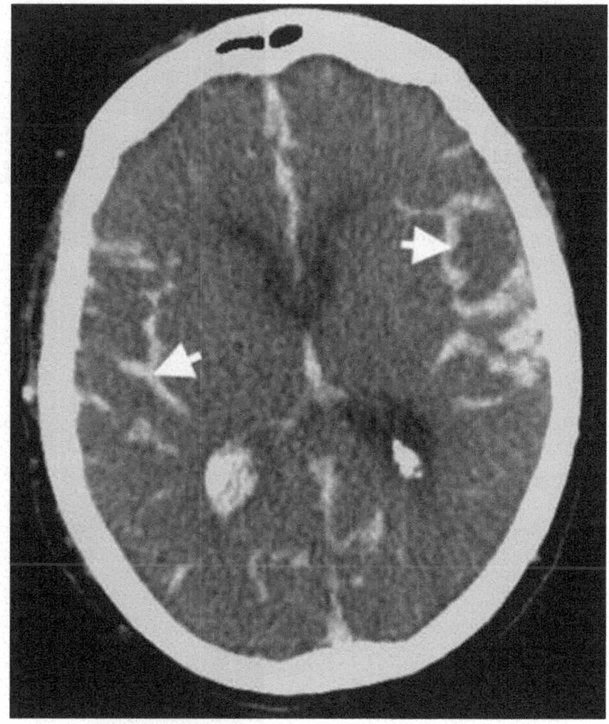

Fig. 5.28 Axial view of the brain on brain windows shows striking high-density haemorrhage in multiple bilateral cerebral sulci (example arrows) in keeping with acute subarachnoid haemorrhage with asymmetric right occipital horn intraventricular extension, the patient was taking anticoagulation

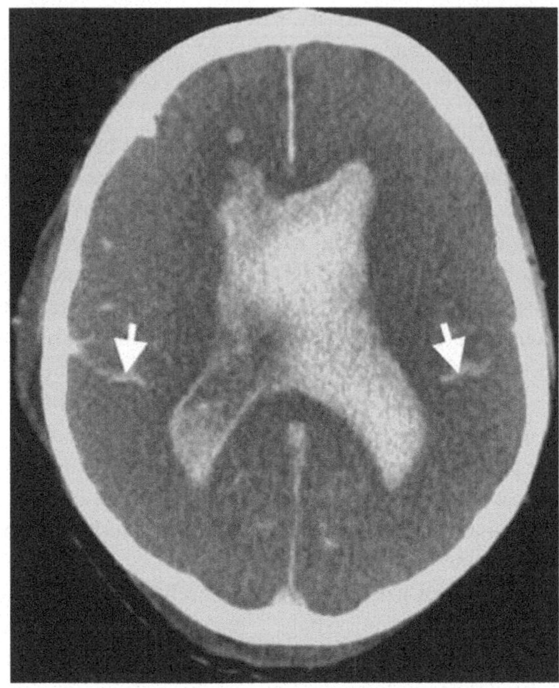

Fig. 5.29 Axial view of the brain on brain windows shows extensive hyperdense intraventricular and subarachnoid haemorrhages (arrows)

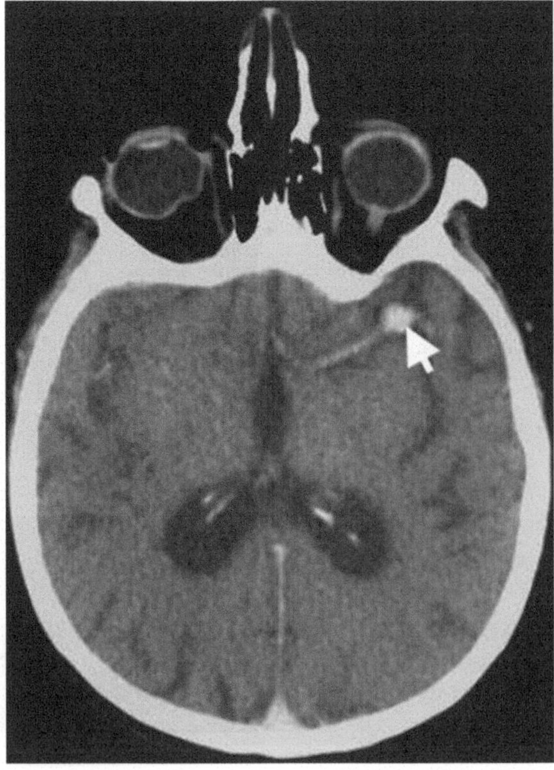

Fig. 5.30 Axial view of the brain on brain windows shows a focal rounded hyperdense mass in relation to the left middle cerebral artery in keeping with an incidental aneurysm. No feature of subarachnoid haemorrhage was seen on this scan

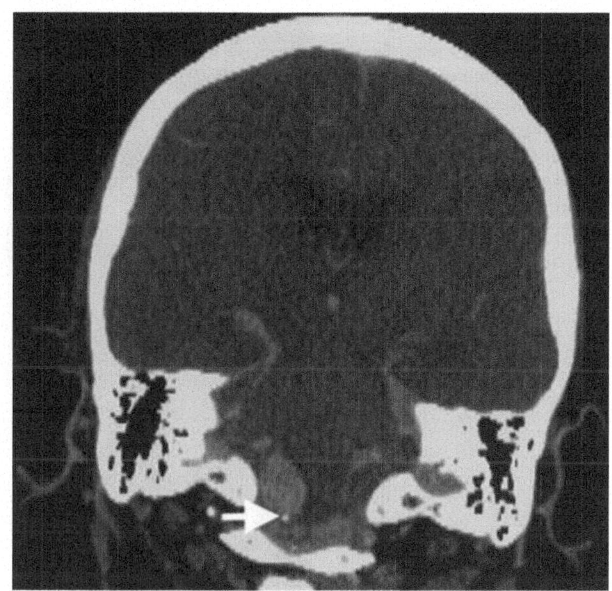

Fig. 5.31 Coronal view of the brainstem, windowed to demonstrate an ovoid hyperdense mass, suspected to be an aneurysm in the setting of acute subarachnoid haemorrhage (a tiny focus of calcification at its inferior margin (arrow) suggests this to be a vascular structure). There is associated mass effect distorting the brainstem

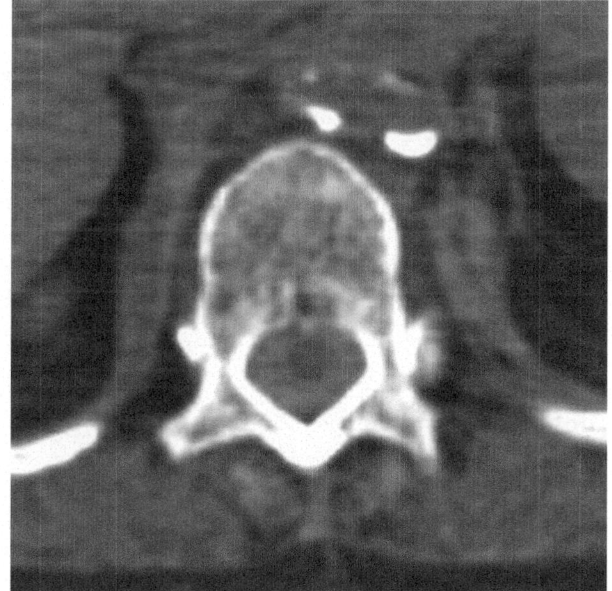

Fig. 5.32 Axial view of a thoracic vertebral body on soft tissue windows shows high-density vertebral canal haematoma outlining the centrally placed, relatively low density thoracic spinal cord. This blood was an extension of a large intracranial subarachnoid haemorrhage in a hypertensive patient who had a sudden collapse

Cerebral Infarction

Small hyper-acute infarcts can be easily be missed on PMCT, just as in routine clinical practice. The hyperdense vessel sign is generally less helpful, as high-density vessels are a common finding and PMCT cannot differentiate ante mortem from post mortem clot [22].

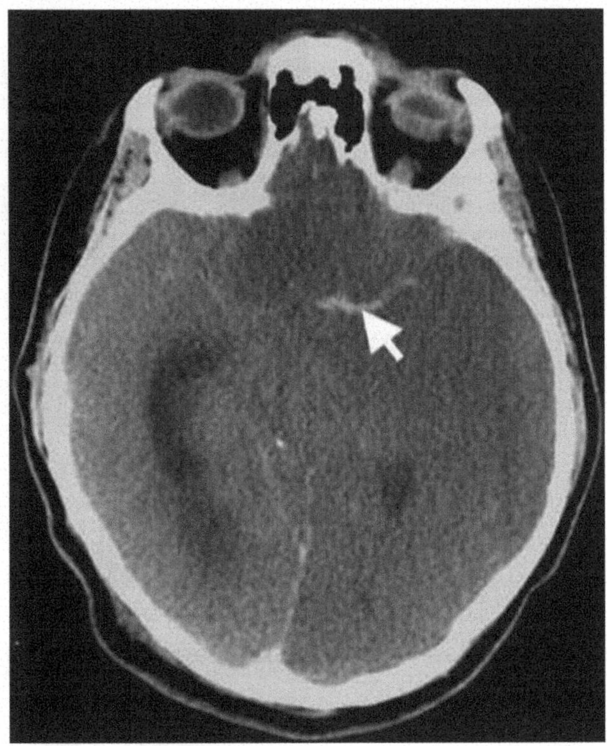

Fig. 5.33 Axial view of the brain on brain windows shows an asymmetric hyperdense left middle cerebral artery (arrow) and associated extensive surrounding parenchymal hypodensity with mass effect, consistent with acute territory infarct

However, if there is asymmetric vessel hyperdensity and/or vascular territory hypodense parenchyma, along with a suitable history, then the diagnosis of infarction can be made with confidence (Figs. 5.33, 5.34, 5.35, and 5.36). In such cases, if the PMCT does not show any other significant extracranial pathological events, it can usually be taken that the extensive cerebral infarction is the cause of death.

Global Ischaemia

In cases where there has been prolonged attempted cardiopulmonary resuscitation, evidence of global hypoxic ischaemic injury can sometimes be identified (Fig. 5.37). The radiologist needs to realise that, in these circumstances, hypoxic damage is not automatically the cause of death but is rather a consequence of the arrest. Conversely, for example, those deaths with a history such as epilepsy and fitting should receive special consideration, as this may indeed be a relevant finding in this setting.

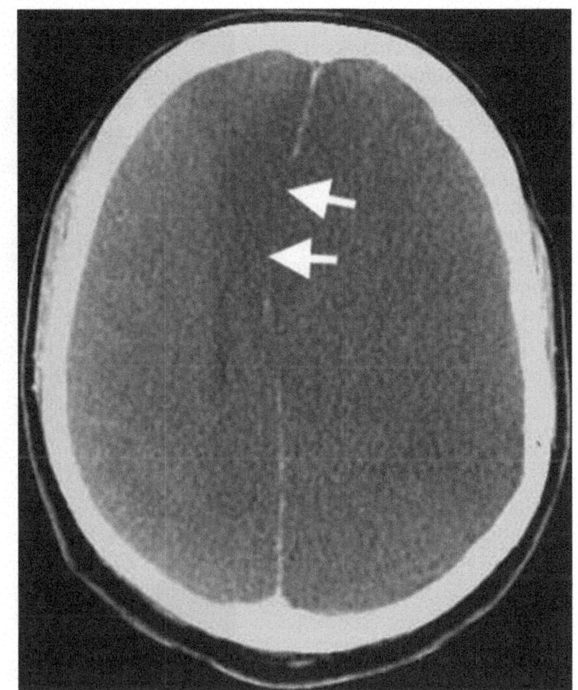

Fig. 5.34 Same case as Fig. 5.30, an axial view more toward the vertex demonstrates the extensive hypodense parenchyma and mass effect, with midline shift bowing the falx toward the right (arrows)

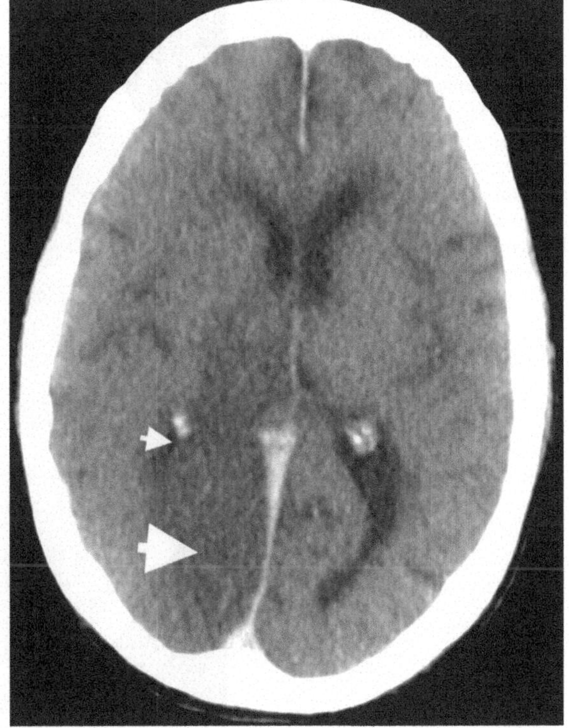

Fig. 5.35 Axial view of the brain on brain windows shows right occipital hypodensity (large arrow) with mild mass effect effacing the occipital horn of the right lateral ventricle (small arrow), in keeping with acute/recent infarct. Note the normal hyperdensity of the choroid plexus in both lateral ventricles and posterior superior sagittal sinus

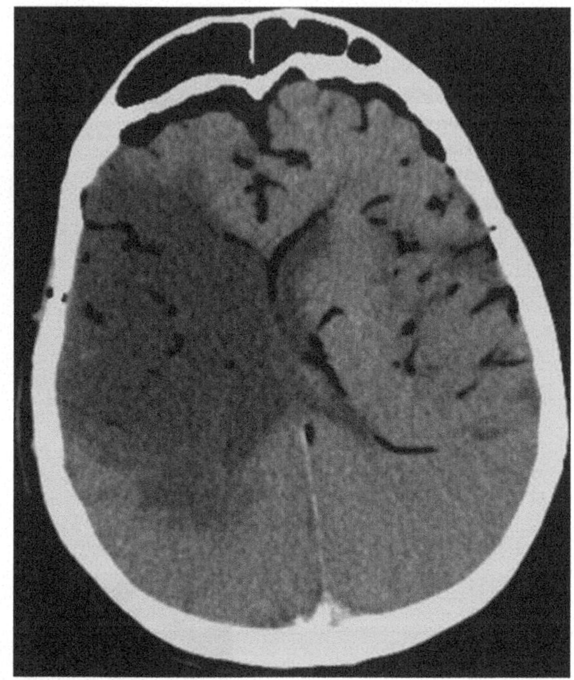

Fig. 5.36 Axial view of the brain on brain windows shows a right middle cerebral artery territory hypodensity with no significant overall positive or negative mass effect, in keeping with an evolving/subacute infarct. The vascular gas and small pneumocephalus are from decomposition changes

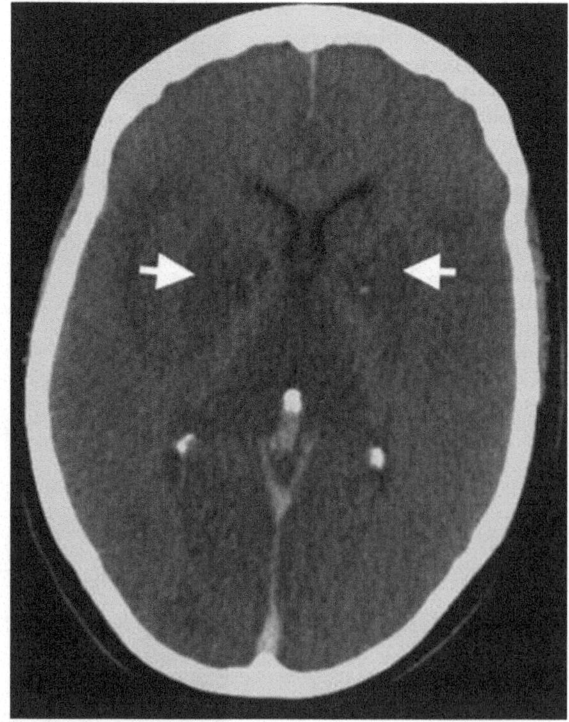

Fig. 5.37 Axial view of the brain on brain windows shows features of global hypoxic ischaemic injury with markedly hypodense basal ganglia (arrows) and insular cortex. The diffuse cerebral swelling may be due to a combination of hypoxia and further post mortem change

Ventricular Obstruction and Hydrocephalus

Although mild cerebral swelling is relatively common on PMCT, and evidence of involutional changes may occasionally be noted, dilated ventricles are not a normal finding. If ventricular dilatation cannot be attributed to significant central atrophy, then cerebrospinal fluid (CSF) obstruction needs to be carefully considered, although the underlying cause may be occult.

With such appearances, a rare but important finding in the context of sudden death is a colloid cyst of the third ventricle. These are benign lesions sometimes found following investigation for headaches and pressure symptoms (suggesting raised intracranial pressure) but occasionally first identified at autopsy. As on clinical imaging, they present as a focal rounded hyperdense midline mass (1–2 cm diameter) related to the third ventricle (Fig. 5.38) and can cause acute hydrocephalus and sudden unexpected death. Such secondary hydrocephalus is easier to demonstrate and document on PMCT, compared to open autopsy, where brain retention and prolonged fixation may be required [23].

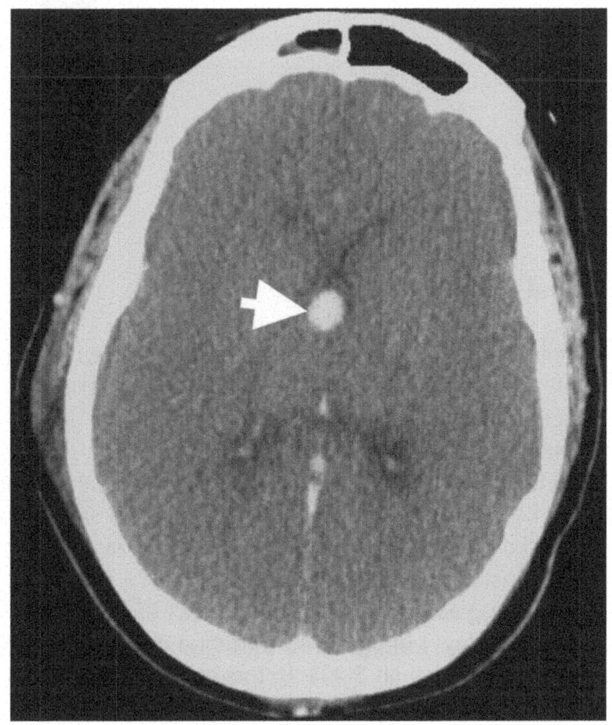

Fig. 5.38 Axial view of the brain on brain windows shows a focal midline hyperdense rounded mass in relation to the third ventricle (arrow) in keeping with a colloid cyst. Hydrocephalus is not seen in this example

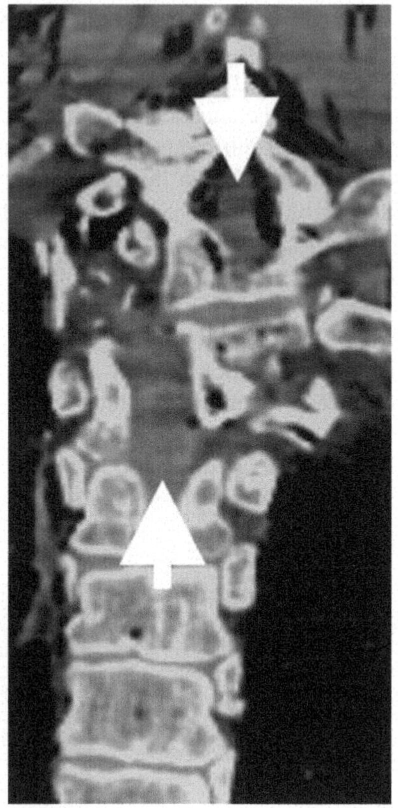

Fig. 5.39 Coronal view of the upper thoracic spine on soft tissue windows shows significant lateral displacement of the vertebral column secondary to traumatic fractures resulting in a transection of the spinal cord (arrows)

Spinal Cord Injury

In general, spinal cord injury may be inferred when vertebral fractures are significantly displaced or there is obliteration of the vertebral canal (Figs. 5.39 and 5.40). Vertebral trauma is also discussed in Chap. 10.

Injuries to the cranio-cervical region and high cervical cord are particularly important due to their potential effect on critical neurological centres. These may prove fatal even when other injuries sustained are not extensive. Injury to the cord should be particularly considered in the setting of chronic spinal stenosis, as this may predispose to cord compression [24].

Following acute trauma, air may enter the vertebral canal and intracranial thecal space from direct injury to the vertebral column or to the chest via a pleural fistula (Figs. 5.40, 5.41, and 5.42). In this context, the air is particularly useful as it may outline a significant spinal cord injury such as transection [25] (Fig. 5.43). Blood can also outline the craniovertebral structures (Figs. 5.18 and 5.32). This effect has been termed the 'pseudo-CT myelogram' sign and may also help reveal significant anatomic distortion or injury [26].

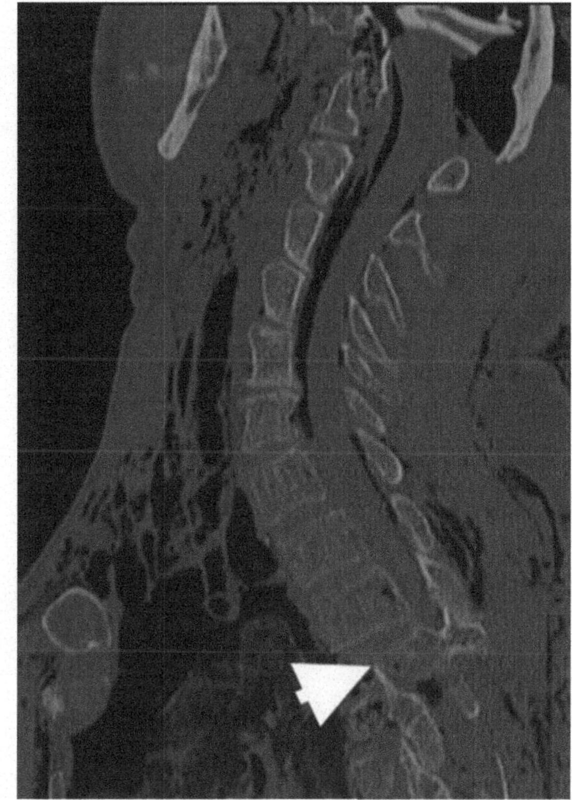

Fig. 5.40 Same case as Fig. 5.39, an oblique sagittal view of the cervicothoracic spine on bone windows again shows the significantly displaced thoracic fracture with obliteration of the vertebral canal (arrow) consistent with inevitable cord injury. Also shown is traumatic pneumorachis, pneumothorax and soft tissue gas

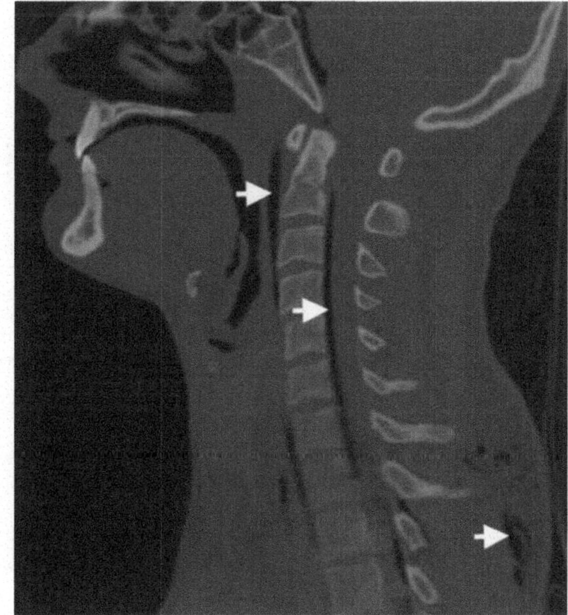

Fig. 5.41 Sagittal view of the cervical spine on bone windows shows (arrows top to bottom) pre-vertebral gas, pneumorachis and dorsal soft tissue gas in the setting of a penetrating chest injury, note the absence of decomposition gas elsewhere

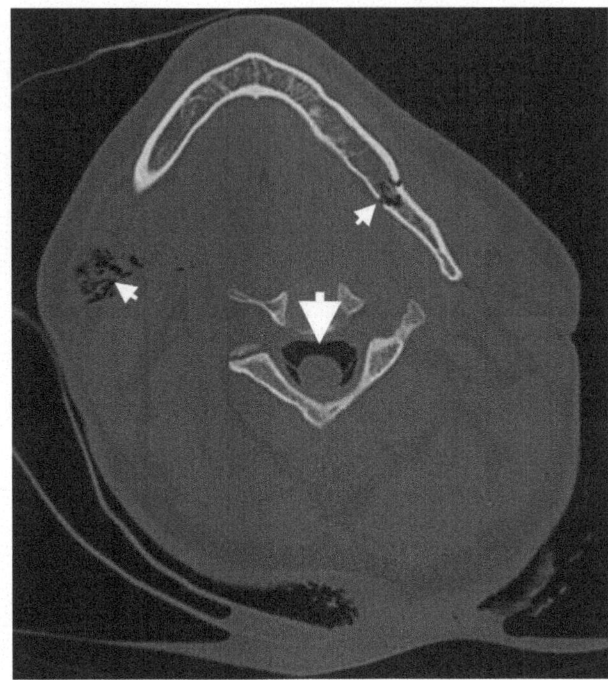

Fig. 5.42 Axial view of the neck on bone windows shows a traumatic pneumorachis (large arrow) outlining the spinal cord and nerve roots. A left mandibular body fracture and focal right submandibular surgical emphysema are also demonstrated (small arrows)

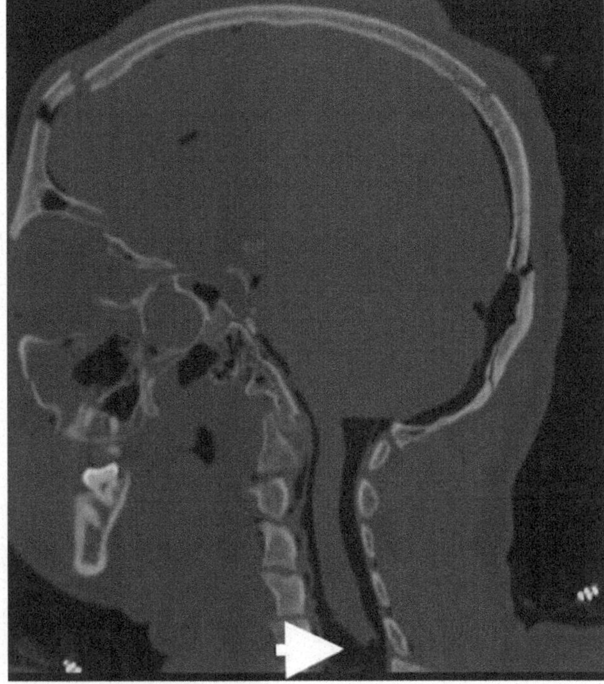

Fig. 5.43 Sagittal view of the head and neck on bone windows showing spinal cord transection outlined by air (arrow), in the setting of trauma. There are extensive additional skull base and skull vault fractures

A small haemorrhage within the brainstem has previously been reported to be visualised on PMCT although not in the context of trauma [27]; such a finding would be important as it may cause central respiratory failure. CT is however not sensitive enough to *exclude* the presence of intrinsic cord haemorrhage, particularly if there is beam hardening due to surrounding bony structures or obesity degrading the images.

In summary, given that there will not always be gas or blood to outline spinal structures, it is important to appreciate that spinal cord injuries cannot be excluded purely based on PMCT [24]. As in the clinical setting, one should be aware that disco-ligamentous injuries and small perivertebral haemorrhages can also remain radiologically occult [28].

Reporting Brain and Spinal Cord Findings: Pearls and Pitfalls

Loss of grey–white matter differentiation, mild cerebral swelling and generally hyperdense vessels should usually be reported as normal post mortem appearances.

Significant haemorrhage, mass effect, major territory infarction, traumatic injury and pathologic gas collections can reliably be visualised or excluded on most PMCT scans, if substantial decomposition has not occurred.

A clear comment regarding the absence of pathology may help avoid the need to open the cranial cavity should open autopsy be required.

If intrinsic spinal cord, malignant or infective pathology is suspected, and no evidence is seen, then the limitations of PMCT should also be expressed.

Example PMCT report phrases:

- Loss of cerebral grey–white matter differentiation with mild diffuse cerebral swelling are considered to be normal post mortem findings.
- Hyperdense appearance of the major dural venous sinuses is a normal post mortem finding.
- Diffuse intravascular gas is judged in keeping with decomposition.
- Large pneumocephalus and loss of normal brain architecture in keeping with advanced decomposition. This significantly limits PMCT assessment of the brain.
- No intracranial haemorrhage, space-occupying mass or large vessel territory infraction. No mass effect, midline shift or hydrocephalus demonstrated.

References

1. Roberts I, Traill Z. The radiological autopsy. In: Suvarna SK, editor. Atlas of adult autopsy [Internet]. Cham: Springer International Publishing; 2016. p. 362. http://link.springer.com/10.1007/978-3-319-27022-7_13.

2. Burton JL, Suvarna SK. The central nervous system, with eye and ear. In: Suvarna SK, editor. Atlas of adult autopsy [Internet]. Cham: Springer International Publishing; 2016. p. 271–97. http://link.springer.com/10.1007/978-3-319-27022-7_9.
3. Burton JL. Health and safety at necropsy. J Clin Pathol [Internet]. 2003;56(4):254–60. http://www.ncbi.nlm.nih.gov/pubmed/12663635.
4. Suvarna SK, McNamara MH, Scholes AL, Strickland SS. Autopsy cranial tissue examination rarely provides valuable information unless there is a specific prompt to open the head. J Clin Pathol [Internet]. 2016;69(7):647–8. http://jcp.bmj.com/lookup/doi/10.1136/jclinpath-2016-203657.
5. Wagensveld IM, Blokker BM, Wielopolski PA, Renken NS, Krestin GP, Hunink MG, et al. Total-body CT and MR features of postmortem change in in-hospital deaths. PLoS One [Internet]. 2017;12(9):e0185115. https://dx.plos.org/10.1371/journal.pone.0185115.
6. Ishida M, Gonoi W, Okuma H, Shirota G, Shintani Y, Abe H, et al. Common postmortem computed tomography findings following atraumatic death: differentiation between normal postmortem changes and pathologic lesions. Korean J Radiol [Internet]. 2015;16(4):798. https://www.kjronline.org/DOIx.php?id=10.3348/kjr.2015.16.4.798.
7. Panda A, Kumar A, Gamanagatti S, Mishra B. Virtopsy computed tomography in trauma: normal postmortem changes and pathologic spectrum of findings. Curr Probl Diagn Radiol [Internet]. 2015;44(5):391–406. https://linkinghub.elsevier.com/retrieve/pii/S0363018815000420.
8. Smith AB, Lattin GE, Berran P, Harcke HT. Common and expected postmortem CT observations involving the brain: mimics of antemortem pathology. Am J Neuroradiol [Internet]. 2012;33(7):1387–91. http://www.ajnr.org/lookup/doi/10.3174/ajnr.A2966.
9. Flach PM, Thali MJ, Germerott T. Times have changed! Forensic radiology—a new challenge for radiology and forensic pathology. Am J Roentgenol [Internet]. 2014;202(4):W325–34. http://www.ajronline.org/doi/10.2214/AJR.12.10283.
10. Wilson AJ. Gunshot injuries: what does a radiologist need to know? RadioGraphics [Internet]. 1999;19(5):1358–68. http://pubs.rsna.org/doi/10.1148/radiographics.19.5.g99se171358.
11. van Kan RAT, Haest IIH, Lahaye MJ, Hofman PAM. The diagnostic value of forensic imaging in fatal gunshot incidents: a review of literature. J Forensic Radiol Imaging [Internet]. 2017;10:9–14. https://linkinghub.elsevier.com/retrieve/pii/S2212478017300527.
12. Abdul Rashid SN, Martinez RM, Ampanozi G, Thali MJ, Bartsch C. A rare case of suicide by gunshot with nasal entry assessed by classical autopsy, post-mortem computed tomography (PMCT) and post-mortem magnetic resonance imaging (PMMR). J Forensic Radiol Imaging [Internet]. 2013;1(2):63–7. https://linkinghub.elsevier.com/retrieve/pii/S2212478013000464.
13. Jeffery AJ, Rutty GN, Robinson C, Morgan B. Computed tomography of projectile injuries. Clin Radiol [Internet]. 2008;63(10):1160–6. https://linkinghub.elsevier.com/retrieve/pii/S000992600800130X.
14. Roberts ISD, Benamore RE, Benbow EW, Lee SH, Harris JN, Jackson A, et al. Post-mortem imaging as an alternative to autopsy in the diagnosis of adult deaths: a validation study. Lancet [Internet]. 2012;379(9811):136–42. https://linkinghub.elsevier.com/retrieve/pii/S0140673611614839.
15. Rutty GN, Morgan B, Robinson C, Raj V, Pakkal M, Amoroso J, et al. Diagnostic accuracy of post-mortem CT with targeted coronary angiography versus autopsy for coroner-requested post-mortem investigations: a prospective, masked, comparison study. Lancet [Internet]. 2017;390(10090):145–54. https://linkinghub.elsevier.com/retrieve/pii/S0140673617303331.
16. Takahashi Y, Sano R, Kominato Y, Takei H, Kobayashi S, Shimada T, et al. Usefulness of post-mortem computed tomography for demonstrating cerebral hemorrhage in a brain too fragile for macroscopic examination. J Forensic Radiol Imaging [Internet]. 2013;1(4):212–4. https://linkinghub.elsevier.com/retrieve/pii/S221247801300083X.
17. Sano R, Hirasawa S, Awata S, Kobayashi S, Shimada T, Takei H, et al. Use of postmortem computed tomography to reveal acute subdural hematoma in a severely decomposed body with advanced skeletonization. Leg Med [Internet]. 2013;15(1):32–4. https://linkinghub.elsevier.com/retrieve/pii/S1344622312001320.

18. Tappero C, Thali MJ, Schweitzer W. The possibility of identifying brain hemorrhage in putrefied bodies with PMCT. Forensic Sci Med Pathol [Internet]. 2020;16(4):571–6. http://link.springer.com/10.1007/s12024-020-00283-8.
19. Ruder TD, Zech W-D, Hatch GM, Ross S, Ampanozi G, Thali MJ, et al. Still frame from the hour of death: acute intracerebral hemorrhage on post-mortem computed tomography in a decomposed corpse. J Forensic Radiol Imaging [Internet]. 2013;1(2):73–6. https://linkinghub.elsevier.com/retrieve/pii/S2212478013000440.
20. Given CA, Burdette JH, Elster AD, Williams DW. Pseudo-subarachnoid hemorrhage: a potential imaging pitfall associated with diffuse cerebral edema. AJNR Am J Neuroradiol [Internet]. 2003;24(2):254–6. http://www.ncbi.nlm.nih.gov/pubmed/12591643.
21. Berger N, Ampanozi G, Schweitzer W, Ross SG, Gascho D, Ruder TD, et al. Racking the brain: detection of cerebral edema on postmortem computed tomography compared with forensic autopsy. Eur J Radiol [Internet]. 2015;84(4):643–51. https://linkinghub.elsevier.com/retrieve/pii/S0720048X15000030.
22. Sutherland T, O'Donnell C. The artefacts of death: CT post-mortem findings. J Med Imaging Radiat Oncol [Internet]. 2018;62(2):203–10. http://doi.wiley.com/10.1111/1754-9485.12691.
23. Andersen AM, Frost L, Thorup Boel LW. Colloid cysts of the third ventricle at post-mortem CT and at autopsy: a report of two cases. J Forensic Radiol Imaging [Internet]. 2015;3(1):96–9. https://linkinghub.elsevier.com/retrieve/pii/S2212478015000088.
24. Makino Y, Yokota H, Hayakawa M, Yajima D, Inokuchi G, Nakatani E, et al. Spinal cord injuries with Normal postmortem CT findings: a pitfall of virtual autopsy for detecting traumatic death. Am J Roentgenol [Internet]. 2014;203(2):240–4. http://www.ajronline.org/doi/10.2214/AJR.13.11775.
25. Berger N, Ross SG, Ampanozi G, Majcen R, Schweitzer W, Gascho D, et al. Puzzling over intracranial gas: disclosing a pitfall on postmortem computed tomography in a case of fatal blunt trauma. J Forensic Radiol Imaging [Internet]. 2013;1(3):137–41. https://linkinghub.elsevier.com/retrieve/pii/S2212478013000737.
26. Bolster F, Ali Z, Daly B. The "pseudo-CT myelogram sign": an aid to the diagnosis of underlying brain stem and spinal cord trauma in the presence of major craniocervical region injury on post-mortem CT. Clin Radiol [Internet]. 2017;72(12):1085.e11–1085.e15. https://linkinghub.elsevier.com/retrieve/pii/S0009926017304051.
27. Chatzaraki V, Heimer J, Thali M, Dally A, Schweitzer W. Role of PMCT as a triage tool between external inspection and full autopsy—case series and review. J Forensic Radiol Imaging [Internet]. 2018;15:26–38. https://linkinghub.elsevier.com/retrieve/pii/S2212478018300601.
28. Iwase H, Yamamoto S, Yajima D, Hayakawa M, Kobayashi K, Otsuka K, et al. Can cervical spine injury be correctly diagnosed by postmortem computed tomography? Leg Med [Internet]. 2009;11(4):168–74. https://linkinghub.elsevier.com/retrieve/pii/S1344622309001679.

Post Mortem Computed Tomography of the Extra-Cranial Head and Neck

6

Introduction

Significant fatal pathology in the extracranial head and neck, seen at post mortem computed tomography (PMCT), predominantly deals with trauma from various sources. Of particular note in the autopsy arena is the pathology of hanging. Consequently, this topic is presented in more depth as a specific circumstance. Occasionally, PMCT is performed after an episode of choking, with the scan potentially able to identify airway obstruction.

Other pathologies such as infections or malignancy might also be found in PMCT, often as part of systemic disease. However, in terms of being the cause of death, they are infrequent findings compared to cardiac and lung disease.

The extracranial head and neck includes the deep facial tissues and paranasal sinuses. These structures are rarely examined during an invasive autopsy (see below), as they have a low yield of unexpected relevant positive findings. PMCT has the advantage of being able to readily visualise the entirety of this anatomic region and may occasionally reveal surprising pathology. Clearly, it also has the advantage of avoiding destructive facial interactions.

As with most CT, the depiction of bony detail and gas distribution is excellent, but soft tissue evaluation is limited unless structures are outlined by contrast or clear fat planes. Streak artefact from jewellery, dental appliances or amalgam can significantly obscure the neck and oral cavity views (Figs. 6.1 and 6.2). Where possible, before the scan commences, such items should be removed to enhance imaging. As with all PMCT, discussed earlier in this book, the changes of decomposition can also significantly limit assessment (see Chap. 3).

A. Shenton et al., *Post Mortem CT for Non-Suspicious Adult Deaths*,
https://doi.org/10.1007/978-3-030-70829-0_6

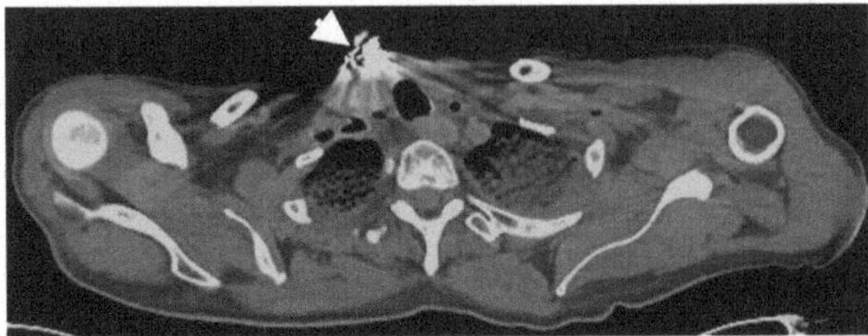

Fig. 6.1 Axial view at the level of the thyroid on soft tissue windows shows streak artefact from metallic jewellery (arrow) obscuring the neck tissues

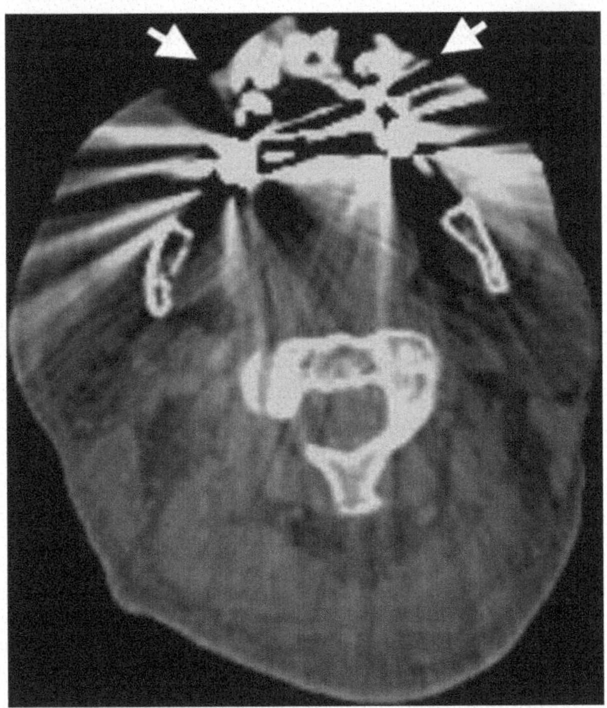

Fig. 6.2 Axial view of the neck at the level of the oral cavity shows multiple streak artefacts from dental amalgam (arrows) which obscure the tissues

Autopsy of the Extracranial Head and Neck: The Pathologist's Perspective

The pathologist is aware that the face is one of the few areas commonly viewed by relatives after death. It causes distress to the family and friends if there are disfiguring marks or sutures. Consequently, many pathologists prefer not to open the head tissues, particularly if PMCT has excluded any pathology at these sites.

However, if required, the dissection of the head and neck is normally accomplished by a Y-shaped incision running across the upper chest up towards both mastoid processes. This allows the skin and underlying fatty soft tissue to be reflected upwards. It exposes the strap muscles, blood vessels, airway, thyroid, parathyroids, salivary glands and oesophagus, up to the angle of the mandible [1].

In a conventional autopsy, the knife incision runs along the inner aspect of the mandible and then allows incision onto the front of the cervical spine to release/remove the neck contents.

Conventionally, the neck arteries are explored up to the bifurcation of the carotid vessels but only after the neck tissues had been removed from the body. Rarely, the vertebral bodies are removed in order to consider the spinal cord as discussed in the previous chapter. Confirmation of the course and tissue interaction for artificial airways, long lines and electronic devices should be undertaken as part of the routine assessment.

In forensic cases, close attention to the strap muscles, hyoid bone and laryngeal cartilages is undertaken in order to look for bruising and fractures of the airway framework tissues.

Exposure of the facial tissues is not normally undertaken unless an assault is under consideration, again in a forensic setting.

The inner nose (exposed via the soft and hard palate), the inner ear (examined by means of focused temporal bone resection and decalcification) and eye (often approached from the bone of the anterior cranial fossa) are not normally seen in routine cranial practice [2].

It would be fair to say that there is rarely significant natural pathology in any of these anatomic areas unless there is airway obstruction, primary/metastatic disease or infection.

Normal PMCT Findings

Soft Tissues

If sufficient fat planes are present, a reasonable assessment of the soft tissues can be made compared to those individuals lacking in body fat (Figs. 6.3 and 6.4). This allows the exclusion of significant masses (that obstruct the airway) or substantial haemorrhage. The outlines of the thyroid, salivary glands and muscles also allow for a gross assessment.

The thyroid is readily visualised due to its inherent hyperdensity (Fig. 6.5) but is rarely of significance unless a neoplastic or a large goitre narrows the airway. The laryngeal cartilages are generally non-calcified when young (Fig. 6.6) but become variably calcified with increasing age.

As the face is often exposed in the open, compared to other body parts, earlier decomposition and maggot infestation may be present (see Chap. 3). Maggots are seen on PMCT as multiple tiny soft tissue densities in and around the facial tissues, nasal cavities, orbits, ears and paranasal sinuses and may destroy much of the soft tissues of the head and neck (Figs. 6.7 and 6.8).

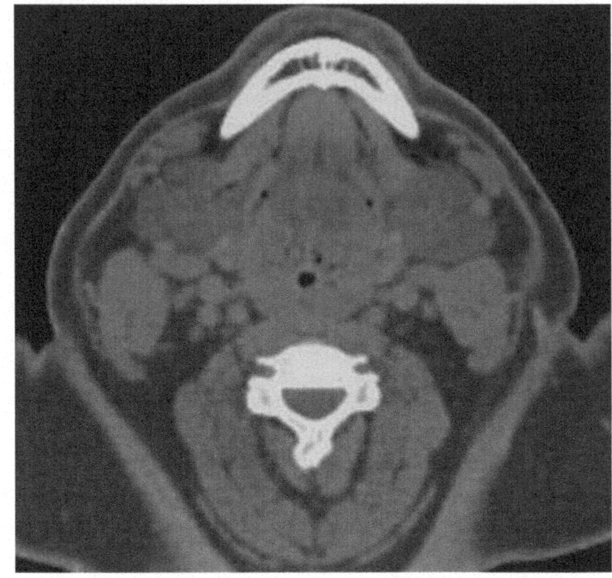

Fig. 6.3 Axial view of the neck on soft tissue windows at the level of the submandibular glands showing good soft tissue structure definition due to the prominent fat planes in this obese body, despite the absence of intravenous contrast

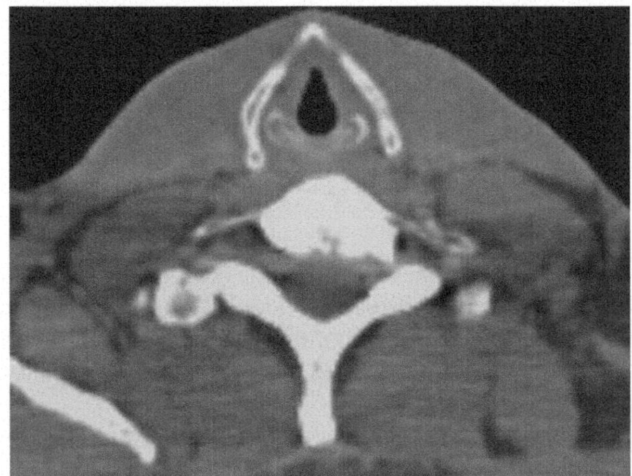

Fig. 6.4 Axial view of the neck at the level of the larynx in this body with minimal body fat shows poor definition of the anterior neck structures and tissue planes but no gross asymmetry or hyperdense haemorrhage

Orbits

In the post mortem state, over time there is loss of ocular volume leading to crumpling of the globes (Figs. 6.9 and 6.10), with vascular gas accumulation (Fig. 6.11) and occasionally dislocation of the lens (Fig. 6.12). With more advanced decomposition, the globes become unrecognisable (Fig. 6.13), but one should also be aware that corneal tissues may have been harvested for tissue donation (Fig. 6.14).

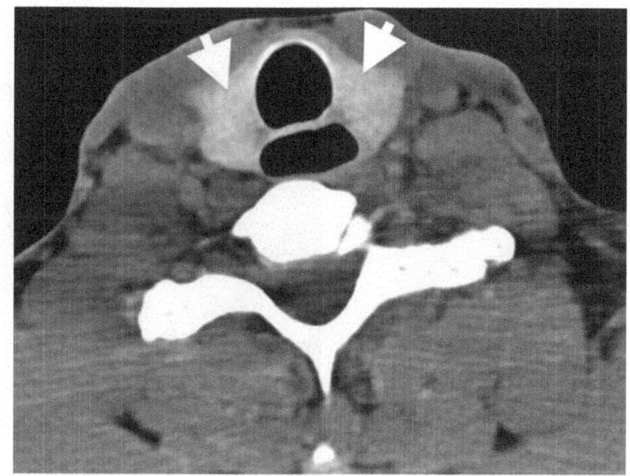

Fig. 6.5 Axial view of the neck on soft tissue windows shows a normal size and morphology of the thyroid (arrows), which has increased density relative to surrounding tissues owing to its intrinsic iodine content

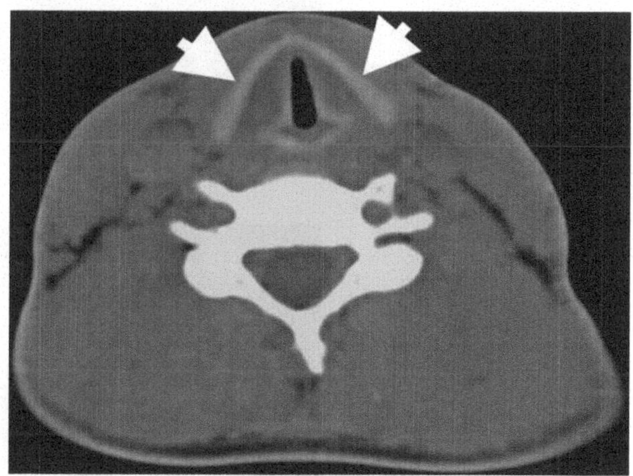

Fig. 6.6 Axial view of the neck at the level of the larynx shows normal, non-calcified thyroid cartilage (arrows) in a 16-year-old

It has been shown that body fluids such as vitreous humour and cerebrospinal fluid slightly increase in density over time [3] but only by a few Hounsfield units. This may in the future help forensic investigation with estimation of an unknown post mortem interval (PMI). If frankly high-density intra-ocular fluid is seen, it is more likely to relate to haemorrhage [4]. Orbital implants and retinal detachments are also occasionally seen (Figs. 6.15 and 6.16), usually reflected in the past medical history. These are often unrelated to the cause of death, particularly if there is no history of trauma.

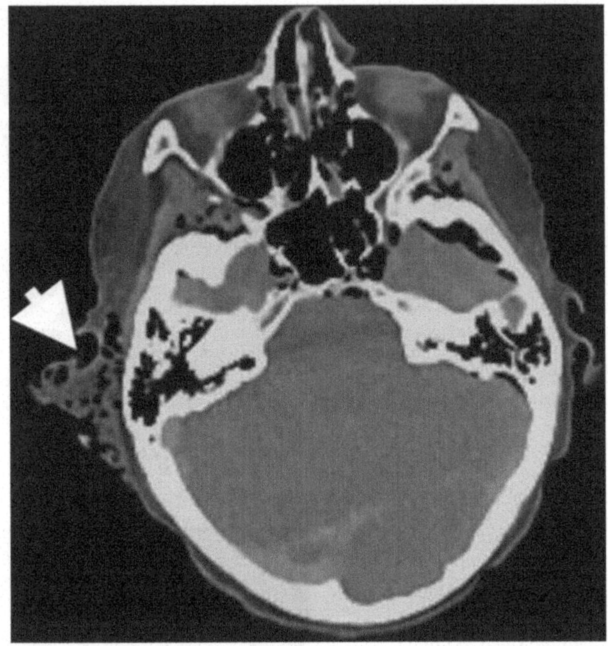

Fig. 6.7 Axial view of the head on soft tissue windows shows soft tissue destruction of the right pinna (arrow) secondary to maggot activity, note also a small decomposition pneumocephalus

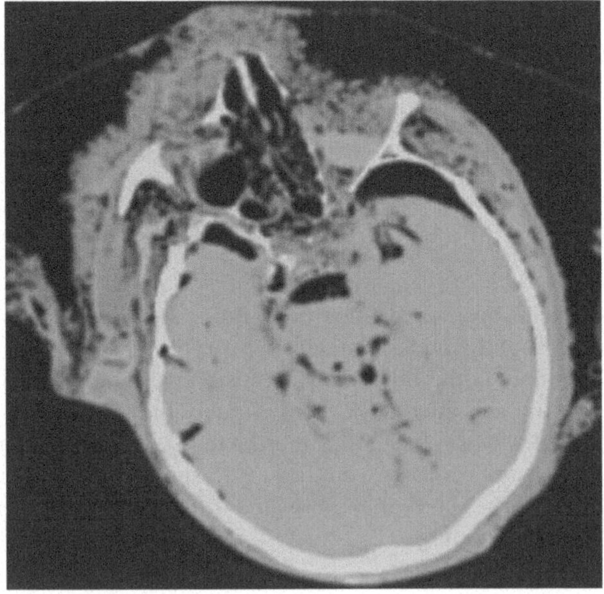

Fig. 6.8 Axial view at the level of the paranasal sinuses on lung windows shows multiple discrete soft tissue densities in-and-around the facial tissues in keeping with maggot infestation and soft tissue destruction. Small decomposition pneumocephalus also present

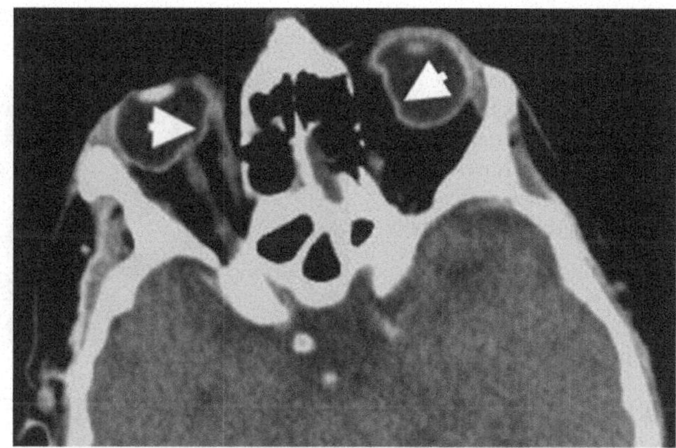

Fig. 6.9 Axial view of the orbits windowed to show normal post mortem crumpling of the globe margins (arrows)

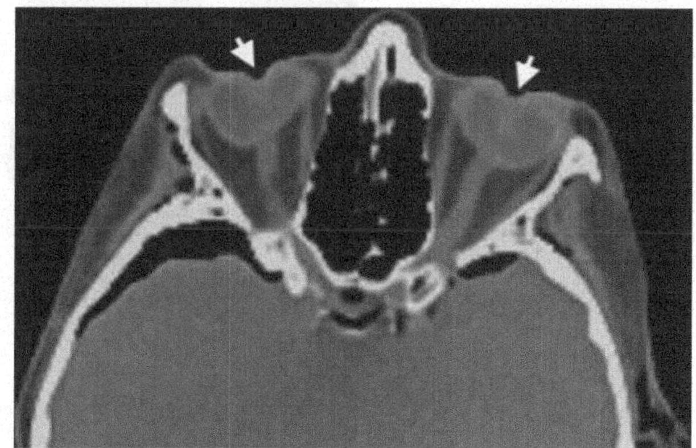

Fig. 6.10 Axial view of the orbits on soft tissue windows shows normal post mortem ocular collapse (arrows) and small pneumocephalus due to decomposition

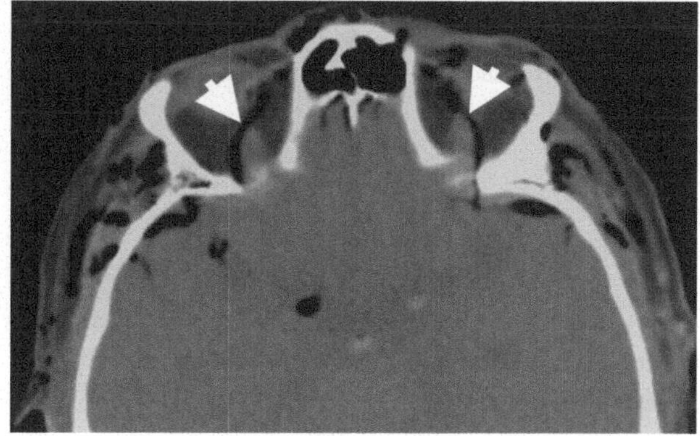

Fig. 6.11 Axial view of the orbits on soft tissue windows shows vascular gas due to decomposition in the superior ophthalmic veins (arrows)

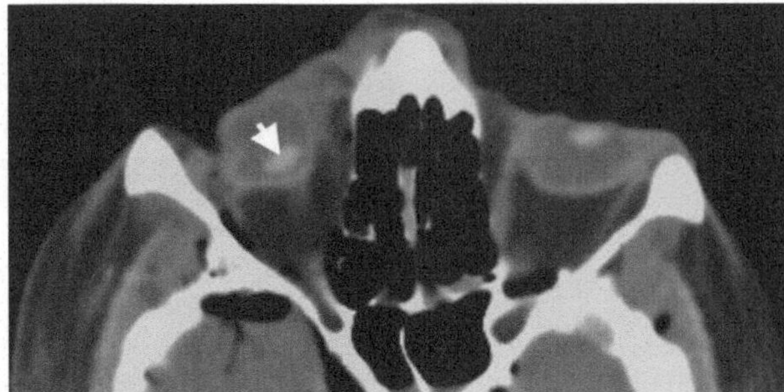

Fig. 6.12 Axial view of the orbits on soft tissue windows shows post mortem dislocation of the right globe lens (arrow) and partially collapsed globes. Note also soft tissue decomposition gas

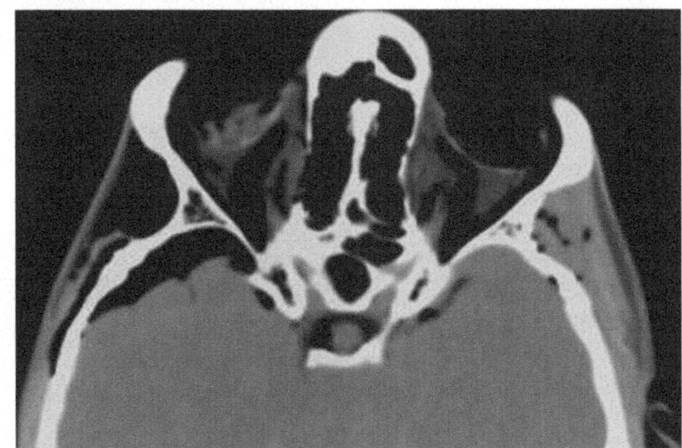

Fig. 6.13 Axial view of the orbits windowed to show almost complete loss of globe tissue and surrounding soft tissue decomposition gas

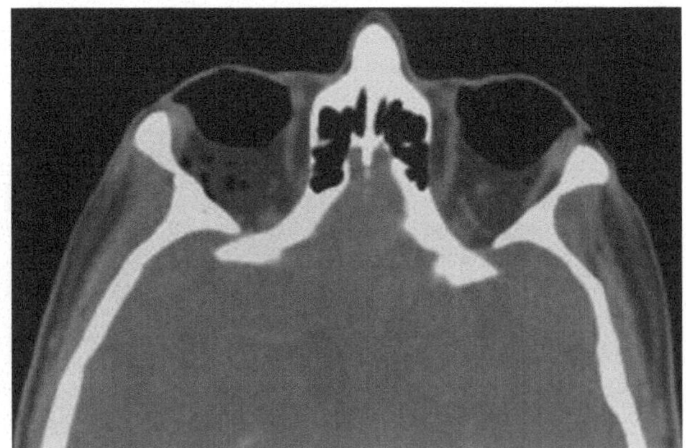

Fig. 6.14 Axial view of the orbits showing absence of both globes, harvested for transplant with post-procedure orbital gas yet no surrounding evidence of soft tissue decomposition

Paranasal Sinuses

Fluid in the paranasal sinuses and nasopharynx is a common finding on PMCT [5] and should usually be considered as normal (Figs. 6.16 and 6.17). One can speculate whether unilateral collections point to localised infection or neoplasia, but the origin and density of such fluid is often multifactorial. Indeed, collections may relate

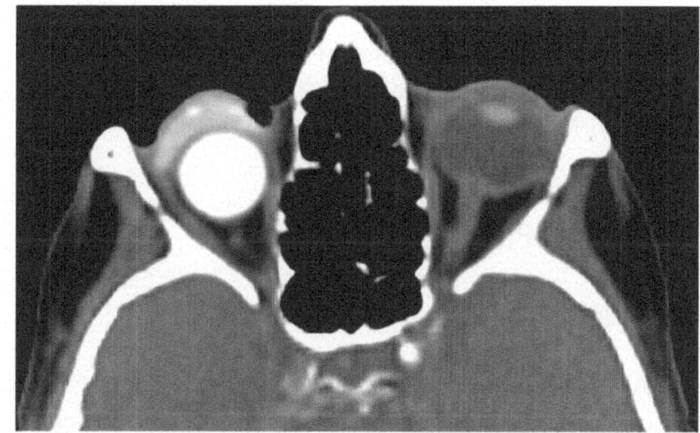

Fig. 6.15 Axial view of the orbits showing a dense (white) spherical right orbital implant and anterior eye prosthesis

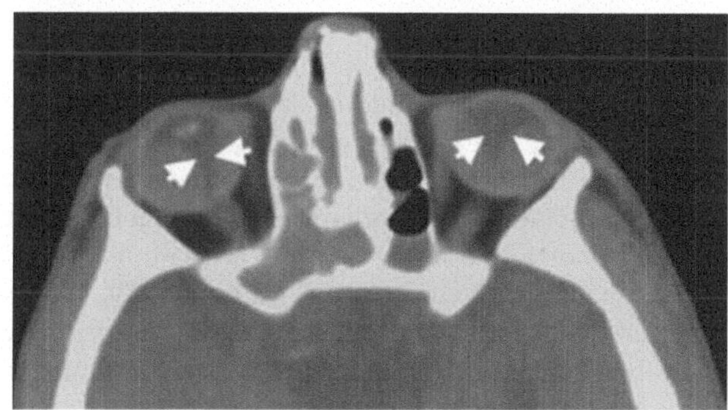

Fig. 6.16 Axial view of the orbits windowed to show chronic bilateral hyperdense retinal detachments (arrows) and right-side cataract in a person who was registered blind. Incidental partial opacification of the paranasal sinuses is also demonstrated

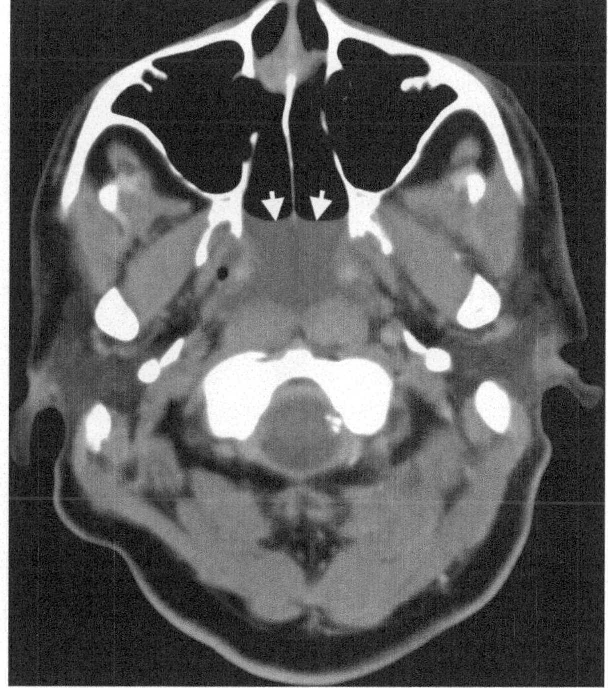

Fig. 6.17 Axial view at the level of the nasopharynx showing a homogenous, gravity-dependent fluid level in the nasopharynx (arrows), generally considered to be a normal post mortem finding

to respiratory secretions, decomposition, regurgitated stomach contents, haemorrhage and/or aspirated material to name a few. Without prior imaging, or a relevant clinical history, it may well be impossible to differentiate the exact nature of this fluid on PMCT.

Abnormal PMCT Findings

Trauma

Facial, skull vault/base and cervical spine fractures (see also Chaps. 5 and 10) are well demonstrated on PMCT, and they are easier to define compared to open autopsy. Such fractures range from the trivial through to the fatal; particularly, if the airway is compromised, there is significant neurological injury or massive haemorrhage.

The cervical spine should always be examined for fracture, dislocation or subluxation (bearing in mind that post mortem muscular laxity or rigor may result in unusual positioning such as a cervical rotational subluxation). Whilst the spectrum of trauma includes that similar to clinical practice, in the post mortem setting it is more common to see severe fractures with implied cord injury which might be considered incompatible with life (Figs. 6.18, 6.19, 6.20, and 6.21). One should note that bone fragments, haemorrhage or debris may be actively or passively transferred from the head and neck into the lower airways, acting either as pathology or as artefacts.

Following trauma, surgical emphysema (Fig. 6.22) or non-decomposition vascular air (Fig. 6.23) is readily visualised on PMCT. Significant soft tissue disruption

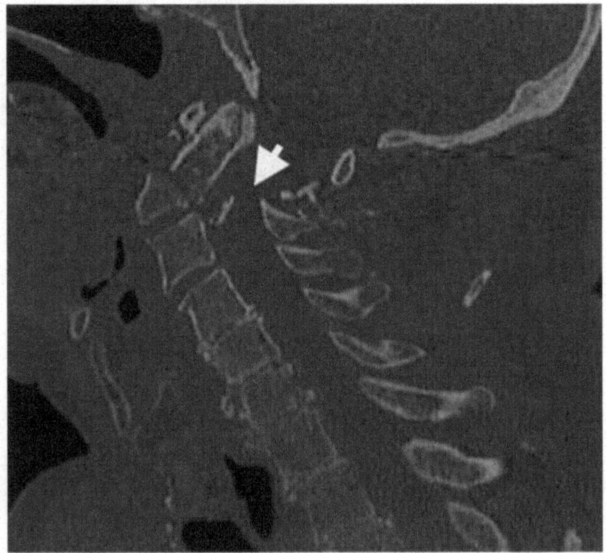

Fig. 6.18 Sagittal view of the cervical spine on bone windows showing significantly displaced, comminuted fractures of C2 resulting in bony cervical canal stenosis (arrow) and therefore potential cord injury. A background of degenerative change is noted

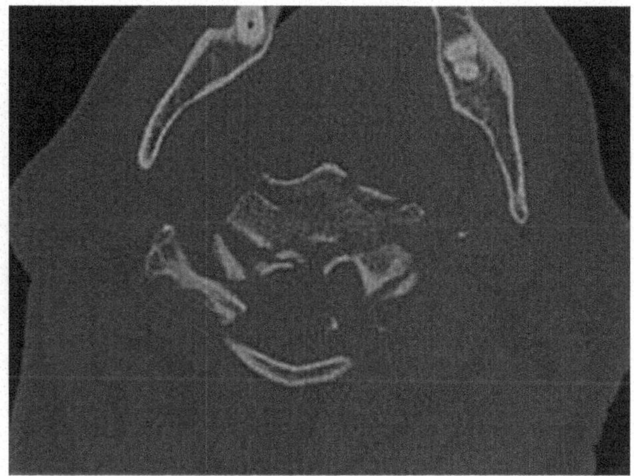

Fig. 6.19 Same case as Fig. 6.18, an axial view again shows the severely comminuted C2 fracture with multiple bony fragments

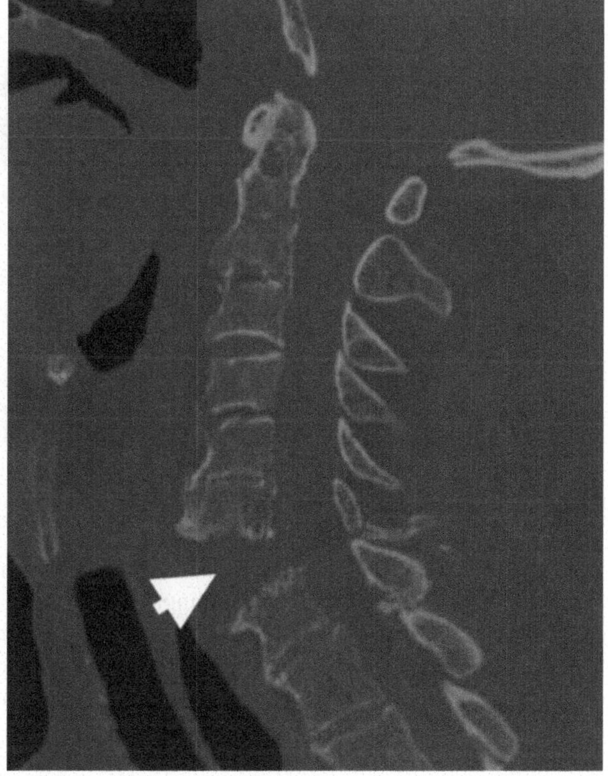

Fig. 6.20 Sagittal view of the cervical spine on bone windows showing an extension-type fracture through the C6/7 disc-space (arrow) and C6/C7 posterior elements with significant residual fracture distraction. A background of degenerative change is noted

and haematoma will also be visualised, but the reporter should be aware that superficial bruising or small volumes of haemorrhage are much more difficult to appreciate and cannot be excluded on the basis of PMCT alone, demonstrating the need for additional, good-quality external examination.

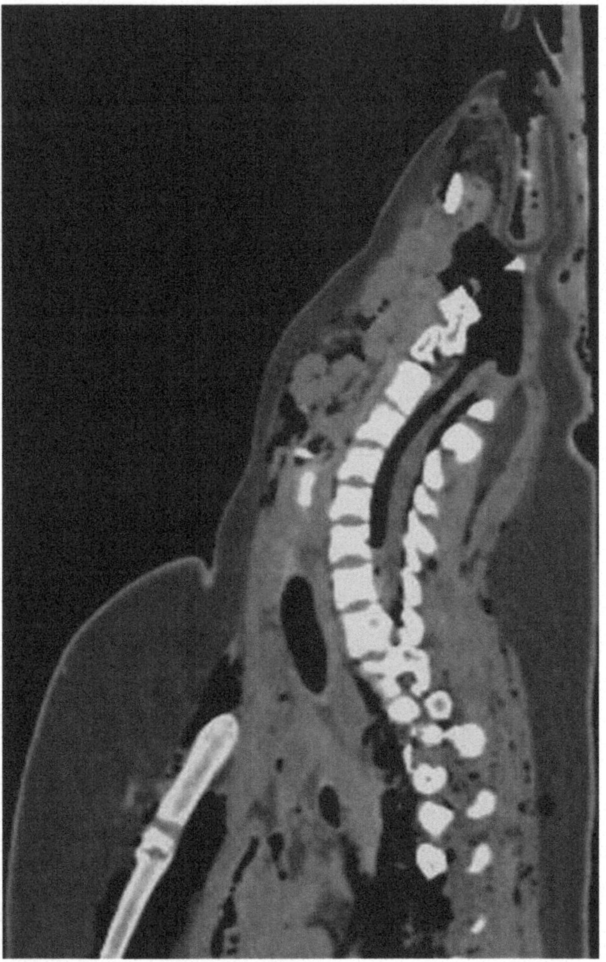

Fig. 6.21 Sagittal view of the head, neck and upper chest on soft tissue windows showing extensive cranio-cervical trauma, incompatible with life

Choking and Aspiration

Whilst, as discussed earlier, fluid in the nasopharynx, paranasal sinuses and airways is usually a normal post mortem finding, in the setting of a witnessed episode of coughing or choking, the presence of mixed density debris (potential food matrix) in the upper aerodigestive tract raises the possibility of fatal airway obstruction (Figs. 6.24, 6.25, 6.26, 6.27, and 6.28). Other findings linked to (potentially chronic) aspiration include lung changes reflecting the foreign matter and/or secondary inflammation with pneumonia, these may add confidence to the diagnosis (see also Chap. 7). Nevertheless, it is stressed that without an appropriate history, any such PMCT findings are probably best regarded as indeterminate.

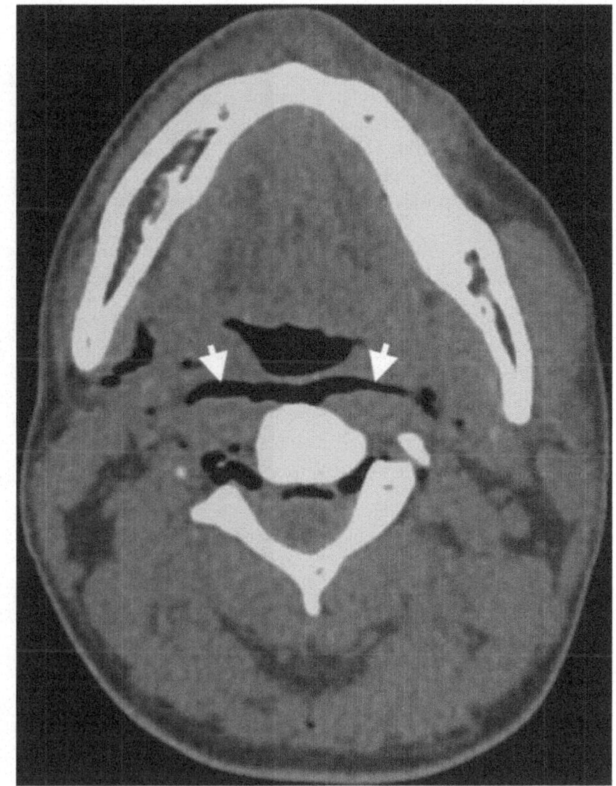

Fig. 6.22 Axial view of the neck on soft tissue windows showing pre-vertebral surgical emphysema (arrows) and a small pneumorachis from cranial trauma (not seen on this slice). Note the lack of decomposition gas elsewhere indicating that these gas collections are traumatic in nature

Infections of the Head and Neck

One appreciates that there are many systemic consequences of infective processes that may result in death. Considering the head and neck specifically, infections can be implicated in the person's death directly by means of airway compromise and large infective processes damaging normal tissue function. The external clues of sepsis such as generalised erythema, skin necrosis, a greenish tinge or marbling (see Chap. 3) cannot be seen on PMCT. Consequently, any ante mortem data should always be considered from a potential infection perspective. When reviewing the PMCT, the possibility of microbial pathology may be considered when there is a focal mass, inflammatory stranding, lymphadenopathy (reactive) and localised gas production, causing surgical emphysema [6].

Potential sites of infective pathology include the tonsils, salivary glands, teeth/gums with extension to the para- or retro-pharyngeal space, the floor of mouth or upper mediastinum. Spondylodiscitis may also present with upper aerodigestive tract swelling [7], further increasing the importance of reviewing the spine.

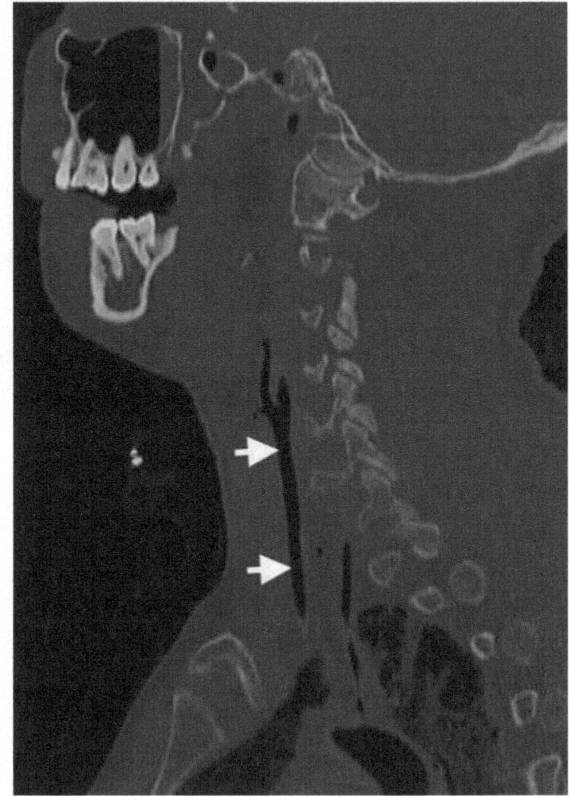

Fig. 6.23 Sagittal view of the neck on bone windows showing gas embolus in the carotid artery lumen (arrow) resulting from a chest injury sustained in a road traffic collision. Note the lack of decomposition gas elsewhere

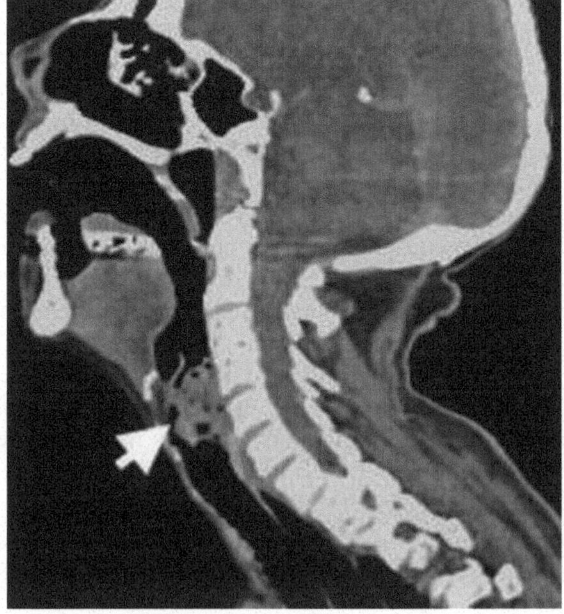

Fig. 6.24 Sagittal view of the neck on soft tissue windows showing a discrete mixed density suspected food bolus in the hypopharynx and laryngeal inlet (arrow) in a case of witnessed choking

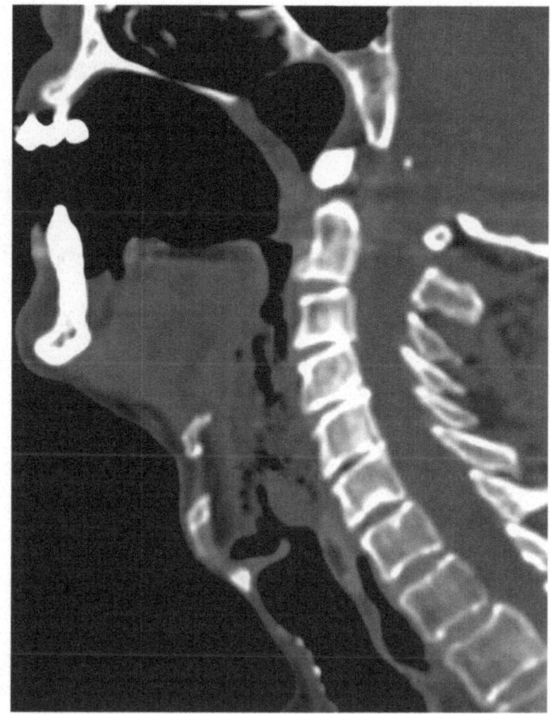

Fig. 6.25 Sagittal view of the neck on soft tissue windows showing mixed density debris in the hypopharynx. This was a case of witnessed choking on food in patient with a history of Parkinson's disease

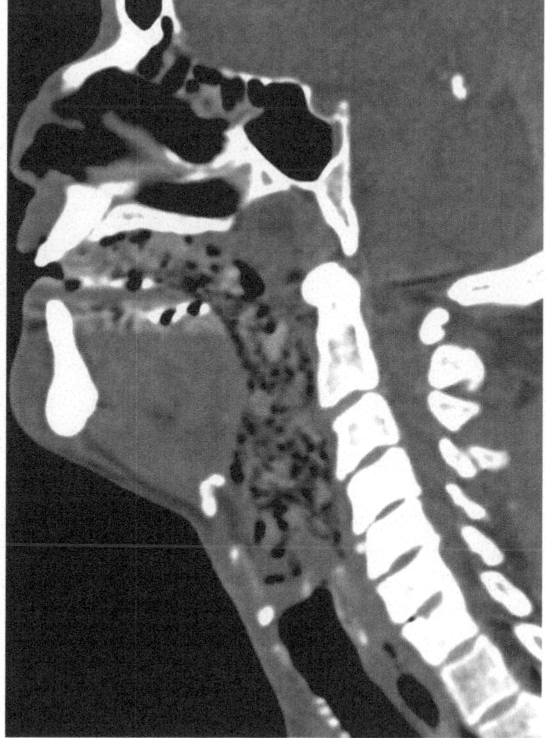

Fig. 6.26 Sagittal view of the neck on soft tissue windows showing mixed density suspected food or vomit in the upper aerodigestive tract in a patient found deceased at home. The lack of a supporting history makes the imaging finding alone less reliable

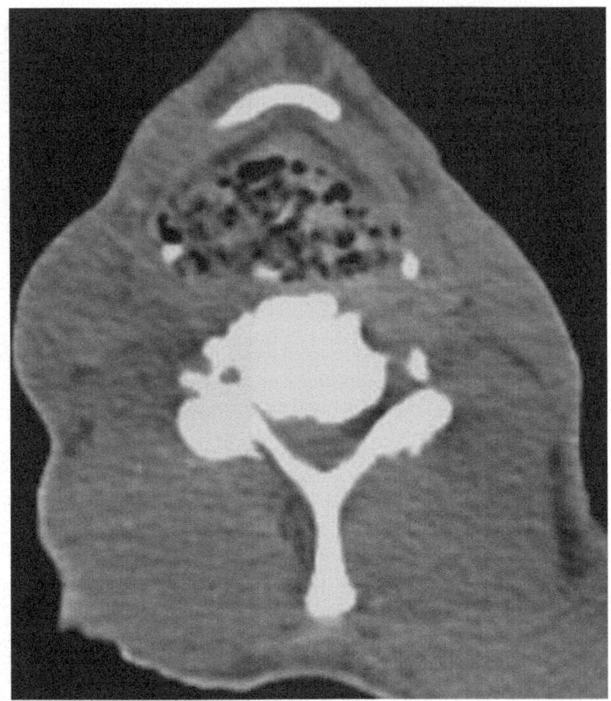

Fig. 6.27 Same case as Fig. 6.26, the axial view of the neck shows that the mixed density debris slightly distends and obstructs the airway

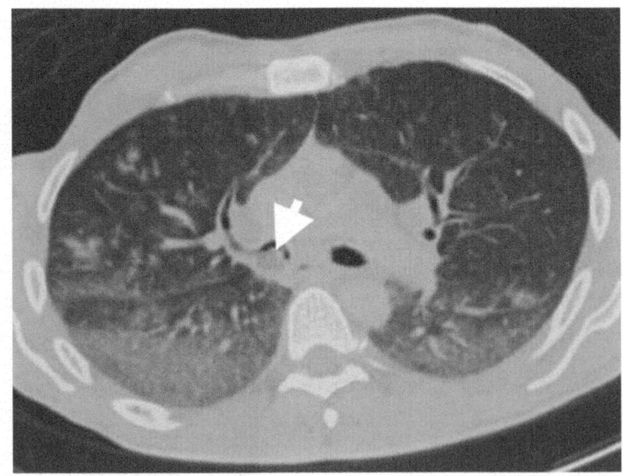

Fig. 6.28 Same case as Fig. 6.26, axial view of the chest on lung windows shows similar debris partially filling the right main bronchus (arrow) and patchy nodular lung opacities due to aspiration (as well as normal hypostasis)

A rare complication of sinusitis or oto-mastoiditis is of bone destruction and intracranial extension of infection. This may lead to meningitis, empyema or abscess. The latter two may be appreciated on non-contrast PMCT if sizeable [8]. As with clinical imaging, meningitis alone would not be appreciated on PMCT (see Chap. 5).

It would be nearly impossible on PMCT alone to exclude a previously unknown tumour as a potential cause of infection or haemorrhage or indeed to exclude secondary vascular thrombosis. If such pathology is suspected, then a limited open autopsy or needle biopsy may be indicated, with the PMCT used to comprehensively assess the bones and exclude pathology in the other body compartments.

Special Circumstances: Hanging

Suicide by hanging is unfortunately a common cause of death across the world. This distressing reality for the relatives is potentially made worse if they have concerns about an open autopsy. A detailed PMCT may be sufficient to avoid such investigation. The role of the radiologist is to assess the neck for hanging-related injury and to consider the body for other injuries, disorders, and alternate causes of death or co-existing pathology.

Where possible, owing to the complexity and small size of neck structures, thin-slice CT should be acquired in a small field of view, with both bone and soft tissue algorithms applied. This may occasionally require additional acquisitions performed specifically for these circumstances.

One should be mindful that if subsequent open autopsy is performed, then the scan provides a permanent record of appearances before potentially difficult and/or destructive pathological examination.

Types of Hanging

Hanging may vary in format. First, hanging can involve a body dropped from a height with a noose applied around the neck. In this circumstance, the sudden halt of the fall causes a violent jerking of the head at the neck. This can lead to cervical spine fracture dislocations (C1/C2 level), with spinal cord injury compromising brainstem vital centres and causing death almost instantly.

Second, hanging can involve the application of a noose around the neck without any drop. This latter reality may involve full or partial suspension of the body. Full suspension implies that no body parts are in contact with the ground as implied with a rope/noose holding the body aloft. Partial suspension implies some contact of the body with the ground. Commonly, the body is partly suspended with a neck ligature attached to a door handle, coat hook or other room structure. This partial suspension still causes compression of neck structures and death. It involves interference with blood flow to/from the brain as well as impeding gas flow in/out of the trachea [9]. There is also an effect from the direct pressure on carotid baroreceptors, which may drop heart rate and blood pressure. Furthermore, there may also be a surge in catecholamine release, which can exacerbate the risk of arrhythmia and subsequent cardiac arrest.

Imaging Findings

Looking at suicidal hangings, the radiologist will often note that the standard PMCT is normal. The absence of other abnormal findings, along with appropriate circumstances, will support the interpretation of hanging as the cause of death. The pathologist will arrange toxicology assessment and a thorough external assessment to exclude other injuries and features of third-party involvement. It is tempting for the radiologist to declare suicidal death directly after PMCT, but it is advised that this be left to the pathologist in case additional data later becomes available.

Many cases of hanging have skin or soft tissue distortion and compression from a ligature. The ligature/noose may still be attached to the body and evident on PMCT (Fig. 6.29) but often with the tension released. Scanning with the ligature in maintained tension is helpful, as it allows assessment of any anatomic distortion or airway narrowing that may be present (Figs. 6.30, 6.31, 6.32, and 6.33). There may be cranial displacement of the hyoid or larynx, resulting in occlusion of the soft tissues of the pharynx. Constriction of these soft tissues is more likely than compression of the stronger laryngeal or tracheal cartilage [9], but there may also be injury to these structures.

Even if removed, the ligature may have left an externally visible mark on the body. If causing deformity of the tissues, this can be seen on volume-rendered surface imaging or multiplanar reconstructions. When a body is found in full suspension, the ligature mark is usually symmetrical and slopes cranially toward the back of the neck [10]. This contrasts with partial suspension [11], where the head may be turned or flexed to one side, with asymmetry of the ligature marks.

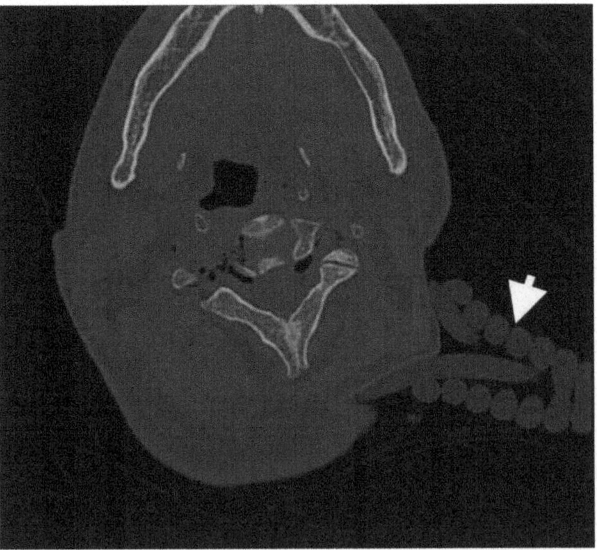

Fig. 6.29 Axial view of the neck on bone windows following a hanging in suspension. The thick rope ligature remains in place externally (arrow)

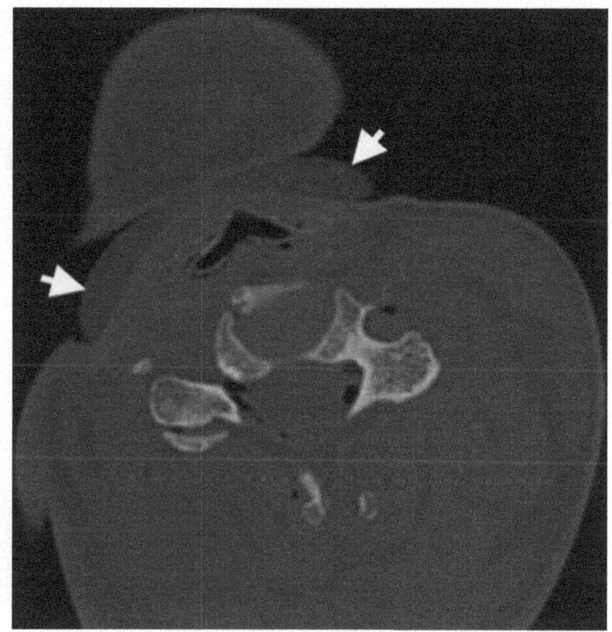

Fig. 6.30 Axial view of the neck on bone windows following a hanging in suspension shows an external rope ligature (arrows) in tension between the chin and neck tissues. There is anteroposterior compression of the cricoid cartilage and airway

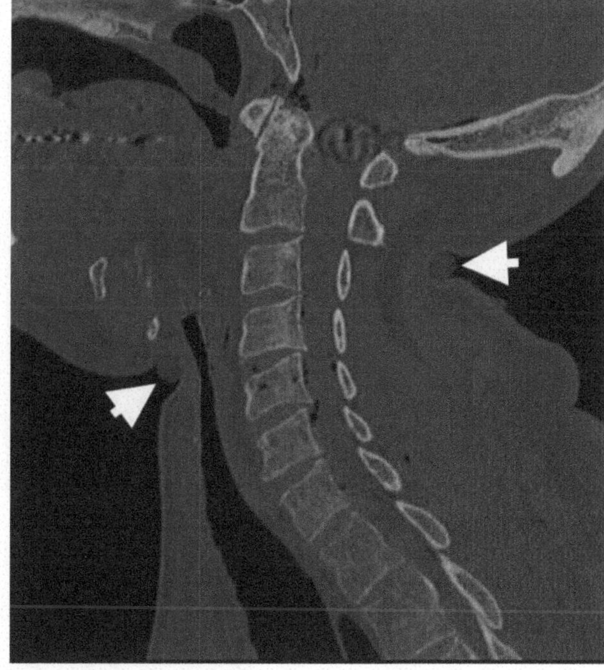

Fig. 6.31 Same case as Fig. 6.30, the sagittal view of the neck shows the external rope ligature anteriorly and posteriorly around the neck (arrows) in tension. There is resultant airway narrowing at the level of the ligature and cranial displacement of the larynx causing soft tissue occlusion of the oropharynx

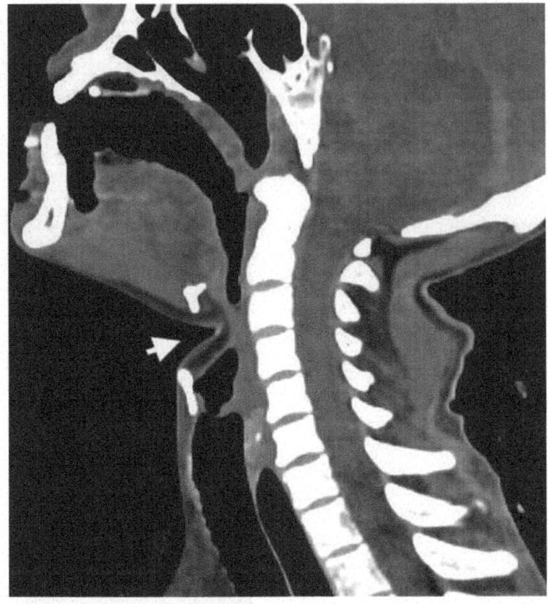

Fig. 6.32 Sagittal view of the neck on soft tissue windows in a case of hanging by shoelace (still in place but not well seen due to a thin calibre). This lies at the level of the thyrohyoid membrane (arrow) and is causing airway occlusion at the same level

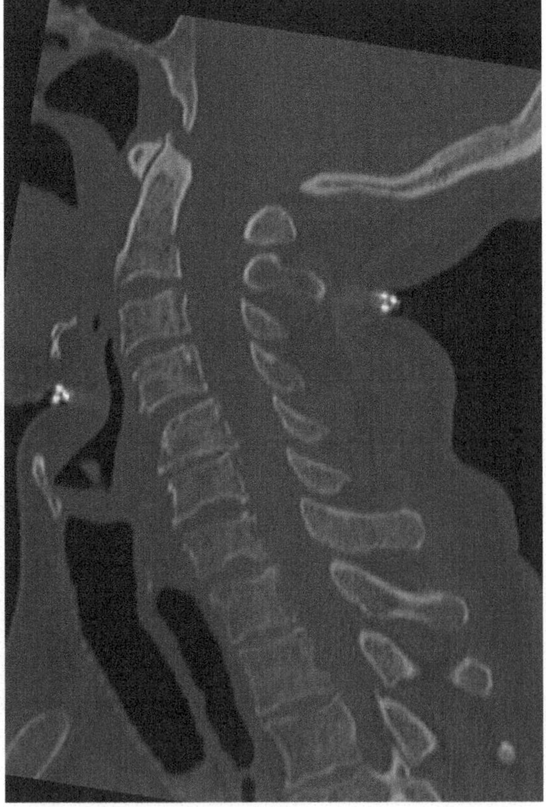

Fig. 6.33 Sagittal view of the neck on bone windows showing an electrical cable ligature (metallic density) in tension at the level of the thyrohyoid membrane. There is upward displacement of the hyoid bone with soft tissue airway occlusion at the level of the oropharynx

Fractures and Dislocations

It is unusual for suicidal hangings to result in cervical spine fractures, unless jumping or falling from a height [9]. In full suspension hangings, fractures may be symmetrical or asymmetrical in pattern. In contrast, in partial suspension hangings there a more likely to be asymmetry in any fractures. While interesting to correlate with the hanging mechanism, in the non-suspicious post mortem setting, extensive detail regarding the fracture pattern is not necessary as might be the case for clinical management or forensic cases.

When present, vertebral fractures and dislocations should be described with the same terminology as for clinical CT, with consideration whether this has led to spinal cord trauma (Figs. 6.34 and 6.35).

In addition, evidence of fracture or distortion of the laryngeal cartilages (Figs. 6.36, 6.37, 6.38, 6.39, and 6.40) and hyoid bone (Figs. 6.41, 6.42, 6.43, and 6.44) should be sought as part of the overall review. Injuries to the superior horns of the thyroid cartilage are generally most common in cases of hanging [11]. When the hyoid is fractured this generally involves the greater horns [11].

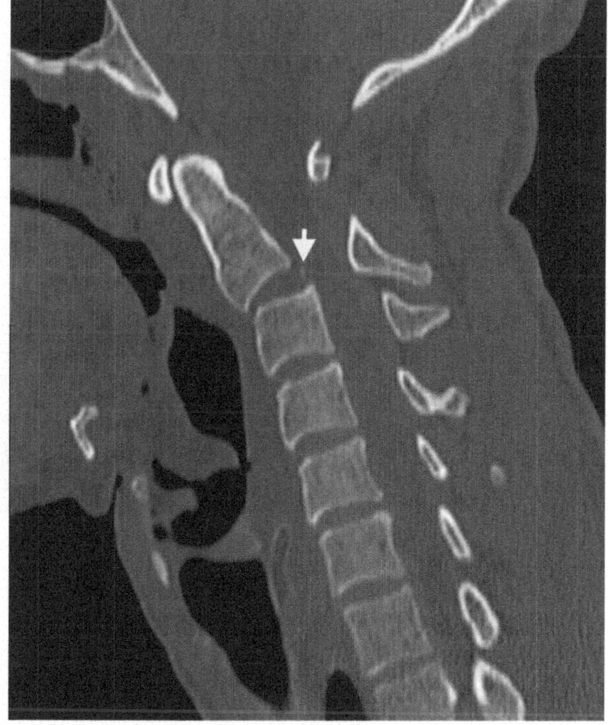

Fig. 6.34 Sagittal view of the neck on bone windows showing angulation and disc space widening at C2/3 and a tiny displaced postero-inferior corner fracture of C2 (arrow) suggesting ligamentous disruption. These injuries resulted from a hanging in suspension

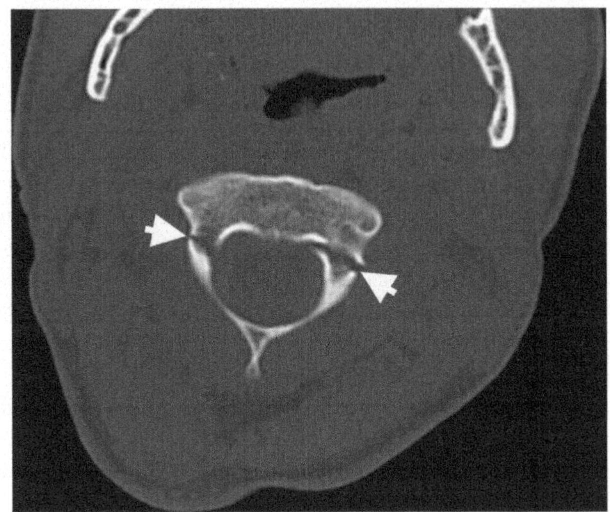

Fig. 6.35 Same case as Fig. 6.34, the axial view of C2 shows bilateral transverse fractures through the pedicles (arrows) also known as a 'Hangman type fracture'

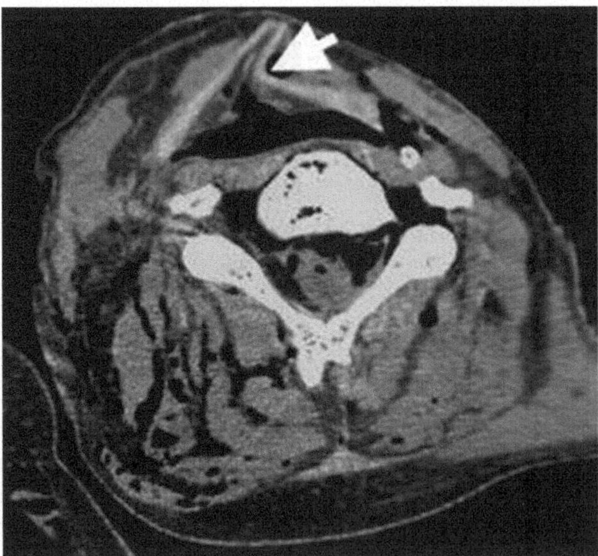

Fig. 6.36 Axial view of the neck on soft tissue windows shows a buckled, non-calcified thyroid cartilage following hanging (arrow). There is also decomposition gas in the soft tissues

Other Findings Resulting from Hanging

Soft tissue injury may be subtle at PMCT, with open autopsy and PMMRI being considered more sensitive in detecting strap muscle trauma [12, 13]. However, even with open autopsy there may also be surprisingly little to find macroscopically [9], although there may be histological changes if sampled.

Subcutaneous gas collections in the head and neck, out of proportion to decomposition changes, might possibly be caused by airway rupture from gasps for breath

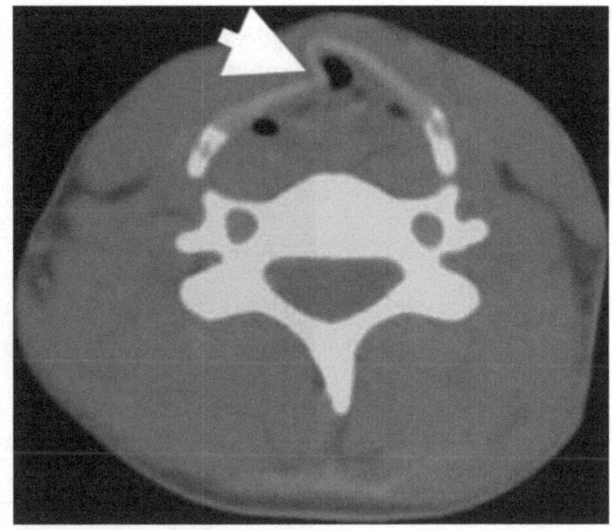

Fig. 6.37 Axial view of the neck windowed to show a minimally calcified thyroid cartilage in a young adult, buckled from hanging injury (arrow)

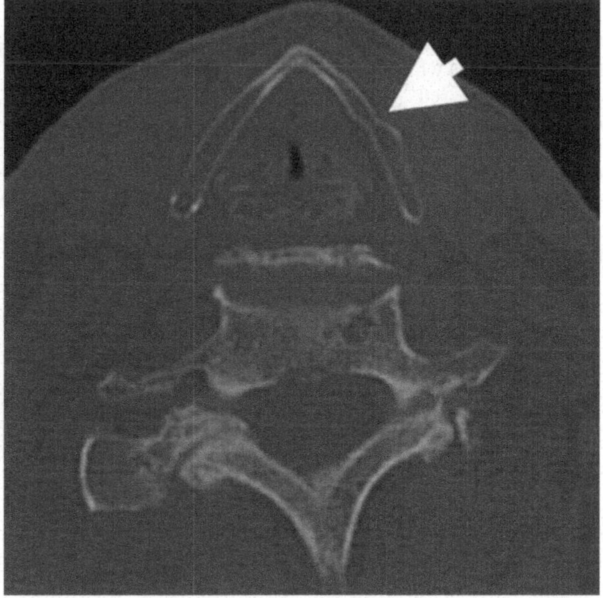

Fig. 6.38 Axial view of the neck on bone windows shows a subtle buckle injury of a calcified left thyroid cartilage lamina (arrow) secondary to hanging in full suspension. Additional facet joint and vertebral degenerative changes are noted

[12] and are better demonstrated on PMCT than open autopsy. This may just be a subtle 'gas bubble sign', a very tiny focus of gas in the peri-laryngeal soft tissues indicative of adjacent laryngeal fracture [11] or a small volume of gas within the cartilage itself (Fig. 6.40).

When hanging vertically for some time, the effects of post mortem hypostasis may be seen 'dependently' in the lower torso and legs [9]. There may be a

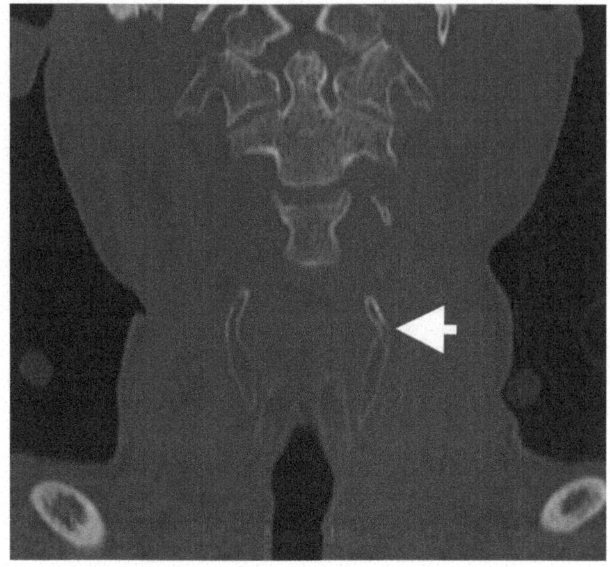

Fig. 6.39 Coronal view of the neck on bone windows showing the thyroid cartilage with a buckle fracture of the left greater horn (arrow) and a loose rope ligature externally around the neck

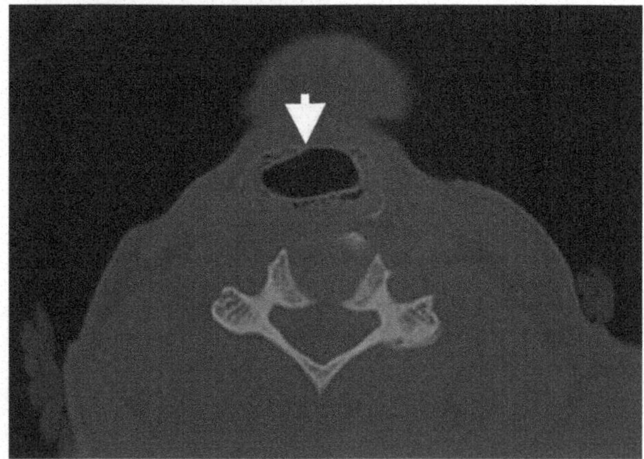

Fig. 6.40 Axial view of the neck on bone windows shows a compressed cricoid cartilage (arrow) following hanging injury. Gas within the cartilage (and not elsewhere) suggests possible barotrauma

craniocaudal gradient of ground-glass change in the lungs, although with later supine positioning of the body this may partly or wholly redistribute. In younger people with no significant co-morbidities, the lungs may be almost completely clear, which is generally unusual for PMCT (Fig. 6.45).

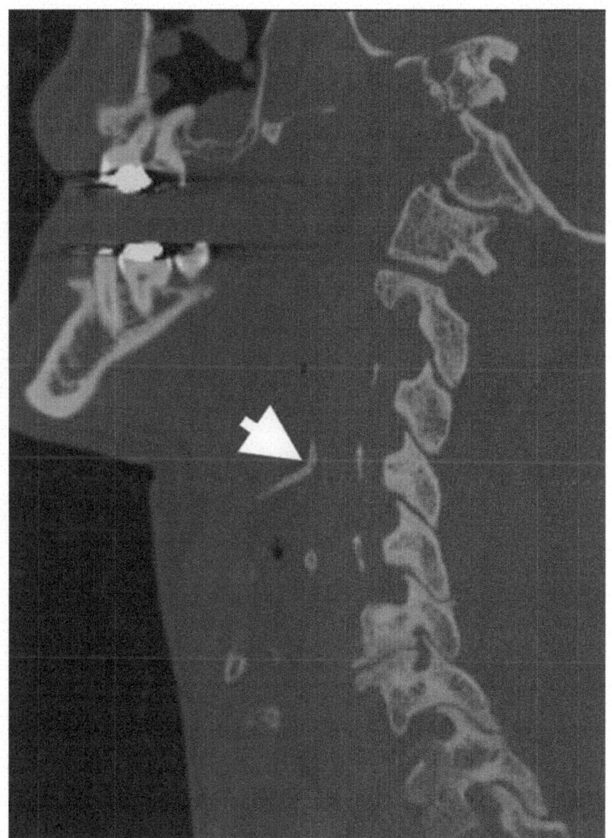

Fig. 6.41 Sagittal view of the neck on bone windows showing a cranially orientated fracture of the greater horn of the hyoid (arrow) following hanging

Hanging or Strangulation?

In the declared 'non-suspicious' setting, radiologists rely on the history supplied regarding circumstances and how the body was found in order to interpret the findings. The findings of hanging on PMCT may be difficult to differentiate from ligature strangulation or manual compression (i.e. homicide, caused by another person). On external inspection, there may be more superficial abrasion or bruising present in such cases, as the forces involved are likely to have been higher. This highlights the need for an experienced pathologist external assessment and questioning of the information provided in cases of hanging.

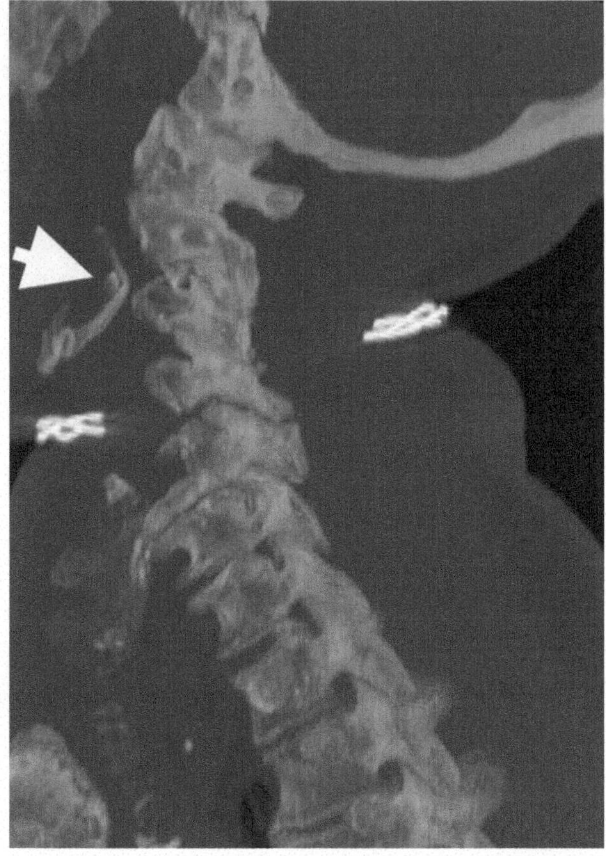

Fig. 6.42 Sagittal maximum intensity projection reconstruction on bone windows showing fracture of the greater horn of the hyoid from hanging in full suspension (arrow). The metallic high-density electrical cable ligature remains present with visible soft tissue indentation

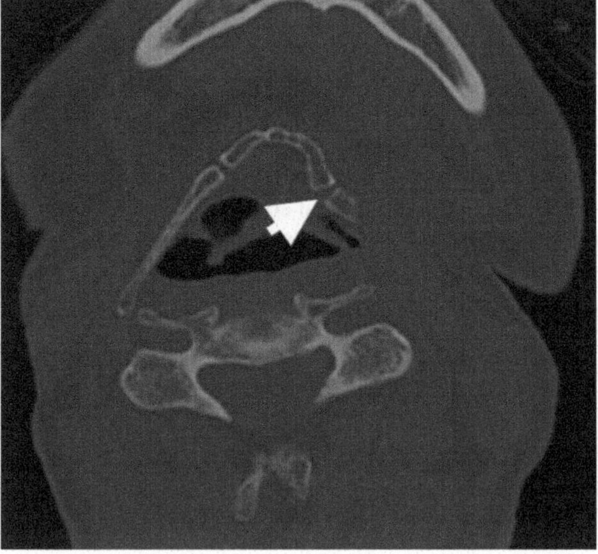

Fig. 6.43 Axial view of the neck on bone windows shows a traumatic disruption at the fibrocartilaginous joint (which is sometimes fused) between the greater horn and body of hyoid (arrow) following hanging. Note the left greater horn is angled out-of-plane

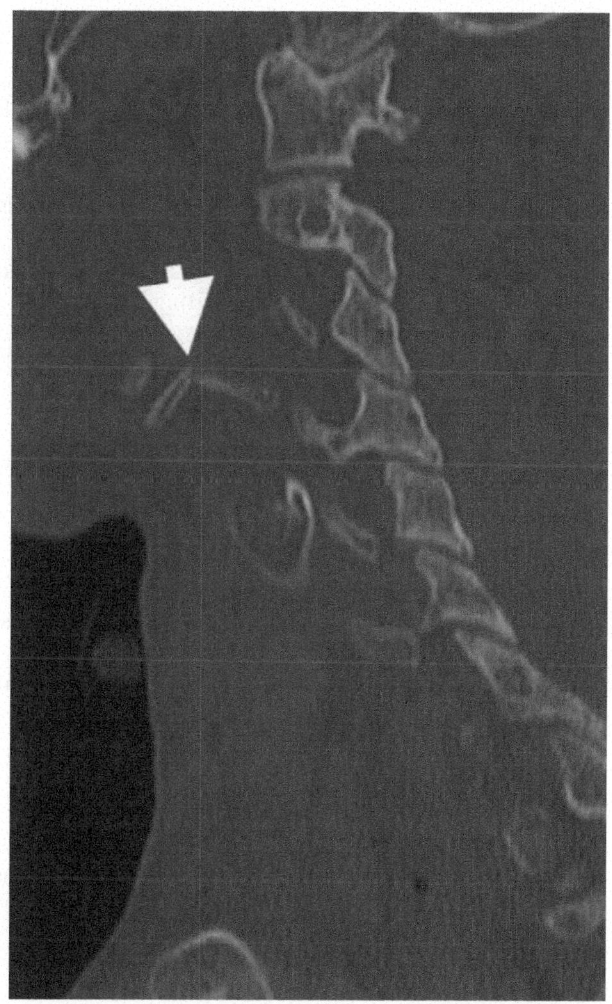

Fig. 6.44 Sagittal view of the neck on bone windows showing a caudally orientated fracture of the greater horn of the hyoid (arrow) following a hanging in suspension

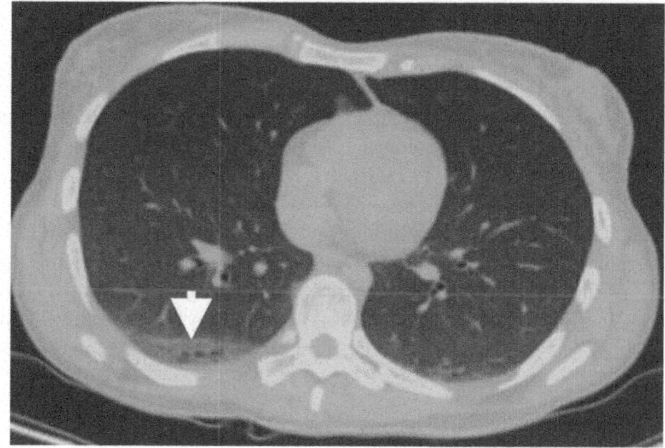

Fig. 6.45 Axial view of the chest on lung windows shows very minimal dependent ground glass change (arrow) in keeping with hypostasis, in the lungs of a young adult following hanging

Reporting Head and Neck Findings: Pearls and Pitfalls

The soft tissues and bones of the head and neck should be routinely reviewed to ensure there is no significant mass, airway occlusion or trauma in all PMCT cases.

Fluid in the paranasal sinuses and nasopharynx is a common finding on PMCT and should usually be considered as normal.

Findings consistent with choking and airway occlusion may be correlated when there is an appropriate supporting history.

In cases of hanging, assessment should be made of the cervical spine, hyoid, laryngeal cartilages, trachea and surrounding soft tissues. A description of any injuries, with relevant negative findings should be included. In many cases, there may be no specific findings on imaging to confirm, or refute, hanging as the cause of death other than the supplied history. This conclusion should be made clear in the report.

Example PMCT report phrases:

- Fluid in the nasopharynx and paranasal sinuses is judged to be a normal post mortem finding.
- No cervical spine fractures. Normal alignment of the cranio-cervical junction, cervical vertebral bodies and facet joints.
- A ligature remains in place, with tension released.
- Anteroposterior compression of the neck by a ligature at the level of the thyrohyoid membrane is causing complete airway obstruction.
- No fractures of the cervical spine, hyoid or laryngeal cartilages.
- No surgical emphysema or large soft tissue haematoma.

References

1. Coe MS, Suvarna SK. Evisceration. In: Suvarna S, editor. Atlas of adult autopsy [Internet]. Cham: Springer International Publishing; 2016. p. 47–63. http://link.springer.com/10.1007/978-3-319-27022-7_3.
2. Burton JL, Suvarna SK. The central nervous system, with eye and ear. In: Suvarna SK, editor. Atlas of adult autopsy [Internet]. Cham: Springer International Publishing; 2016. p. 271–97. http://link.springer.com/10.1007/978-3-319-27022-7_9.
3. Klein WM, Kunz T, Hermans K, Bayat AR, Koopmanschap DHJLM. The common pattern of postmortem changes on whole body CT scans. J Forensic Radiol Imaging [Internet]. 2016;4:47–52. https://linkinghub.elsevier.com/retrieve/pii/S2212478015300289.
4. Panda A, Kumar A, Gamanagatti S, Mishra B. Virtopsy computed tomography in trauma: normal postmortem changes and pathologic spectrum of findings. Curr Probl Diagn Radiol [Internet]. 2015;44(5):391–406. https://linkinghub.elsevier.com/retrieve/pii/S0363018815000420.

5. Biljardt S, Brummel A, Tijhuis R, Sieswerda-Hoogendoorn T, Beenen LF, van Rijn RR. Post-mortem fluid stasis in the sinus, trachea and mainstem bronchi; a computed tomography study in adults and children. J Forensic Radiol Imaging [Internet]. 2015;3(3):162–6. https://linkinghub.elsevier.com/retrieve/pii/S2212478015300046.
6. Baumeister R, Gauthier S, Schweitzer W, Thali MJ, Mauf S. Small—but fatal: postmortem computed tomography indicated acute tonsillitis. J Forensic Radiol Imaging [Internet]. 2016;6:52–6. https://linkinghub.elsevier.com/retrieve/pii/S2212478015300332.
7. Clarke M, McGregor A, Robinson C, Amoroso J, Morgan B, Rutty GN. Identifying the correct cause of death: the role of post-mortem computed tomography in sudden unexplained death. J Forensic Radiol Imaging [Internet]. 2014;2(4):210–2. https://linkinghub.elsevier.com/retrieve/pii/S2212478014001075.
8. Hyodoh H, Matoba K, Murakami M, Saito A, Okuya N, Matoba T. Lethal complication in Pott's puffy tumor: a case report. J Forensic Radiol Imaging [Internet]. 2018;14:12–5. https://linkinghub.elsevier.com/retrieve/pii/S2212478018300510.
9. Saukko P, Knight B. Knight's forensic pathology [Internet]. 4th ed. Boca Raton: CRC Press; 2015. https://www.routledge.com/Knights-Forensic-Pathology/Saukko-Knight/p/book/9780340972533.
10. Kawasumi Y, Hosokai Y, Usui A, Sato M, Takane Y, Saito H, et al. Hanging: postmortem computed tomography. Poster session presented at: European Congress of Radiology; 2011 March 3–7; Vienna, Austria. [Internet]. https://doi.org/10.1594/ecr2011/C-1846.
11. Schulze K, Ebert LC, Ruder TD, Fliss B, Poschmann SA, Gascho D, et al. The gas bubble sign—a reliable indicator of laryngeal fractures in hanging on post-mortem CT. Br J Radiol [Internet]. 2018;20170479. http://www.birpublications.org/doi/10.1259/bjr.20170479.
12. Elifritz J, Hatch GM, Kastenbaum H, Gerrard C, Lathrop SL, Nolte KB. 1.8. PMCT findings in hanging. J Forensic Radiol Imaging [Internet]. 2014;2(2):97. https://linkinghub.elsevier.com/retrieve/pii/S2212478014000227.
13. Gascho D, Heimer J, Tappero C, Schaerli S. Relevant findings on postmortem CT and postmortem MRI in hanging, ligature strangulation and manual strangulation and their additional value compared to autopsy—a systematic review. Forensic Sci Med Pathol [Internet]. 2019;15(1):84–92. http://link.springer.com/10.1007/s12024-018-0070-z.

Post Mortem Computed Tomography of the Chest

7

Introduction

The causes of sudden death in an adult often relate to the chest, making this a crucial cavity to thoroughly examine. As this is an important region and a large topic, it is split over two chapters. This first chapter covers non-cardiac findings in the lungs and mediastinum, with the heart being covered in its own right in the subsequent chapter.

The lungs can be challenging to interpret on post mortem computed tomography (PMCT). Despite the absence of movement artefact, there may be partial lung collapse due to a non-inspiratory phase and variable 'ground-glass' parenchymal opacity due to normal fluid hypostasis after death. In addition, there are a myriad of background pathologies that may be encountered as incidental, contributory and/or directly relevant to the cause of death.

This chapter discusses various normal and pathological chest findings and also covers drowning as a special circumstance, which may be unfamiliar to those who work in general clinical practice.

Autopsy of the Chest: The Pathologist's Perspective

It would be fair to state that the majority of pathologies causing death reside within the thorax, affecting the heart and/or lungs.

The pathologist approaches the thorax initially from the external perspective, examining the chest for features of hyper-expansion, deformity, injuries, scars and symmetry. The internal aspects of the chest are considered by reflecting the skin and soft tissues from the rib cage and then removing the chest plate of anterior ribs and sternum in one piece.

A. Shenton et al., *Post Mortem CT for Non-Suspicious Adult Deaths*,
https://doi.org/10.1007/978-3-030-70829-0_7

Fluid collections in the pleural cavities and pericardium can easily be identified and measured. At this point, the examination should also consider features of congenital anatomy variation, particularly with regard to the heart (see Chap. 8).

One can remove the chest content either with the mouth, pharynx and neck structures and/or the abdominal tissues down to the pelvic compartment in one or multiple fragments. Alternatively, one can transect the mediastinal tissues at the thoracic inlet and cut across the superior aspect of the diaphragm to assist release of the heart and lungs with the mediastinal component. Once removed, the thorax should be considered, looking for fractures, metastatic neoplasia and infections, with additional usually brief review of the vertebral body alignment.

After opening the pericardium and removing the heart (see Chap. 8), the lungs are normally removed separately by cutting through the pulmonary hilum (vessels, airways) so that the lungs may be examined sequentially. As the cardiac tissues are removed, it is important to check for pulmonary embolism by direct palpation of the pulmonary artery content and visual inspection of the vasculature.

Once isolated, the lung tissues can be examined in two ways. They can be sliced longitudinally (in the parasagittal plane) to provide an overview of the architecture, somewhat akin to sequential radiological slices. Many pathologists also have an alternate approach that is initially to dissect along the pulmonary artery to exclude small pulmonary emboli and then to turn the lung tissues over and dissect along the bronchi to exclude obstructions, infections and neoplasia. If these two sequential examinations are performed, then the lung tissues would have been thoroughly examined and samples can be reserved for histology as deemed appropriate.

The mediastinum rarely poses any pathological process for consideration of a cause of death, although tumours of the thymus and mediastinal lymph nodes should always be considered at the same time as pathology of the major airways and large vessels are being reviewed.

Normal PMCT Findings

Thoracic Airways

The upper respiratory tract (pharynx, larynx, trachea and main bronchi) is normally well preserved following death and easy to identify on PMCT. Quite often there is fluid in the trachea and main bronchi which may partially or completely fill these structures (Figs. 7.1 and 7.2). When low-density and homogenous, this should usually be considered a normal finding [1].

More unusually, in cases found in warmer months or exposed circumstances, maggots may have crawled down the airways from the nose and mouth and appear as filling defects or an irregular soft tissue mass [2]. This must be considered in cases of decomposition in order to avoid misinterpretation as pathological airway obstruction (see Chap. 3).

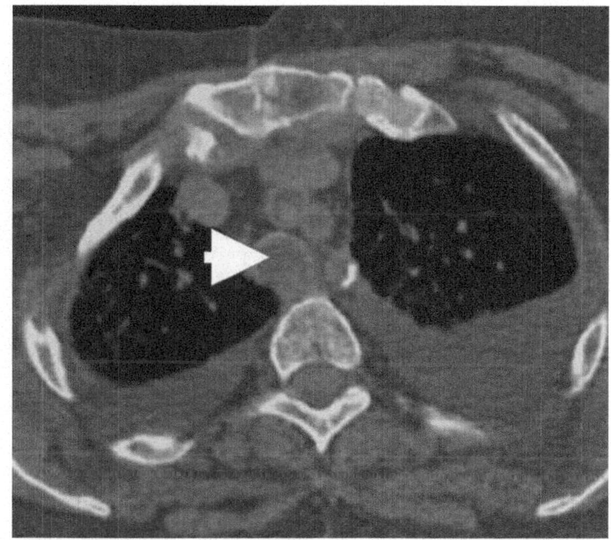

Fig. 7.1 Axial view of the upper chest on soft tissue windows shows fluid filling the upper trachea (arrow) and moderate bilateral pleural effusions

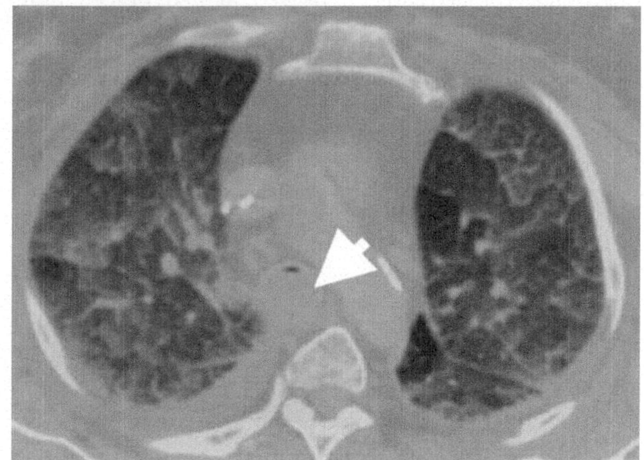

Fig. 7.2 Axial view of the chest on lung windows shows a fluid filled trachea (arrow) with a tiny locule of gas anteriorly. Note also small pleural effusions and patchy ground-glass opacity

Lungs

On PMCT, the lungs almost always appear 'abnormal', compared to clinical imaging. Ideally, the lungs are best examined as soon after death as possible in order to reduce the effects of fluid accumulation, hypostasis and decomposition, which increase over time.

Hypostasis is a commonly encountered post mortem change affecting the lung parenchyma. Generally, it presents as approximately symmetrical ground-glass opacification with a gradient of increasing density toward the dependent area. Often, this gradient has a distinct horizontal 'fluid-level' demarcation (Figs. 7.3, 7.4, 7.5, 7.6, and 7.7). If the body has been lying in a position other than supine, then the

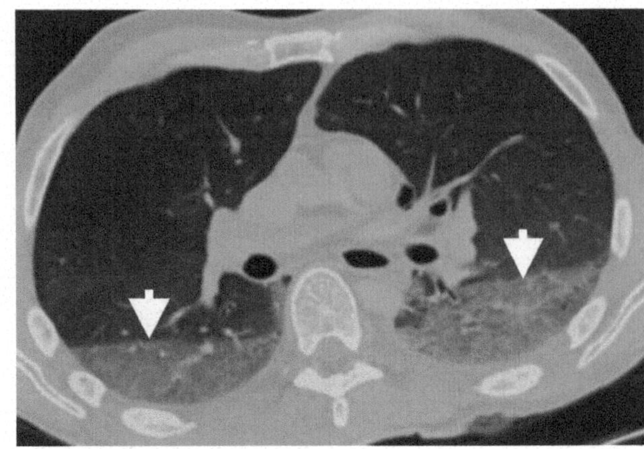

Fig. 7.3 Axial view of the chest on lung windows showing dependent, bilateral ground-glass lung opacity with horizontal demarcation (arrows) in keeping with normal post mortem fluid hypostasis

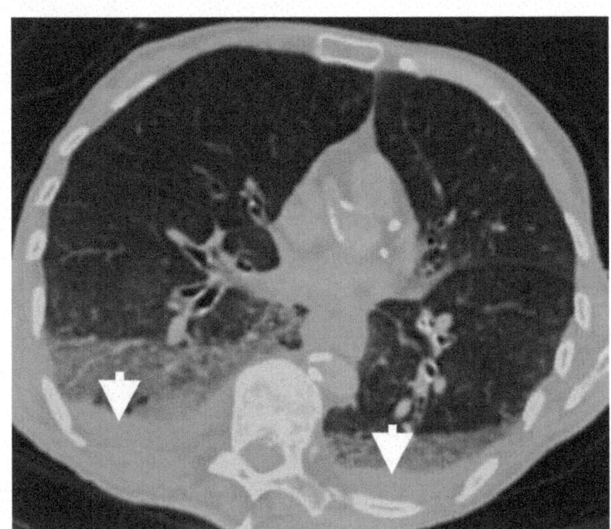

Fig. 7.4 Axial view of the chest on lung windows showing dependent, bilateral fluid hypostasis and additional normal post mortem tiny pleural effusions (arrows)

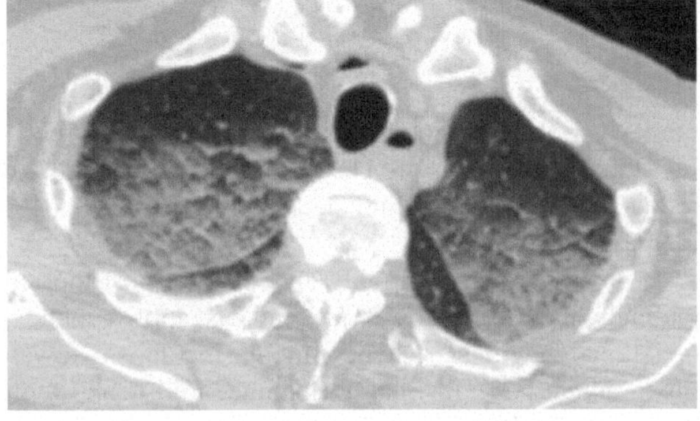

Fig. 7.5 Axial view of the upper chest on lung windows shows more extensive post mortem fluid hypostasis in the lungs compared to previous examples

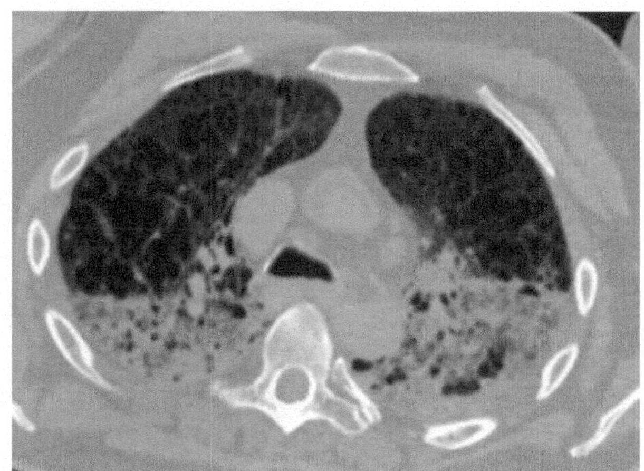

Fig. 7.6 Axial view of the chest on lung windows shows normal post mortem fluid hypostasis of the lungs on a background of emphysema

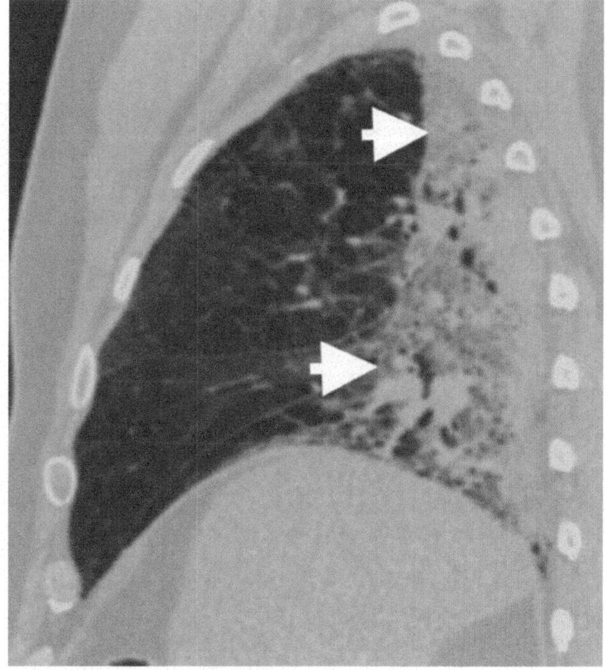

Fig. 7.7 Same case as Fig. 7.6, a sagittal view again shows the dependent (given the supine position of the body) fluid hypostasis of the lung (arrows) on a background of emphysema

direction of the gradient may reflect the position of the body at death (Figs. 7.8, 7.9, 7.10, and 7.11). With ground-glass changes, the vessels are seen 'through' the density.

In some cases, the lung parenchyma may be partially collapsed at the bases. Factors increasing this basal lung density include passive atelectasis from small effusions and a variable 'pushing' effect from the diaphragm, as intra-abdominal organs decompose and expand against the diaphragm. Paradoxically, this same

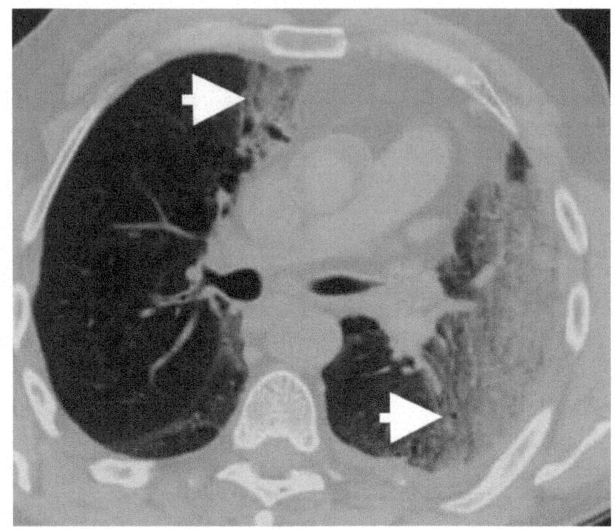

Fig. 7.8 Axial view of the chest on lung windows shows left lateral ground-glass lung density (arrows) in keeping with fluid hypostasis which has settled whilst the body was in a left lateral position

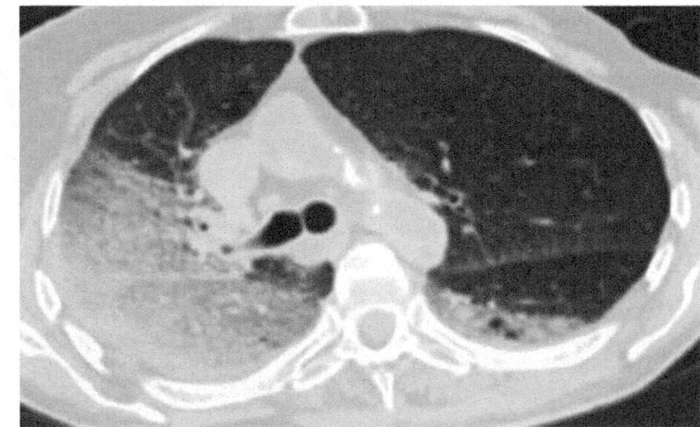

Fig. 7.9 Axial view of the chest on lung windows showing right postero-lateral lung hypostasis. The body was found lying on the right side and then moved supine

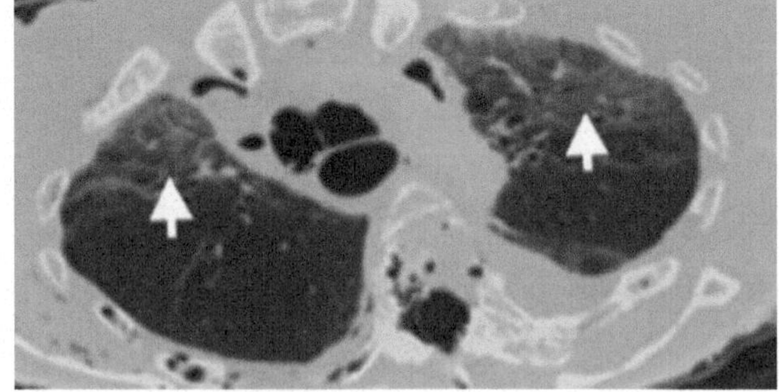

Fig. 7.10 Axial view of the chest on lung windows shows anterior lung hypostasis (arrows) in a body found face down. Vascular gas and pneumorachis are noted, resulting from decomposition

abdominal expansion may occasionally push the sternum ventrally and result in lung volumes that apparently increase with decomposition [3].

In order to improve the diagnostic quality of PMCT for lung pathology, techniques for mechanically expanding the lungs by means of external ventilation have

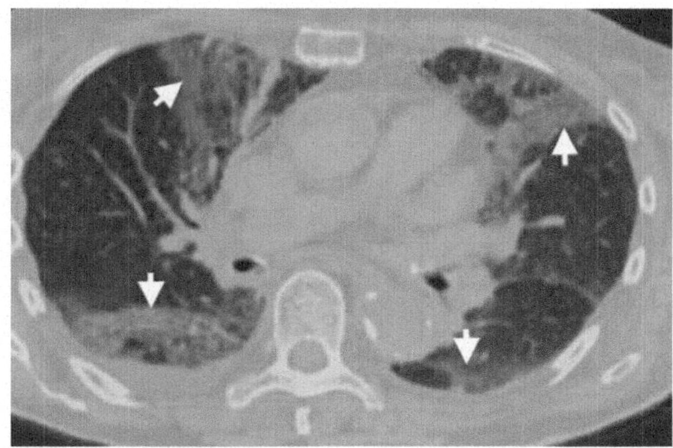

Fig. 7.11 Axial view of the chest on lung windows shows both anterior and posterior hypostasis of the lungs (arrows) in a body found face down and then turned supine. There is a small right and tiny left pleural fluid collection

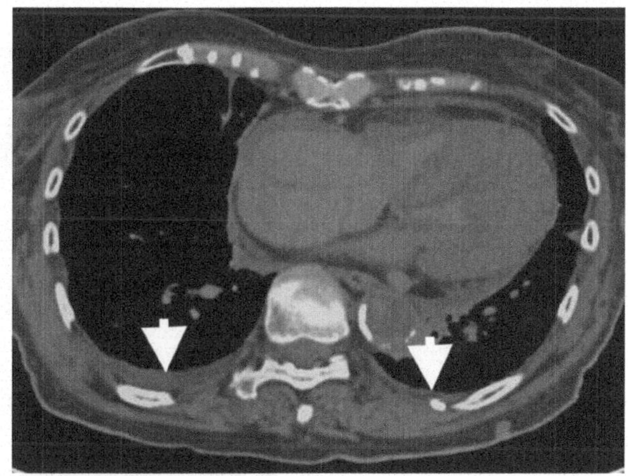

Fig. 7.12 Axial view of the chest on soft tissue windows shows bilateral, small volumes of pleural fluid (arrows), commonly seen post mortem and considered to be normal

been described [4]. These should be considered where feasible, although this technique is not within our practice.

Pleural Spaces

Early post mortem changes include the appearance of small volumes of pleural fluid (Figs. 7.4, 7.11, and 7.12) which increase slightly in volume over the first few days [5]. These should usually be considered as normal. Any large or asymmetric effusions should raise the suspicion of infection, traumatic or neoplastic pathology. Apparent large pleural fluid collections should be carefully reviewed, as they can be difficult to separate from the similar density of densely consolidated lung bases, when fluid also obliterates the expected air bronchograms (Figs. 7.13 and 7.14).

Pneumothoraces are easily detected on PMCT and are usually associated with advanced decomposition (Fig. 7.15). They are also sometimes seen following cardiopulmonary resuscitation (CPR) attempts with or without rib fractures (Fig. 7.16, see also Chap. 11).

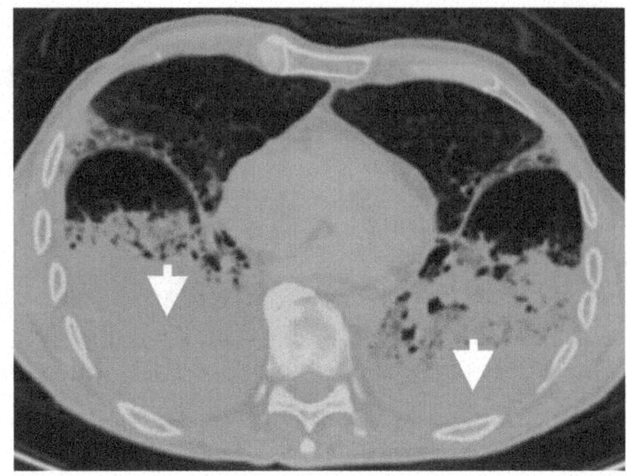

Fig. 7.13 Axial view of the chest on lung windows initially suggests a large right and moderate left pleural effusion (arrows)

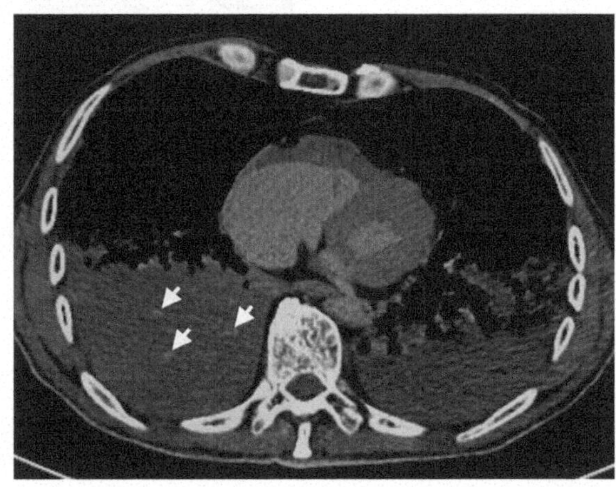

Fig. 7.14 Same case as Fig. 7.13d, careful inspection of the soft tissue windows shows subtle hyperdense vessels in the right lung base (arrows) indicative of right lower lobe consolidation. Note that an expected 'air bronchogram' appearance is obscured by fluid in the distal airways

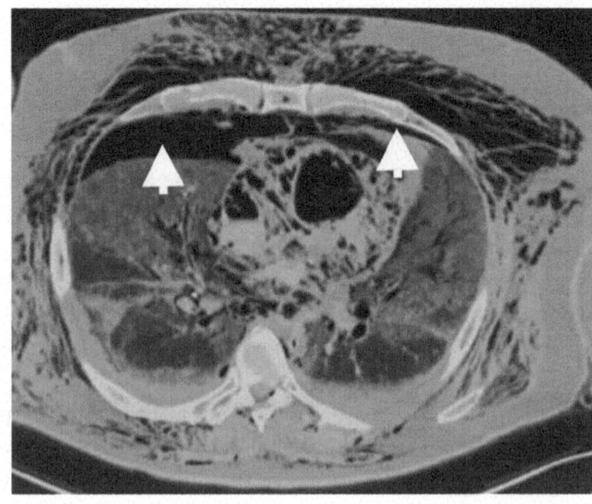

Fig. 7.15 Axial view of the chest on lung windows showing bilateral pneumothoraces (arrows) secondary to advancing decomposition (significant volume of gas seen throughout the body tissues)

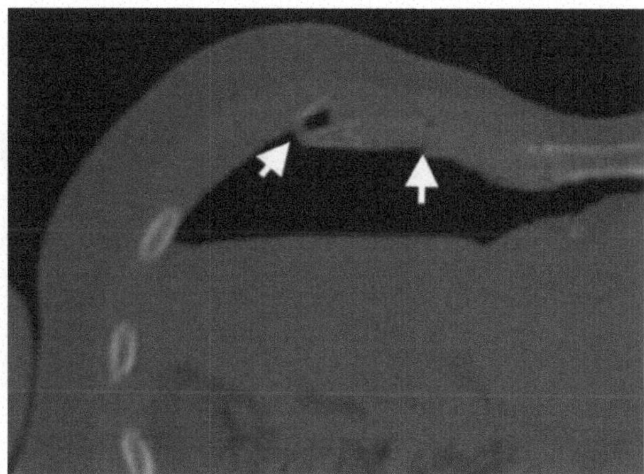

Fig. 7.16 Axial view of the right anterior chest wall on bone windows shows a pneumothorax secondary to rib and costal cartilage fractures (arrows) sustained during chest compressions as part of cardiopulmonary resuscitation attempts

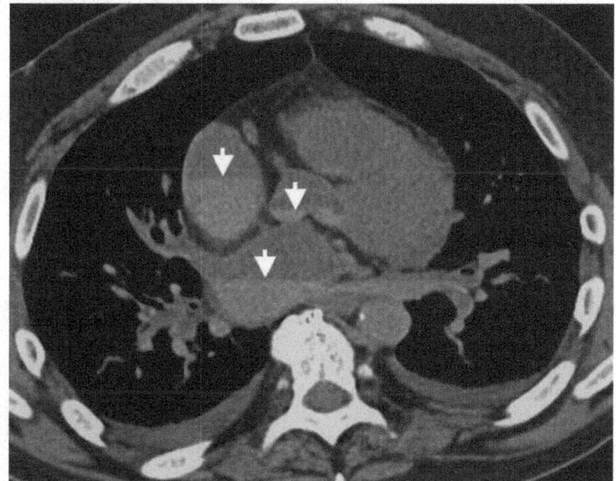

Fig. 7.17 Axial view of the chest on soft tissue windows shows normal post mortem layered separation of the blood components in the heart and great vessels (arrows)

Mediastinal Vessels

Early post mortem changes include the sedimentation or 'layering' of blood in the heart and great vessels (Fig. 7.17) due to the separation of cellular blood components (erythrocytes, leukocytes and platelets, below the plasma) resulting in a 'fluid–fluid' level [6]. This pattern of sedimentation is notable in the main pulmonary arteries and the aorta, but it is not the only recognised post mortem appearance. A heterogeneous appearance representing normal post mortem clot formation is possible; this may be more pronounced in cases with a longer agonal period.

The aortic wall often appears noticeably 'hyperdense' on PMCT compared to clinical imaging (Fig. 7.18). This is thought to reflect the lack of movement artefact of the wall itself and a relatively lower density of its contained, often separated, blood products. The aorta is sometimes partly collapsed or crumpled (Fig. 7.19), and if severe enough it may be difficult to assess for aneurysms or dissection flaps.

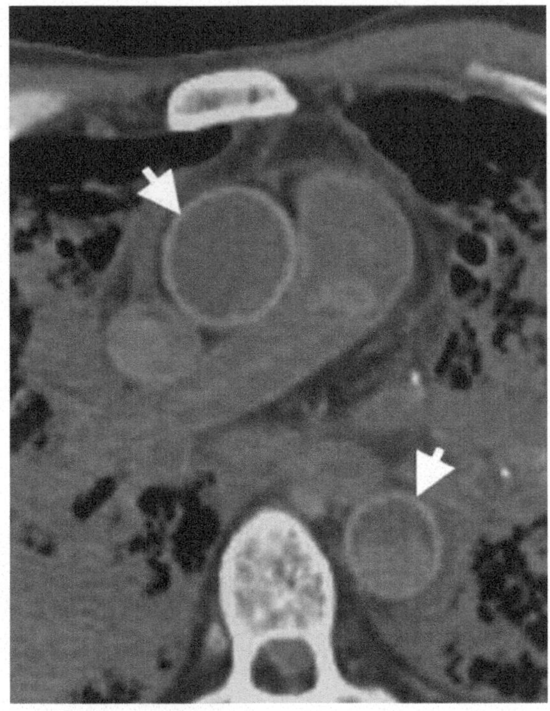

Fig. 7.18 Axial view of the mediastinum on soft tissue windows shows the normal hyperdensity of the motionless aortic wall on PMCT (arrows)

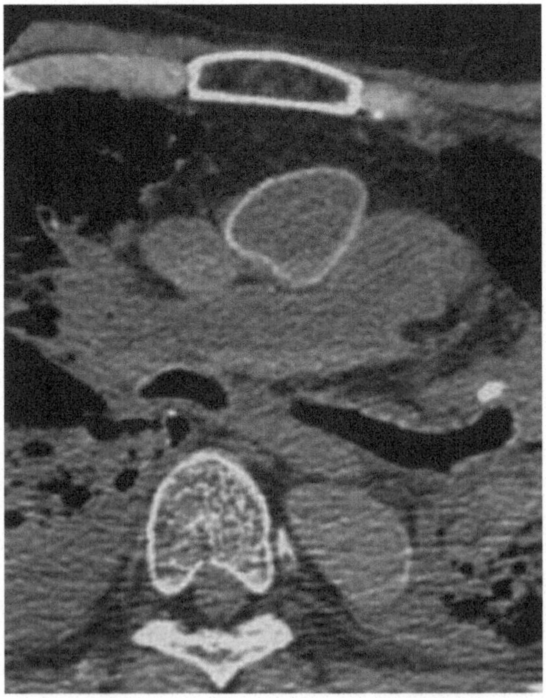

Fig. 7.19 Axial view of the mediastinum showing a slightly collapsed ascending aorta, considered to be normal post mortem, with normal hyperdense wall

Abnormal PMCT Findings

Acute Airway Obstruction

This term usually refers to blockage of the airway, between the pharynx and the bifurcation of the trachea. Choking, with obstruction of the upper aerodigestive tract, is also considered in Chap. 6. This obstruction leads to hypoxia, although death may be caused by neurogenic cardiac arrest [7].

In sudden death cases, the obstructing item is typically a food bolus. On PMCT, this may be difficult to separate from commonly regurgitated stomach content or may even be partially obscured by dental streak artefact [8]. Upper airway obstruction is often supported by a history of choking and/or background neurological disorder, and the diagnosis may be reached when there is a discrete, heterogeneous 'mass' within the upper airway or heterogeneous debris filling the trachea and main bronchi (Figs. 7.20, 7.21, and 7.22). Lung findings may also be present and indirectly support the diagnosis of aspiration (Figs. 7.23 and 7.24).

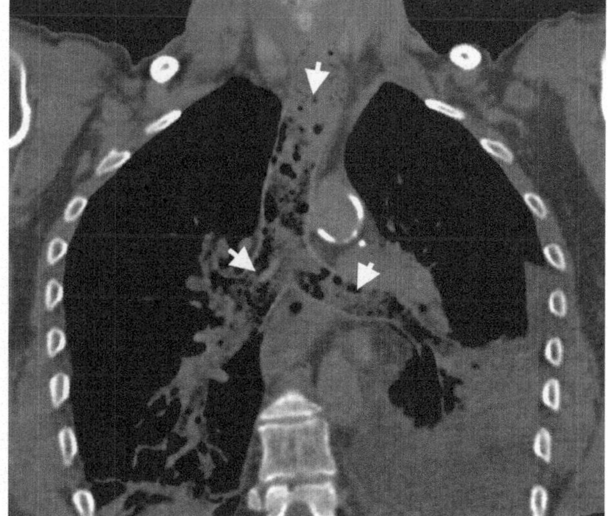

Fig. 7.20 Coronal view of the chest on soft tissue windows showing mixed density debris in the trachea and main bronchi (arrows), extending into the peripheral bronchi of the lower lobes. There was a witnessed episode of choking in a patient with dementia and known swallowing difficulty

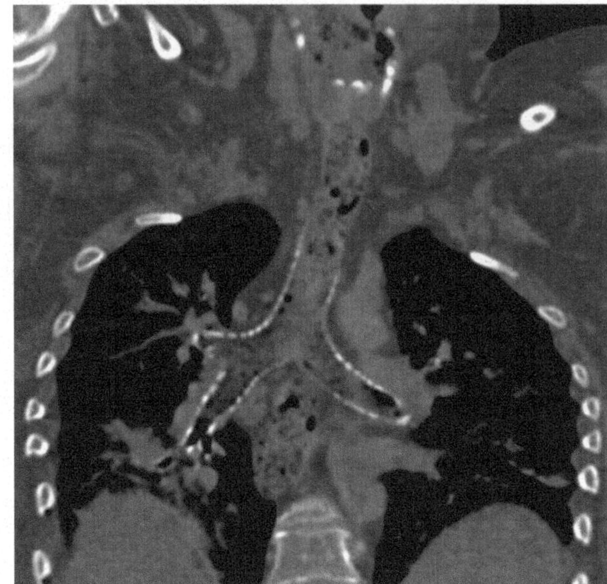

Fig. 7.21 Coronal view of the chest of an epileptic person found deceased at home with food in the mouth, there is similar heterogeneous debris in both the trachea and the oesophagus

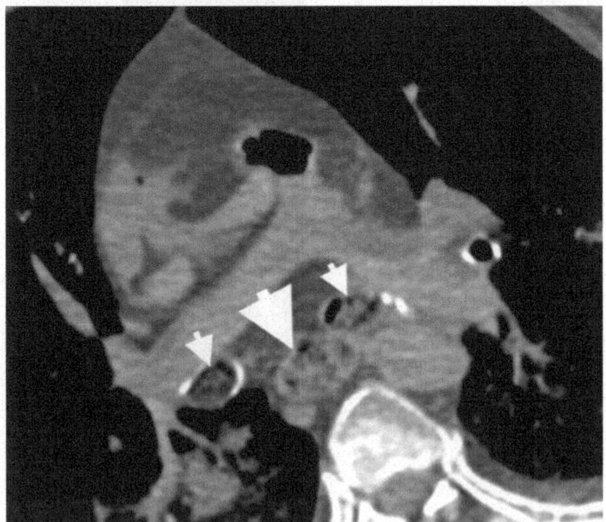

Fig. 7.22 Same case as Fig. 7.21, axial view of the mediastinum again shows similar heterogeneous debris in the airways (small arrows) and the oesophagus (large arrow)

Chest Trauma

A wide range of thoracic traumatic injury may be readily demonstrated on PMCT, including chest wall injuries, haemothorax/pneumothorax, lung and cardiac injury [9] (Figs. 7.25, 7.26, 7.27, and 7.28).

On routine PMCT, it can be difficult to determine the exact origin of haemorrhage when there is extensive haematoma or haemothorax obscuring the anatomy.

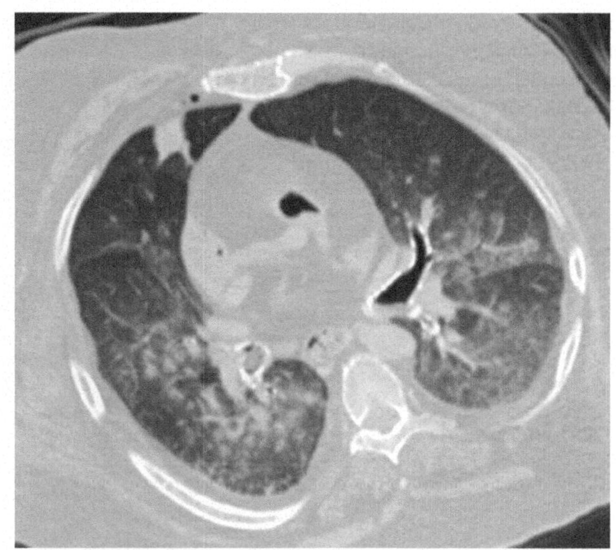

Fig. 7.23 Same case as Fig. 7.22, an axial view of the chest on lung windows more clearly shows the nodular and ground-glass density lung changes, bilateral but more at the right base and consistent with aspiration

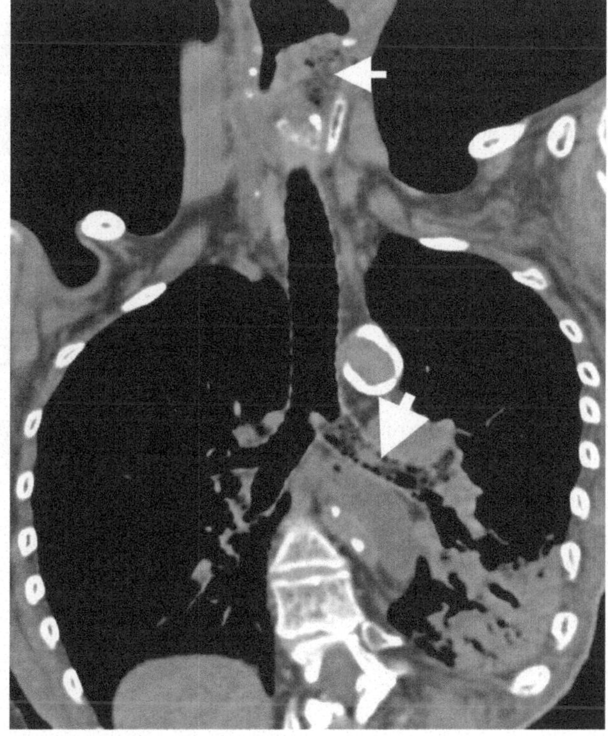

Fig. 7.24 Coronal view of the neck and chest on soft tissue windows showing mixed density debris in the left main bronchus (large arrow) and left basal consolidation, in a patient with dementia and known recurrent aspiration pneumonia. Note also similar debris lodged in the left pyriform fossa (small arrow) which could be due to swallow dysfunction

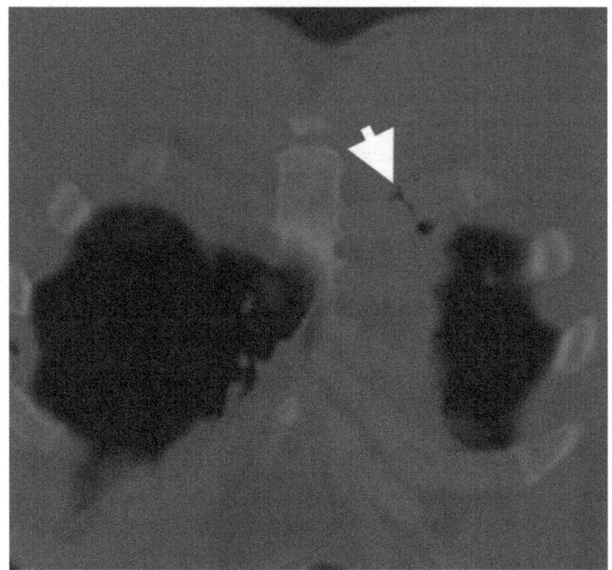

Fig. 7.25 Coronal view of the chest on bone windows shows a left costal cartilage fracture (arrow) following a road traffic collision. These are also sometimes seen following CPR attempts

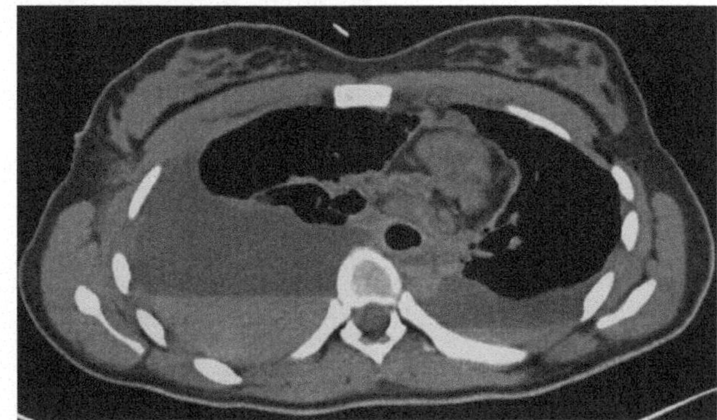

Fig. 7.26 Axial view of the chest on soft tissue windows shows large, bilateral haemothoraces (with separation of blood products due to hypostasis) following a fatal thoracic crush injury

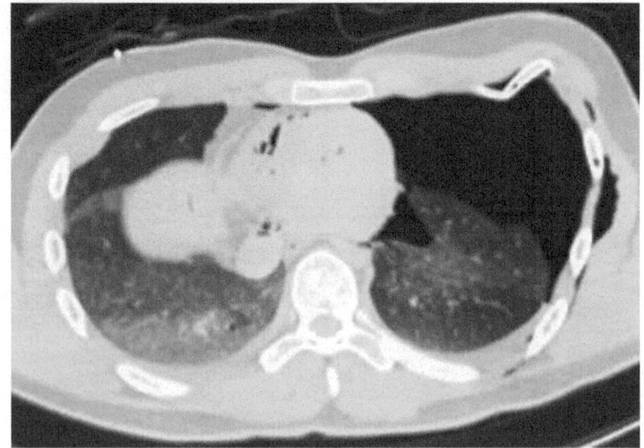

Fig. 7.27 Axial view of the chest on lung windows shows displaced left rib fractures, a large left pneumothorax and mediastinal shift toward the right following a road traffic collision

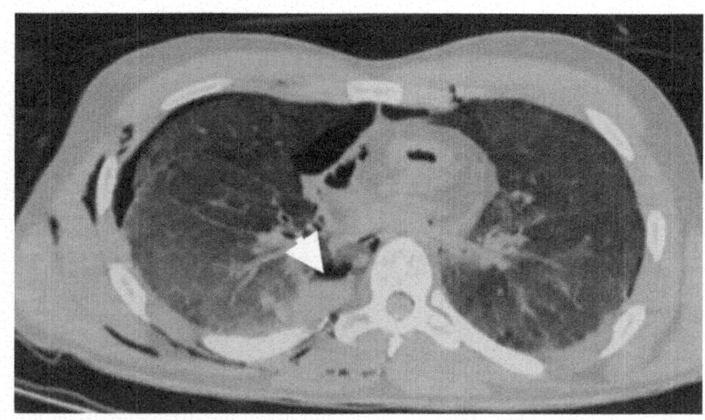

Fig. 7.28 Axial view of the chest on lung windows shows right pneumothorax and haemorrhagic pneumatocoele (arrow) following a road traffic collision

In such traumatic cases, the cause of death is generally either a great vessel or a cardiac injury. A potential source of bleeding may be directly identified on angiography or, more simply, by correlation 'on the balance of probabilities' of the mechanism of trauma and likely site of injury.

Significant chest trauma often presents a constellation of findings. Lung contusions may manifest as focal areas of increased lung density, akin to consolidation, with surrounding ground-glass change. Contusions or lacerations can also lead to venous fistulae and gas entering the systemic circulation. This may be suspected when there is gas in the heart and systemic arteries, without other decomposition changes. Caution should be taken with this interpretation in the setting of attempted CPR (especially after positive pressure ventilation), or onset of decomposition, as these can also explain the presence of vascular gas.

Rib Fractures

In a routine autopsy, the individual ribs are often not dissected/separated or closely examined, unlike the assessment that normally accompanies forensic testing. By contrast, PMCT offers a more thorough routine skeletal assessment and can be used to give a broad suggestion of fracture age (acute, sub-acute or healed). It cannot however reliably distinguish between recent ante mortem, agonal/CPR or post mortem rib fractures.

Rib fractures should be described as incomplete (such as buckle or single cortex, Fig. 7.29) or complete (Fig. 7.16). Fractures consistent with CPR attempts (anterolateral and bilateral) are further discussed in Chap. 11. Lateral and posterior rib fractures suggest an alternate trauma.

Thoracic Aortic Rupture

Sudden death can be caused by aortic rupture, with rapid blood loss into the pericardial sac (see Chap. 8) or pleural spaces (Figs. 7.30, 7.31, and 7.32). Aortic rupture

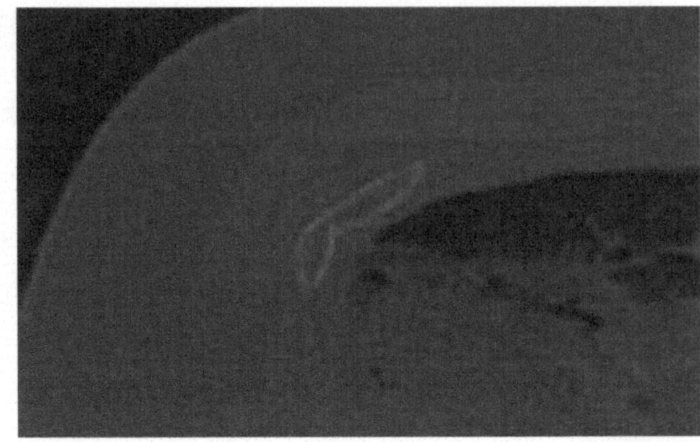

Fig. 7.29 Axial view of the right anterolateral chest wall on bone windows shows an incomplete rib fracture, commonly seen following chest compressions/CPR

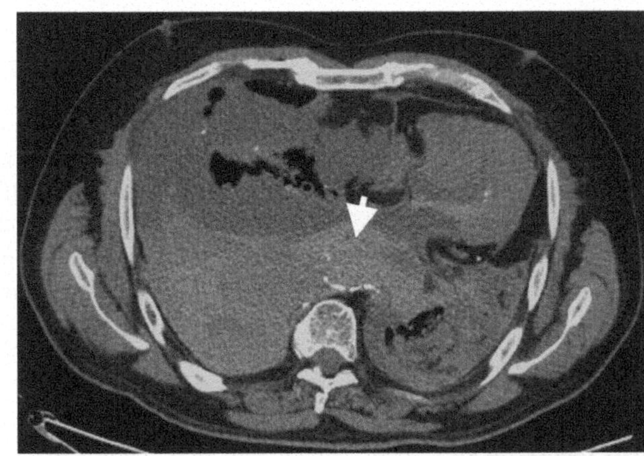

Fig. 7.30 Axial view of the chest on soft tissue windows shows a ruptured thoracic aorta (arrow) with large haemothoraces. The aortic wall is difficult to visually separate from the haematoma but is partially identified by mural calcification

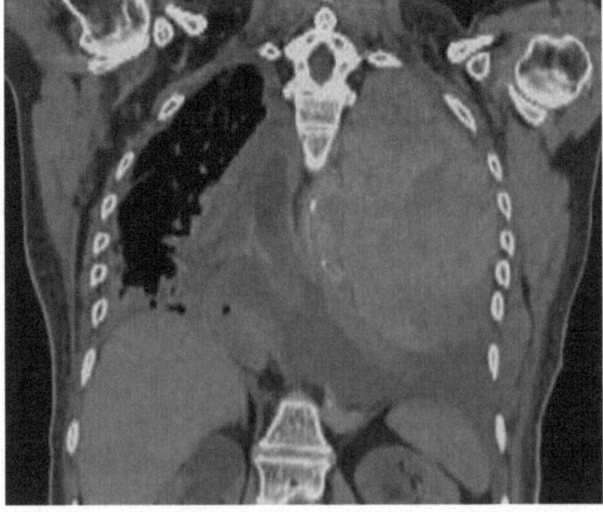

Fig. 7.31 Coronal view of the chest on soft tissue windows shows a fatal aortic rupture with massive left side mixed density haemothorax and secondary mediastinal shift toward the right

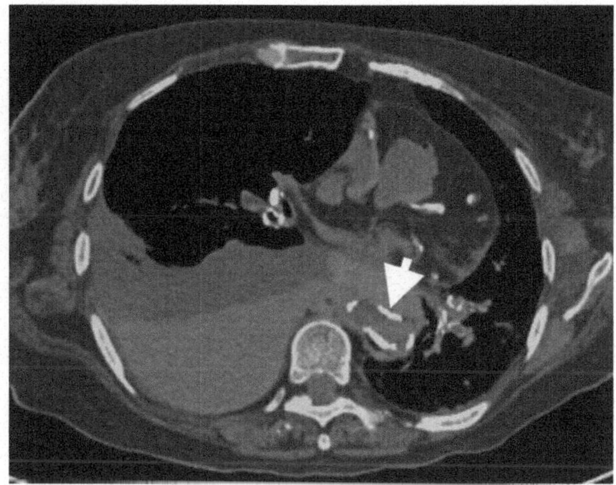

Fig. 7.32 Axial view of the chest on soft tissue windows shows a large, layered right haemothorax with mediastinal shift towards the left. Haematoma is contiguous with the ruptured thoracic aorta, identified by its partially collapsed, calcified wall (arrow)

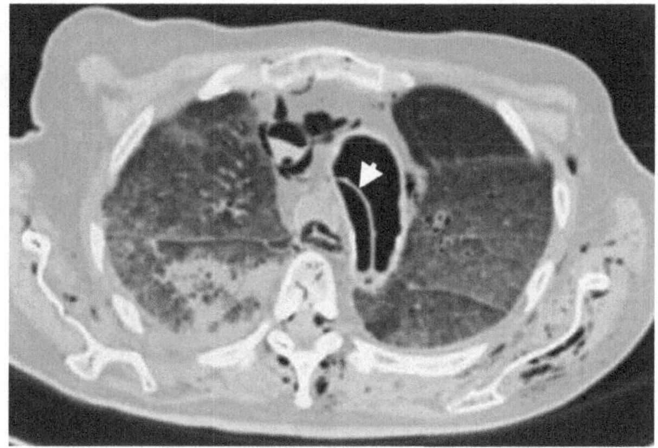

Fig. 7.33 Axial view of the chest on lung windows shows an aortic dissection flap (arrow), outlined by decomposition gas. There was little history available to correlate the finding

may be seen in the setting of hypertension and/or atherosclerosis, but other factors predisposing the condition include dissection, aneurysm, trauma, inflammatory conditions and connective tissue disease.

Aortic dissection, without rupture, may have the blood extend along the middle plane of the vessel wall. This may cause sudden death due occlusion of the coronary or carotid arteries. However, some dissections are chronic and in the absence of appropriate acute symptoms may be judged as incidental (Fig. 7.33).

In cases of fatal aortic rupture, there may be a striking collapse of cardiac chambers and great vessels due to hypovolaemia (Fig. 7.34). The exact point of rupture may not be apparent on non-contrast PMCT, due to the large volume of adjacent haematoma. Angiography in these cases may be helpful, for example using a targeted coronary angiogram technique, if root dissection is suspected [10] with the catheter balloon slightly higher in the ascending aorta than the predicted dissection point. Whole-body angiography [11] and direct cardiac puncture [12] techniques

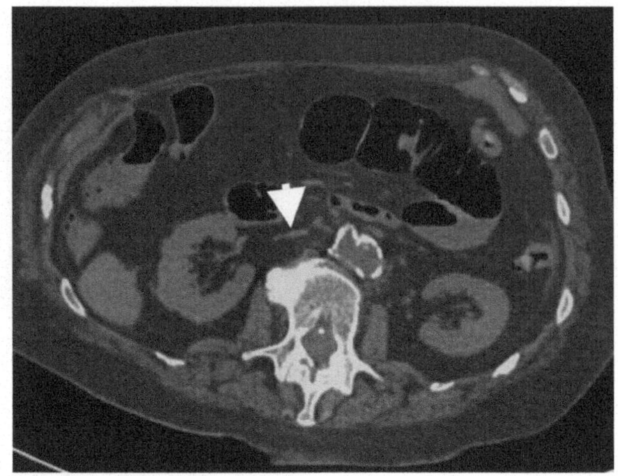

Fig. 7.34 Axial view of the upper abdomen on soft tissue windows shows a flattened IVC (arrow) and partially collapsed abdominal aorta, 'propped' open by calcification, in a case of a ruptured thoracic aorta

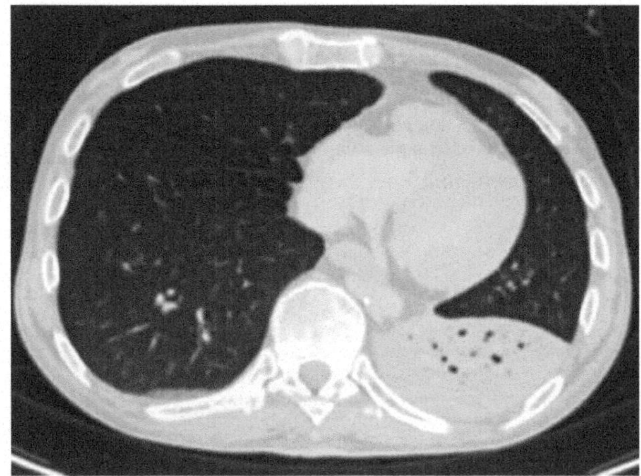

Fig. 7.35 Axial view of the chest on lung windows shows complete left lower lobe consolidation in the setting of a clinical history of chest infection

have also been described for the investigation of thoracic aortic rupture. However, in the context of a non-suspicious sudden death, these additional techniques are not deemed necessary if imaging features are consistent.

Parenchymal Opacity and Consolidation

The lungs are often difficult to confidently assess at PMCT. When post mortem changes are minimal, and the lungs are reasonably aerated, abnormal parenchymal findings may be quite obvious (Fig. 7.35). Asymmetric, patchy or segmental increased density usually indicates a pathologic finding [6] (Figs. 7.36, 7.37, 7.38, and 7.39). Consolidation and other non-hypostatic changes can be reported as seen,

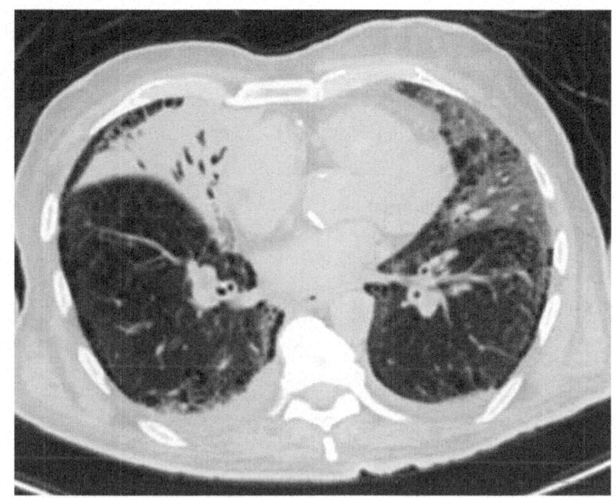

Fig. 7.36 Axial view of the chest on lung windows shows a middle lobe consolidation on a background of emphysema in a known smoker found deceased

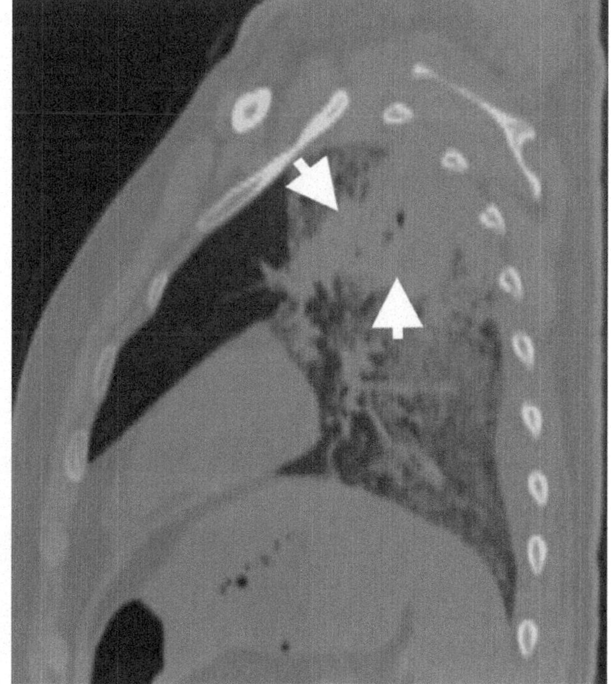

Fig. 7.37 Sagittal view of the chest showing segmental consolidation (arrows) within a region of ground-glass density/fluid hypostasis, in a patient with a clinically diagnosed pneumonia

but in isolation they are of indeterminate aetiology without a correlated history, such as of cough, fever, known malignancy, resuscitation attempts (Fig. 7.40) or trauma.

Difficulty further arises in interpretation, as normal post mortem changes can mask pathology such as inflammation, basal consolidation, nodules, masses or pulmonary oedema. As such, it is possible to miss (or misdiagnose) pneumonia and/or

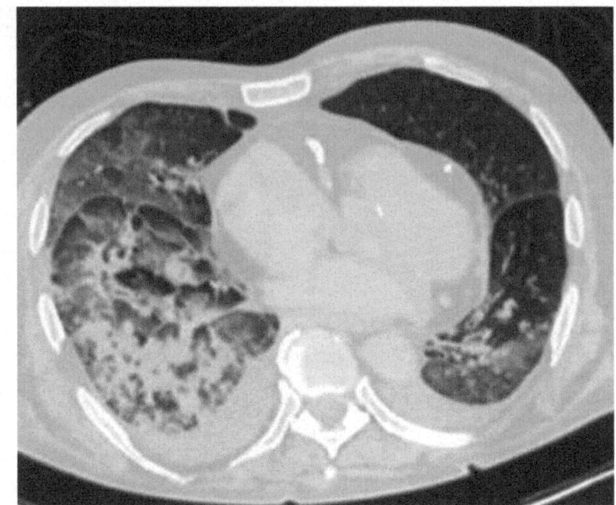

Fig. 7.38 Axial view of the chest on lung windows shows patchy consolidation of the right lung base, in keeping with bronchopneumonia. As there was absent history, this was confirmed at open autopsy

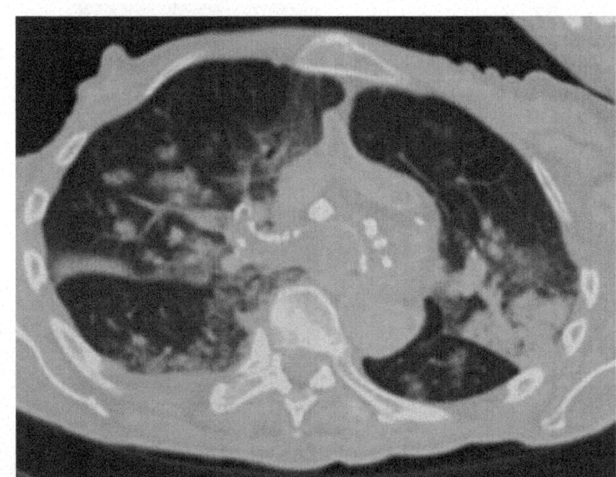

Fig. 7.39 Axial view of the chest on lung windows shows bilateral, patchy consolidation in an unexpected death, therefore indeterminate at PMCT. This was confirmed as pneumonia at open autopsy

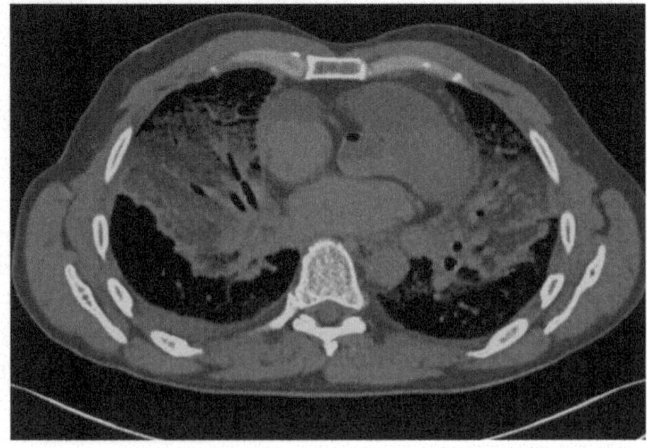

Fig. 7.40 Axial view of the chest on soft tissue windows shows dense symmetrical peri-hilar ground-glass opacity and patchy consolidation following a sudden collapse and prolonged hospital CPR. The lung changes likely relate to CPR and fluid resuscitation but may hide underlying pathology

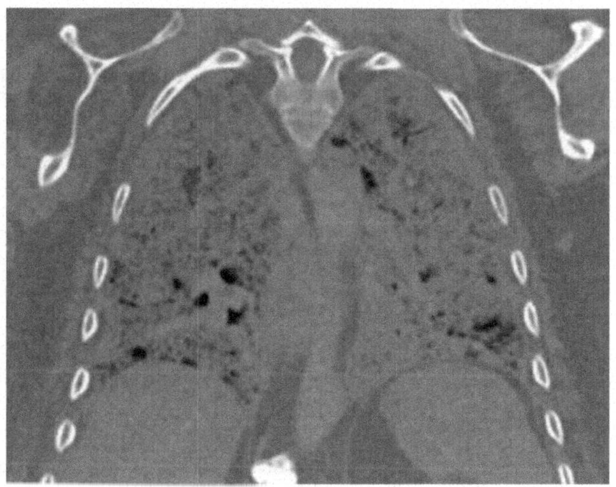

Fig. 7.41 Coronal view of the chest showing near complete lung opacification, considered indeterminate in nature without correlative history

other significant findings on PMCT [13]. Occasionally, the lungs are completely opacified, and it is difficult to radiologically discriminate between infection, oedema, other pathology and background normal post mortem changes (Fig. 7.41).

Pneumothorax and Pneumomediastinum

When considering pathological gas patterns on PMCT, it is imperative to exclude decomposition as the cause, as this is a reasonably common post mortem reality. Pathological pneumothorax and pneumomediastinum have many clinical causes, but in the post mortem setting, these are likely to be seen following trauma, including resuscitation attempts or mechanical ventilation. It has been described that, rarely in a diabetic patient, a pneumomediastinum can be a feature suggestive of a diabetic ketoacidosis (DKA), which is often fatal in cases with a low pH [14].

When a very large or 'tension' type pneumothorax is seen, with lung parenchymal collapse, diaphragmatic depression and mediastinal shift (leading to respiratory and cardiovascular compromise), this is considered to be a reasonable cause for death (Figs. 7.42, 7.43, and 7.44). Nevertheless, correlation data should preferably include a history of trauma, respiratory distress, hypoxia and/or chest pain.

Pulmonary Embolism

Acute pulmonary embolism (PE) is a common cause of a sudden death. PE should always be considered if there are underlying risk factors, such as deep vein thrombosis, recent surgery, obesity, immobility or disseminated malignancy.

It is accepted that PE is a difficult PMCT diagnosis, compared to open autopsy [15], and this is a subject in which further research is required. At open autopsy,

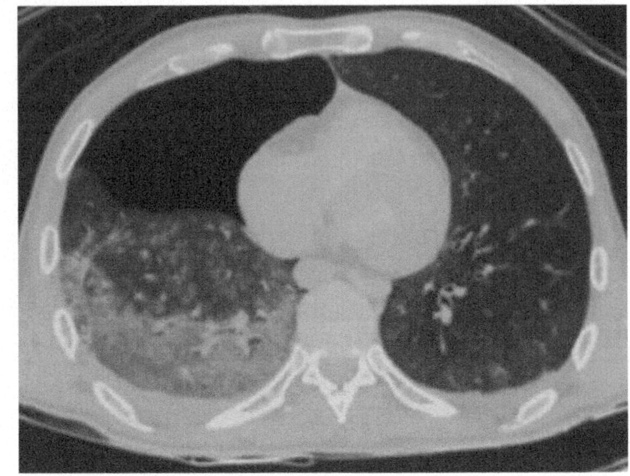

Fig. 7.42 Axial view of the chest on lung windows shows a unilateral, right-side pneumothorax and no significant decomposition change. The deceased was found in bed with no available history

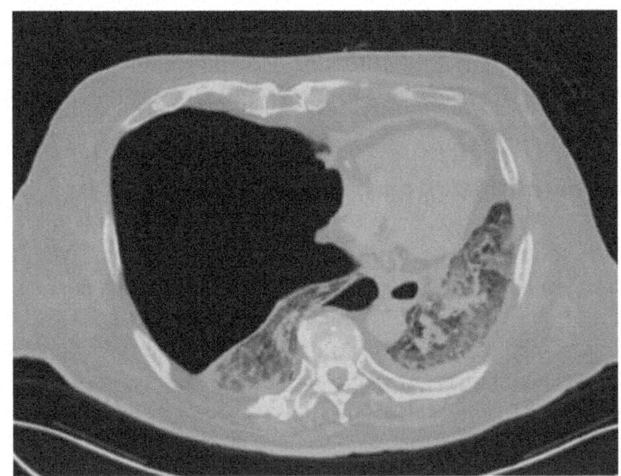

Fig. 7.43 Axial view of the chest on lung windows shows a large right-side pneumothorax, considered to be under tension owing to marked mediastinal shift to the left. The presentation was of sudden collapse

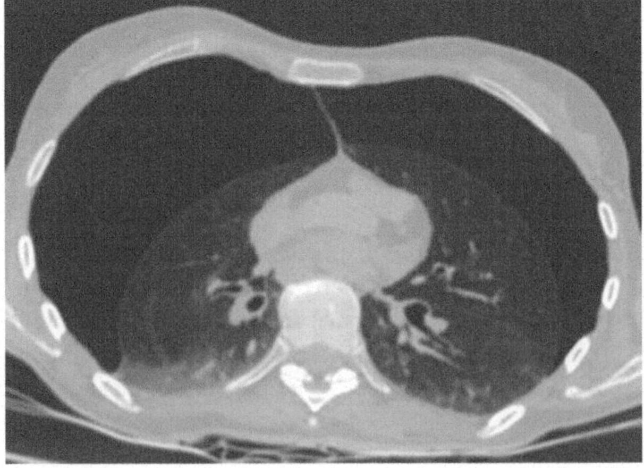

Fig. 7.44 Axial view of the chest on lung windows shows bilateral pneumothoraces and no obvious underlying lung disease. The deceased was found at home

pathological embolus is readily appreciated as being different to normal post mortem clot, which is often described as having a 'chicken-fat' appearance [16], a smooth surface and vascular cast-like shape (replicating the vessel of origin). This post mortem clot may be seen continuously from the right ventricle through into the main pulmonary arteries [17]. At open autopsy, the pulmonary arteries are normally dissected, both centrally and distally, along the pulmonary artery branches.

In comparison, PMCT without contrast is rather limited, as only the larger, central pulmonary arteries are readily assessed, and the appearance of normal post mortem clot is variable. A shower of small emboli into the periphery of the pulmonary artery tissues would almost certainly evade detection. Very early scanning after death may help avoid scan contamination from any central post mortem clot [18], although this may only be achievable for in-hospital deaths with a local PMCT service.

When PE is suspected from the history, the features that support the diagnosis on PMCT include visualisation of discrete central clot/s, with an irregular appearance or attenuation, possibly within a dilated pulmonary artery (Figs. 7.45, 7.46, 7.47, and 7.48). This is different from the layered pattern of blood sedimentation reflecting normal hypostasis. However, such normal layering can still mask peripheral emboli (Fig. 7.49) [19].

Indirect features supportive of PE include right heart dilatation, interventricular septal straightening or bowing into the left ventricle and wedge-shaped pulmonary infarcts. The legs may demonstrate thigh/calf circumference disparity and/or perivascular oedema, possibly indicative of deep vein thrombosis [19]. The inferior vena cava (IVC) is often collapsed at PMCT, so an increased short-axis diameter has been suggested as evidence of PE [20]. However, there are other potential causes for a distended IVC such as right heart failure and acute myocardial infarction. Visualisation of supporting findings along with an appropriate history (or suspicion)

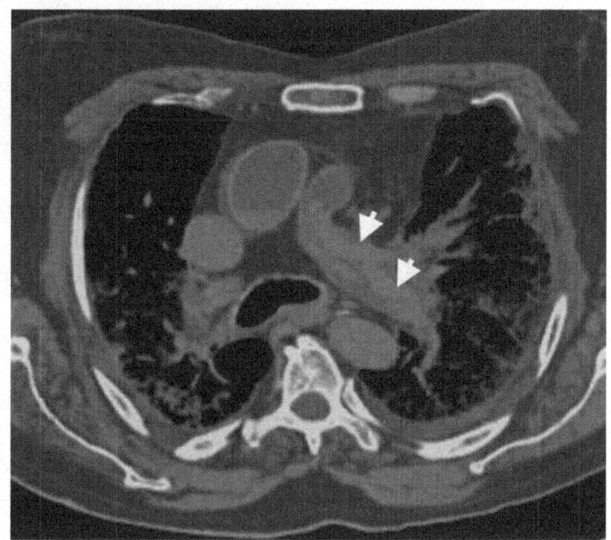

Fig. 7.45 Axial view of the chest on soft tissue windows shows heterogeneous, irregular clots in the main and left pulmonary arteries suggestive of PE (arrows). This was confirmed at a limited chest autopsy. Note the different, simple layered separation of blood products in the ascending aorta

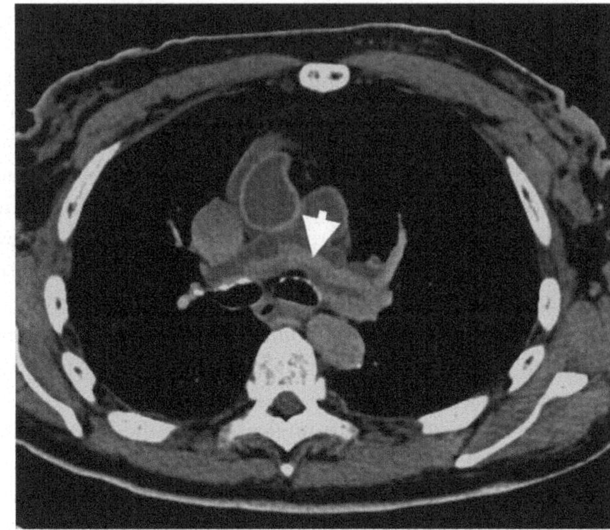

Fig. 7.46 Axial view of the chest on soft tissue windows shows 'saddle type' heterogeneous irregular clot in the main pulmonary arteries (arrow), not contiguous into the pulmonary trunk or right ventricle. Pulmonary thromboembolism was confirmed at limited open autopsy of the chest

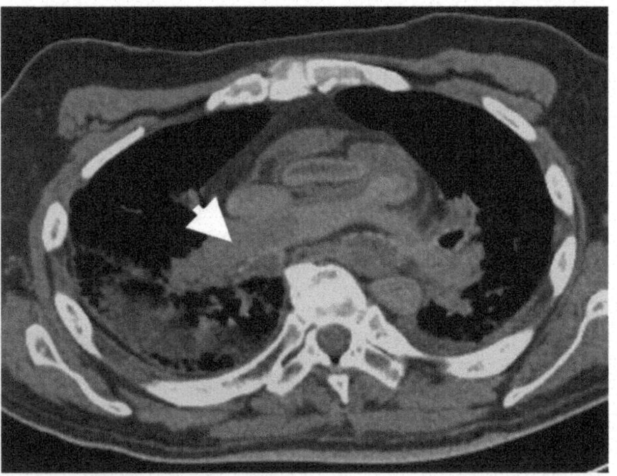

Fig. 7.47 Axial view of the chest on soft tissue windows shows heterogeneous attenuation clot without the normal separation of blood products in a distended right pulmonary artery suggesting a pathological filling defect (arrow). This was confirmed as PE at limited open autopsy. Note that other large vessels appear relatively collapsed

and no other cause of death evident should allow the diagnosis to be made (Figs. 7.50, 7.51, and 7.52), at least 'on the balance of probability'. Depending on confidence levels, a limited open post mortem examination of the pulmonary arteries might still be considered.

Post mortem pulmonary angiography is achievable as part of whole-body techniques [17], or by a peripheral contrast injection with subsequent chest compressions, to opacify the pulmonary arteries [18]. These techniques are recognised to be time-consuming and if performed routinely without a supportive history or other supportive imaging findings may still suffer similar indeterminate results (due to post mortem clot presence) as routine PMCT.

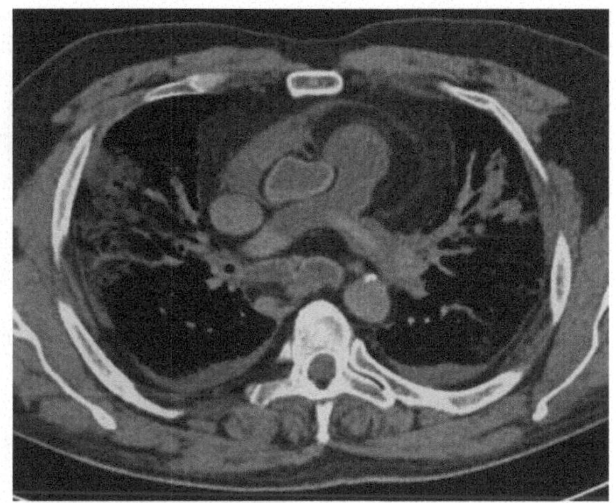

Fig. 7.48 Axial view of the chest on soft tissue windows shows discrete pulmonary arterial clots, confirmed as PE secondary to DVT at open autopsy. Layered separation of blood products in the ascending aorta is noted, representing normal hypostasis

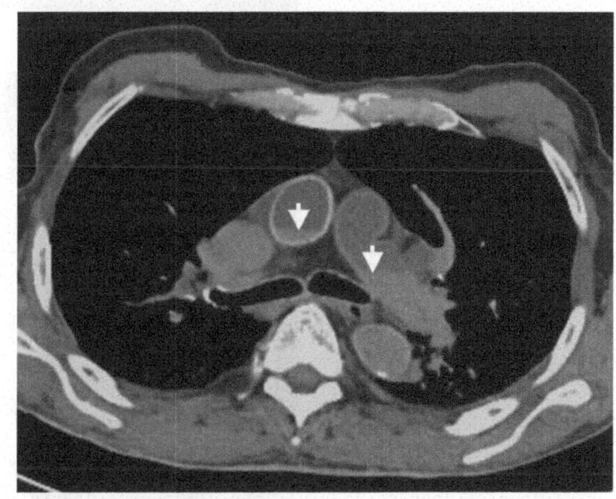

Fig. 7.49 Axial view of the chest on soft tissue windows shows matched horizontal layered sedimentation of blood products in both the aorta and main pulmonary arteries (arrows). PE was not suggested by imaging, yet was revealed to be the cause of death at open autopsy (performed as no cause of death found)

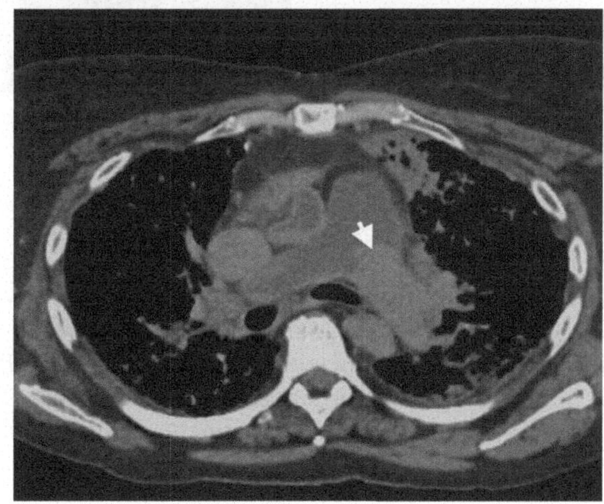

Fig. 7.50 Axial view of the chest on soft tissue windows. There is hyperdense, asymmetric clot distending the left main pulmonary artery (arrow) which was proven to be pathological embolus at open autopsy. The distended main pulmonary artery is different to the partially collapsed aorta which has a normal sedimentation level

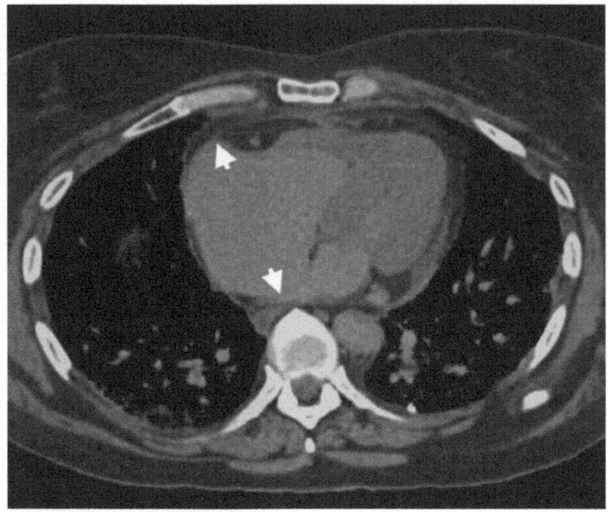

Fig. 7.51 Same case as Fig. 7.50, a case of open autopsy proven PE. Axial view of the chest showing a dilated right atrium (arrows), a supportive feature of PE on PMCT

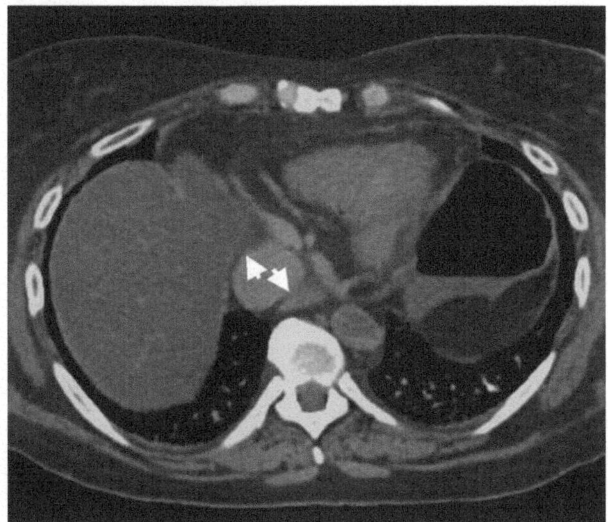

Fig. 7.52 Same case as Fig. 7.50 a case of pathologically proven PE. Axial view of the upper abdomen showing a distended IVC (arrows), a supportive feature of PE on PMCT

Chest Malignancy and Lymphadenopathy

A diagnosis of malignancy will often be known before death and so death certification is normally straightforward. By contrast, incidental primary malignancy in the lungs can be difficult to identify on PMCT, especially if there is post mortem change or other pathology. Yet, sudden deaths are unlikely to relate to malignancy unless associated with complications such as PE (see earlier), haemorrhage (Figs. 7.53, 7.54, 7.55, and 7.56) or airway obstruction (Figs. 7.57 and 7.58). 'Review areas' such as the breasts should be routinely examined for suspicious lesions (Fig. 7.59).

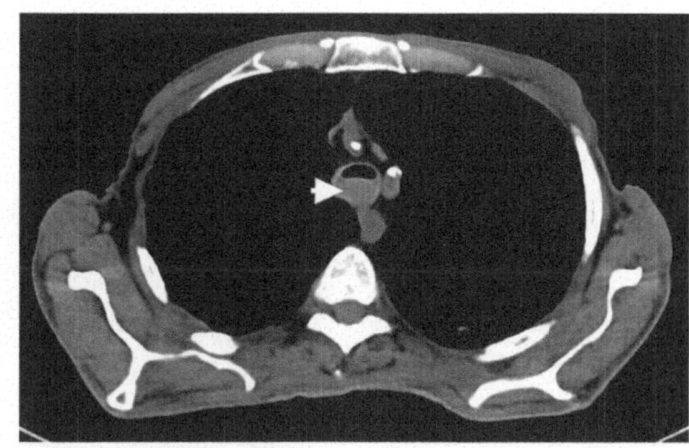

Fig. 7.53 Axial view of the chest on soft tissue windows shows subtle high-density fluid in the trachea (arrow) consistent with haemorrhage/clot. The patient had evidence of haematemesis/haemoptysis when found and a history of recent weight loss

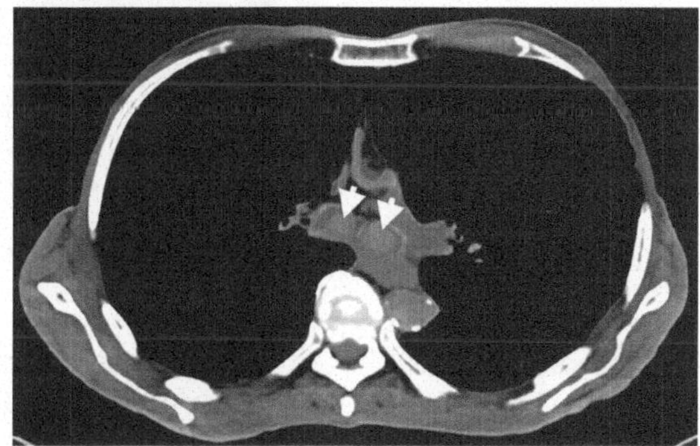

Fig. 7.54 Same case as Fig. 7.53, the high-density clot extends into both main bronchi (arrows)

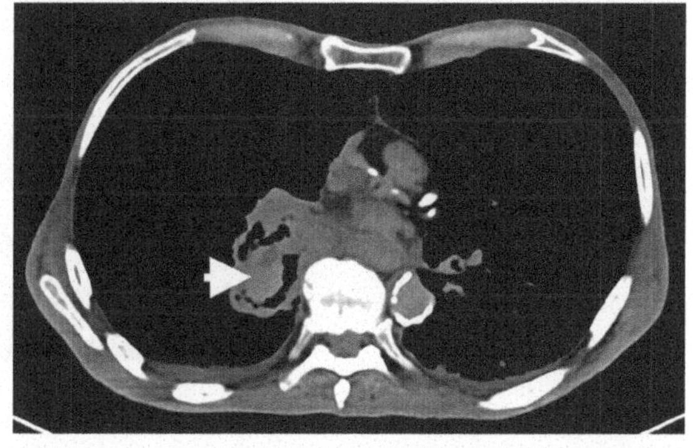

Fig. 7.55 Same case as Fig. 7.53, soft tissue windows reveal a cavitating lung mass in the right lower lobe, consistent with tumour

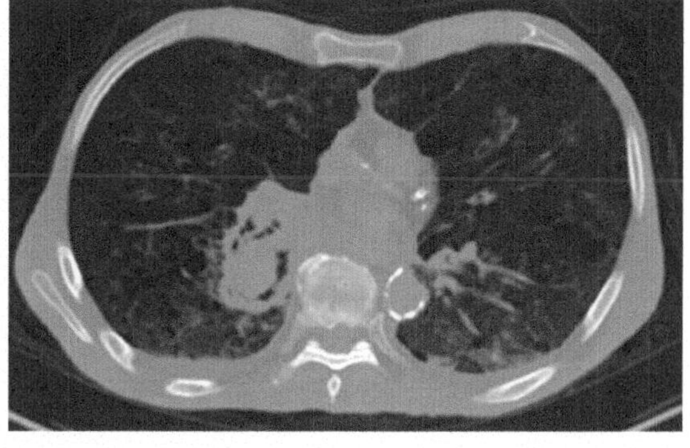

Fig. 7.56 Same case as Fig. 7.53, lung windows reveal background emphysema and the lung mass in right lower lobe, confirmed to be malignancy with vascular invasion and haemorrhage at open autopsy

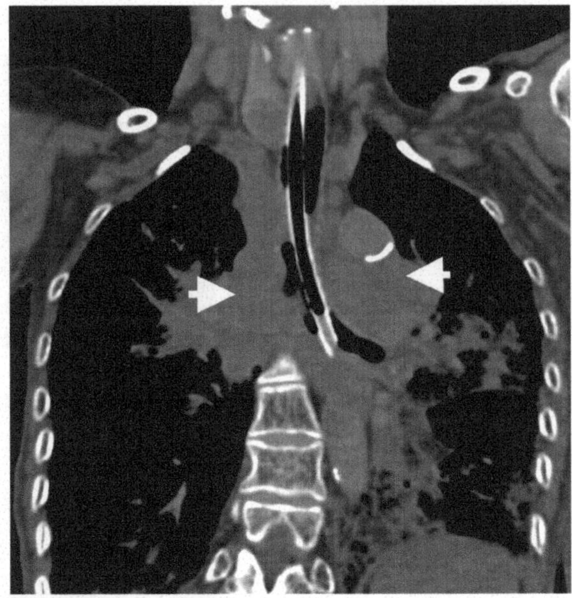

Fig. 7.57 Coronal view of the chest on soft tissue windows showing a large, previously unidentified mediastinal tumour (arrows) with right bronchial obstruction. The patient was intubated after an episode of choking with the endotracheal tube entering the left main bronchus

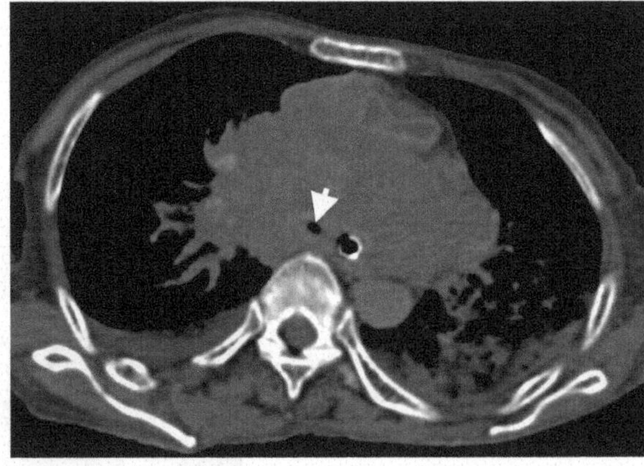

Fig. 7.58 Axial view of same case as Fig. 7.57 showing the large, confluent mediastinal tumour, seen obliterating normal tissue planes without the need for IV contrast. It is causing narrowing of the right bronchus (arrow) and the circular endotracheal tube with radio-dense marker is seen in the left main bronchus

Disseminated neoplasia may be more easily evident. Correlation pathology findings include multiple pulmonary nodules and/or suspicious bone lesions (Fig. 7.60). If there is sufficient body fat, any axillary, aorto-pulmonary window, peri-cardiac and peri-tracheal adenopathy may be seen.

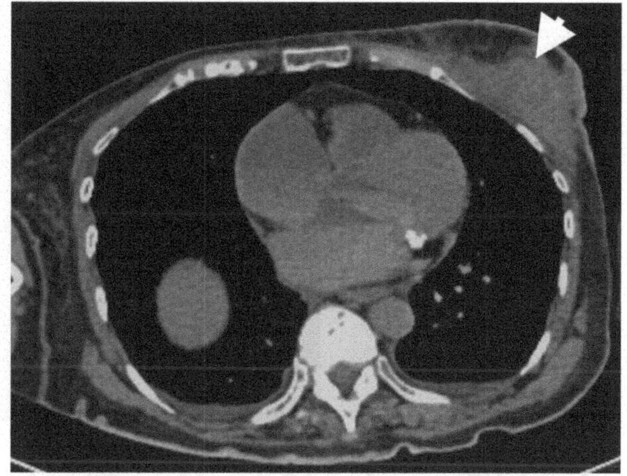

Fig. 7.59 Axial view of the chest on soft tissue windows showing an irregular left side breast mass, consistent with malignancy (arrow). The tiny pleural effusions are considered normal in the post mortem setting

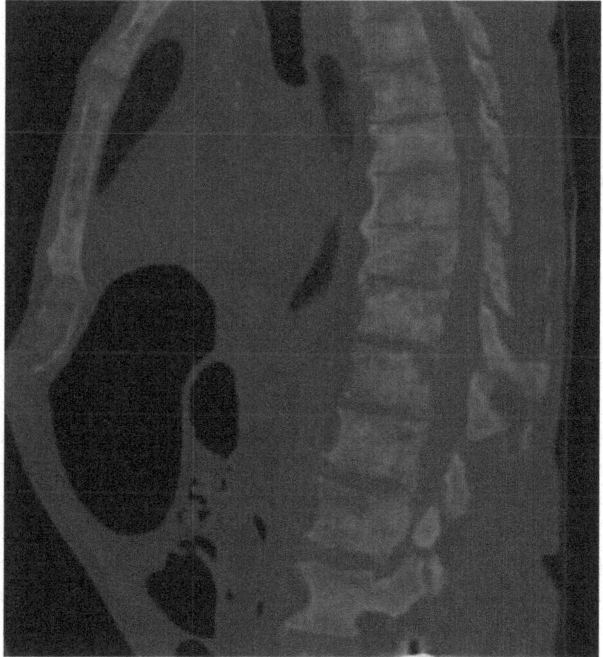

Fig. 7.60 Sagittal view of the chest on bone windows showing widespread sclerotic bony metastases in both the thoracic spine and sternum

Calcified nodes (and lung nodules) are often well demonstrated, potentially pointing to a differential diagnosis of granulomatous disease, for example mycobacterial infection or sarcoid [21]. As with clinical imaging, the cause for any lymphadenopathy should be sought from the medical history.

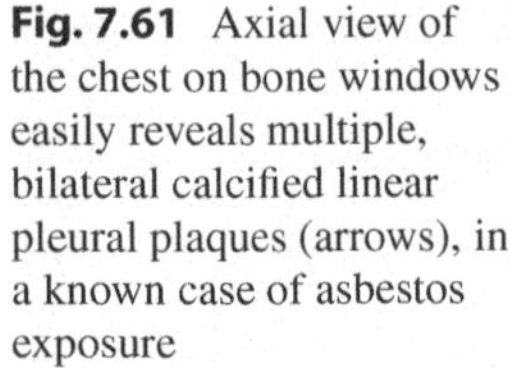

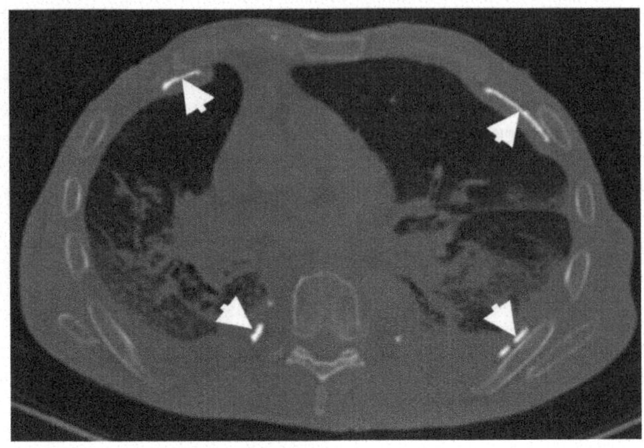

Fig. 7.61 Axial view of the chest on bone windows easily reveals multiple, bilateral calcified linear pleural plaques (arrows), in a known case of asbestos exposure

Industrial/Occupational Related Lung Disease

This mainly reflects asbestos exposures, with silica and coal pathology being less frequent nowadays. One key aspect of the PMCT autopsy in putative industrial disease is to identify any pathology to support such exposures as well as making comment on the extent and severity of the pathology found [22].

Starting with asbestos disease, PMCT can readily reveal calcified pleural plaques (Fig. 7.61), although plaques alone do not normally qualify as supporting a potential post mortem legal claim. In isolation, plaque disease must not be stated as supporting asbestosis, unless there is clear fibrotic change in the scan data. Carcinoma and mesothelioma may also be linked to asbestos exposure, with these often presenting as mass lesions. Persistent pleural effusion and pleural fibrosis are asbestos-linked pathologies, but are very difficult to confirm as not reflecting other disease. Reference to any previous clinical imaging is very helpful.

The changes in coal and silica exposure generally are similar to each other, with small and large parenchymal nodules being found. In coal exposure, there may be dust-related emphysema without significant fibrosis. Contrastingly, silica exposure is variably linked with diffuse fibrosis and may also show calcification of mediastinal nodes.

In almost all cases, and certainly if a claim is being considered, an open autopsy (perhaps limited to the chest) will be necessary. This open autopsy allows histological sampling, with it being recognised that later legal claims and/or defence may run onwards for many years! Overall, in cases of possible industrial disease, PMCT can be helpful in planning targeted tissue sampling as well as excluding alternate pathologies that are wholly or partly responsible for death.

Special Circumstances: Drowning

Not all bodies discovered in water have drowned. Furthermore, drowning may occur away from obvious water sources. In the non-suspicious setting, a history of the mode of death from drowning circumstances should be made available in order to consider this diagnosis and guide how the radiologist considers the case.

In this scenario, PMCT can be used to document findings consistent with drowning and any other injuries present. It may reveal natural disease (which may really be the underlying cause of death, with the body incidentally ending up in water).

The Royal College of Pathologists has issued guidelines on autopsy practice for bodies recovered from water [23]. These guidelines state 'if the history, scene examination, external examination and laboratory results as well as the [PMCT] images support a diagnosis of drowning, then there is no reason that such a cause of death cannot be provided, without the need for an invasive post mortem'. Indeed, many drowning cases do not need open autopsy, although toxicology should always be obtained when bodies are recovered from water. However, toxicology results are rarely available at the time of scanning.

The Mechanism of Death in Drowning Cases

This is complex and multifactorial, involving aspiration, hypoxia, sudden osmolar and electrolyte changes, pulmonary oedema and neural mechanisms (such as the 'diving reflex' and fear). These effects lead to apnoea, bradycardia and peripheral vasoconstriction with the associated risk of developing a fatal arrhythmia. Alternatively, the process of water immersion itself (especially if cold) can, in its own right, precipitate such an arrhythmia. This mechanism cannot be appreciated on a PMCT scan (or open autopsy), and the coronary arteries may appear completely normal.

PMCT Findings

In cases of drowning, PMCT findings are generally non-specific and may not allow a definitive conclusion from the scan alone, especially when there is decomposition, trauma or any animal predation. Open autopsy may also face a similar diagnostic quandary [7]. There may however be a pattern of findings which, together with a clear supporting history, fits the diagnosis [24]. These include the following findings:

Fluid in the Major Airways

Passive regurgitation of fluid into the major airways is common at PMCT, making this finding alone generally indeterminate. In cases of drowning, the fluid in the airways may have a low attenuation (water being generally less dense than respiratory tract secretions or regurgitated stomach content) yet this is considered unreliable as a sign in isolation (Fig. 7.62).

To add to potential confusion, the ingestion of water that contains sediment or debris (such as sand, soil, shell fragments) may paradoxically result in increased airway fluid density [25], although this presence of sediment in the sinuses, airways and stomach may be a helpful sign of drowning if recognised as such [26].

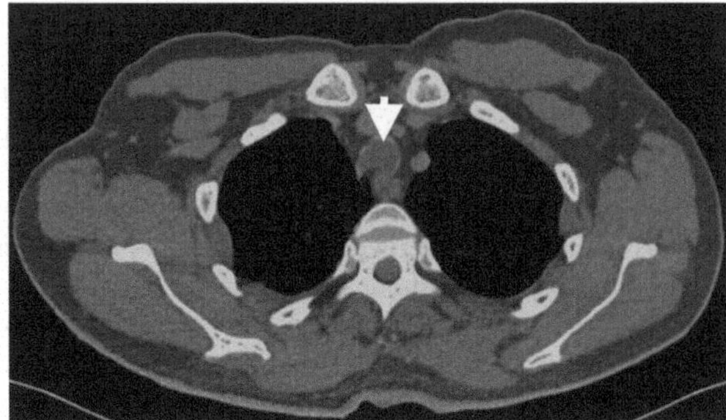

Fig. 7.62 Axial view of the chest on soft tissue windows shows homogenous low-density fluid filling the trachea (arrow), in a case of fresh water drowning. Note how this is essentially no different from Fig. 7.1 which was not a case of drowning

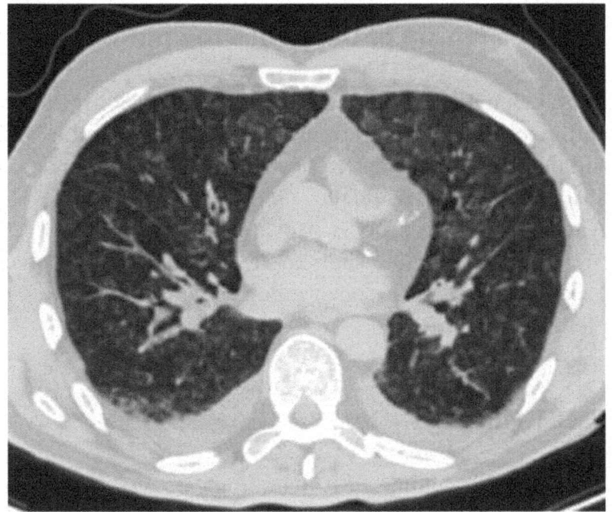

Fig. 7.63 Axial view of the chest on lung windows shows extensive, bilateral nodular ground-glass densities in the lungs. This was a case of fresh water drowning

Occasionally, the fluid in the major airways may have a 'frothy' appearance with a 'plume' from the nose or mouth, although this can also be seen in other circumstances such as drug intoxication or acute cardiac failure. In essence, the fluid pattern in the major airways is highly variable and often non-specific.

Lung Findings in Drowning

A diffuse, mosaic or patchy pattern of ground-glass attenuation may be seen in drowned lungs, sometimes with air space consolidation or nodular densities [24, 25, 27, 28] (Figs. 7.63, 7.64, and 7.65).

There may be an overall increase in lung volume due to air trapping, with a resultant lower position of the diaphragm and a decrease in lung density [29]. At autopsy, the lungs of drowned bodies may appear overinflated and, when cut, are wet with foamy fluid, termed 'emphysema aquosum'.

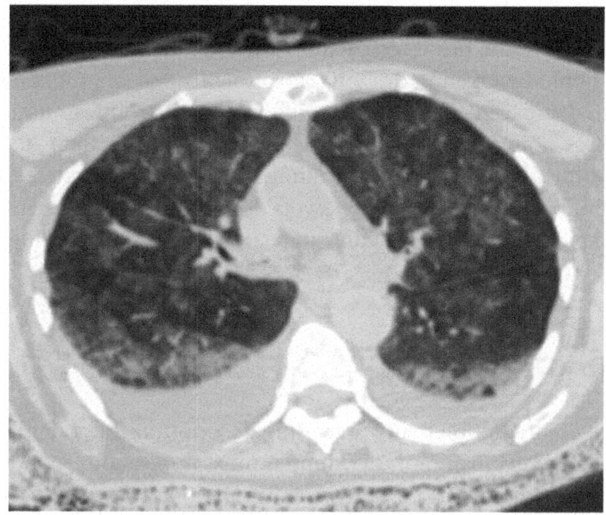

Fig. 7.64 Axial view of the chest on lung windows showing extensive, bilateral patchy and mosaic ground-glass density in a case of known drowning

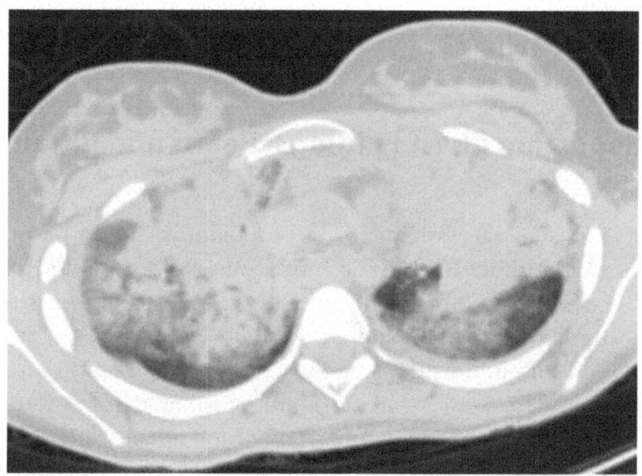

Fig. 7.65 Axial view of the chest on lung windows shows extensive bilateral airspace ground-glass opacity and consolidation in a young epileptic found submerged in bath water

In fresh water drowning, the water is hypotonic and may readily pass into the blood resulting in rapid haemodilution and a reduction in osmolality. The reverse occurs in salt water, resulting in pulmonary oedema. In practice, these factors are difficult to evaluate, given the abundant background variability in lung findings on PMCT, yet fortunately they are also of little practical value in the non-suspicious setting,

Fluid in the Paranasal Sinuses and Gastrointestinal Tract

Generally, more sinus fluid is seen in cases of drowning compared to non-drowning, and fluid in the frontal sinuses (as opposed to than the dependent sphenoid sinuses)

is slightly more supportive of this diagnosis [30]. However, similar to the major airways, the presence of sinus fluid, in isolation, is a non-specific finding. Caution should be taken in drawing any conclusions from its presence.

Increased fluid in the stomach and gastrointestinal tract is also associated with drowning [27]. This may be lower in density than 'usual' stomach content [28], although once again this finding should be interpreted with caution. The absence of fluid in the stomach and bowels does not exclude drowning, as death may have been rapid (before significant ingestion of water) or may have occurred prior to submersion [27].

Dry Drowning

In contradiction to the preceding descriptions of potential PMCT findings, and making the exclusion of drowning almost impossible, is the concept of 'dry drowning'. In this situation, laryngospasm is thought to prevent water entering the major airways and lungs, which consequently remain aerated. An alternate theory maintains that the 'dry' airways are a consequence of fluid being absorbed rapidly through the alveolar walls [7].

Reporting Chest Findings: Pearls and Pitfalls

First, an assessment of decomposition should be made, as this may significantly affect PMCT interpretation. Note should also be made whether resuscitation attempts, with or without chest compressions, were attempted—as these may explain some findings.

Fluid in the airways/sinuses and small pleural effusions can largely be disregarded, as these are common, normal post mortem appearances.

The extent and nature of any lung opacity should be described, and indication made whether the pattern suggests normal post mortem change (symmetrical ground-glass opacity with a dependent gradient) or pathology. When suggested to be pathological, this should ideally correlate with other findings or available history.

Pulmonary embolus is a difficult diagnosis to make on PMCT, although a constellation of findings along with a supporting history may allow the diagnosis to be suggested on the balance of probabilities. It is however much more difficult to *exclude* the diagnosis on PMCT.

Given the difficulties in interpreting PMCT (and open autopsy) in cases of drowning, the history is paramount. It is anticipated that, in the non-suspicious setting, this is already known and that there is no suggestion from the scan otherwise. Correlation with any positive findings can be made, but one should note that their absence does not exclude this diagnosis.

Example PMCT report phrases:

- Fluid seen in the airways is a common and non-specific finding on post mortem imaging.
- Small pleural effusions are considered normal in the post mortem setting. There is no haemothorax or pneumothorax.
- There is a pattern of normal sedimentation of blood in the main pulmonary arteries, with no dilatation of the right heart or IVC to suggest a central pulmonary embolus.
- Symmetrical, ground-glass opacification in both lungs shows a dependent gradient in keeping with normal fluid hypostasis.
- Given the clinical details of infection, superimposed parenchymal consolidation is in keeping with bronchopneumonia.
- Small anterior pneumothorax and multiple anterolateral rib fractures judged secondary to attempted cardiopulmonary resuscitation.
- Almost complete/complete opacification of both lungs. It is not possible to assess the lung parenchyma. Pre-existing/underlying lung pathology could be missed by this study.

References

1. Biljardt S, Brummel A, Tijhuis R, Sieswerda-Hoogendoorn T, Beenen LF, van Rijn RR. Post-mortem fluid stasis in the sinus, trachea and mainstem bronchi; a computed tomography study in adults and children. J Forensic Radiol Imaging [Internet]. 2015;3(3):162–6. https://linkinghub.elsevier.com/retrieve/pii/S2212478015300046.
2. Roberts I, Traill Z. The radiological autopsy. In: Suvarna SK, editor. Atlas of adult autopsy [Internet]. Cham: Springer International Publishing; 2016. p. 362. http://link.springer.com/10.1007/978-3-319-27022-7_13.
3. Klein WM, Kunz T, Hermans K, Bayat AR, Koopmanschap DHJLM. The common pattern of postmortem changes on whole body CT scans. J Forensic Radiol Imaging [Internet]. 2016;4:47–52. https://linkinghub.elsevier.com/retrieve/pii/S2212478015300289.
4. Rutty GN, Morgan B, Germerott T, Thali M, Athurs O. Ventilated post-mortem computed tomography—a historical review. J Forensic Radiol Imaging [Internet]. 2016;4:35–42. https://linkinghub.elsevier.com/retrieve/pii/S2212478016300028.
5. Hyodoh H, Watanabe S, Okazaki S, Mizuo K, Inoue H. Postmortem computed tomography findings in the thorax. J Forensic Radiol Imaging [Internet]. 2014;2(2):100. https://linkinghub.elsevier.com/retrieve/pii/S2212478014000318.
6. Ishida M, Gonoi W, Okuma H, Shirota G, Shintani Y, Abe H, et al. Common postmortem computed tomography findings following atraumatic death: differentiation between normal postmortem changes and pathologic lesions. Korean J Radiol [Internet]. 2015;16(4):798. https://www.kjronline.org/DOIx.php?id=10.3348/kjr.2015.16.4.798.
7. Saukko P, Knight B. Knight's forensic pathology [Internet]. 4th ed. Boca Raton: CRC Press; 2015. https://www.routledge.com/Knights-Forensic-Pathology/Saukko-Knight/p/book/9780340972533.
8. Iino M, Hayakawa H, Kobayashi T, Shiotani S. Asphyxia from choking on a piece of persimmon. J Forensic Radiol Imaging [Internet]. 2015;3(2):139–40. https://linkinghub.elsevier.com/retrieve/pii/S2212478014001257.

9. Panda A, Kumar A, Gamanagatti S, Mishra B. Virtopsy computed tomography in trauma: normal postmortem changes and pathologic Spectrum of findings. Curr Probl Diagn Radiol [Internet]. 2015;44(5):391–406. https://linkinghub.elsevier.com/retrieve/pii/S0363018815000420.
10. Roberts ISD, Benamore RE, Peebles C, Roobottom C, Traill ZC. Diagnosis of coronary artery disease using minimally invasive autopsy: evaluation of a novel method of post-mortem coronary CT angiography. Clin Radiol [Internet]. 2011;66(7):645–50. https://linkinghub.elsevier.com/retrieve/pii/S0009926011000675.
11. Grabherr S, Grimm J, Dominguez A, Vanhaebost J, Mangin P. Advances in post-mortem CT-angiography. Br J Radiol [Internet]. 2014;87(1036):20130488. http://www.birpublications.org/doi/10.1259/bjr.20130488.
12. Zhou S, Wan L, Shao Y, Ying C, Wang Y, Zou D, et al. Detection of aortic rupture using post-mortem computed tomography and post-mortem computed tomography angiography by cardiac puncture. Int J Legal Med [Internet]. 2016;130(2):469–74. http://link.springer.com/10.1007/s00414-015-1171-9.
13. Sonnemans LJP, Kubat B, Prokop M, Klein WM. Can virtual autopsy with postmortem CT improve clinical diagnosis of cause of death? A retrospective observational cohort study in a Dutch tertiary referral centre. BMJ Open [Internet]. 2018;8(3):e018834. http://bmjopen.bmj.com/lookup/doi/10.1136/bmjopen-2017-018834.
14. Yamamoto T, Hayashi T, Murakami T, Hayashi H, Murase T, Abe Y, et al. Postmortem imaging identified pneumomediastinum in two cases of diabetic ketoacidosis. J Forensic Radiol Imaging [Internet]. 2017;10:5–8. https://linkinghub.elsevier.com/retrieve/pii/S2212478017300035.
15. Rutty GN, Morgan B, Robinson C, Raj V, Pakkal M, Amoroso J, et al. Diagnostic accuracy of post-mortem CT with targeted coronary angiography versus autopsy for coroner-requested post-mortem investigations: a prospective, masked, comparison study. Lancet [Internet]. 2017;390(10090):145–54. https://linkinghub.elsevier.com/retrieve/pii/S0140673617303331.
16. O'Donnell C, Woodford N. Post-mortem radiology—a new sub-speciality? Clin Radiol [Internet]. 2008;63(11):1189–94. https://linkinghub.elsevier.com/retrieve/pii/S0009926008002122.
17. Burke MP, Bedford P, Baber Y. Can forensic pathologists diagnose pulmonary thromboembolism on postmortem computed tomography pulmonary angiography? Am J Forensic Med Pathol [Internet]. 2014;35(2):124–31. https://journals.lww.com/00000433-201406000-00013.
18. Pichereau C, Maury E, Monnier-Cholley L, Bourcier S, Lejour G, Alves M, et al. Post-mortem CT scan with contrast injection and chest compression to diagnose pulmonary embolism. Intensive Care Med [Internet]. 2015;41(1):167–8. http://link.springer.com/10.1007/s00134-014-3520-4.
19. Ampanozi G, Held U, Ruder TD, Ross SG, Schweitzer W, Fornaro J, et al. Pulmonary thromboembolism on unenhanced postmortem computed tomography: feasibility and findings. Leg Med [Internet]. 2016;20:68–74. https://linkinghub.elsevier.com/retrieve/pii/S1344622316300293.
20. Mueller SL, Thali Y, Ampanozi G, Flach PM, Thali MJ, Hatch GM, et al. Distended diameter of the inferior vena cava is suggestive of pulmonary thromboembolism on unenhanced post-mortem CT. J Forensic Radiol Imaging [Internet]. 2015;3(1):38–42. https://linkinghub.elsevier.com/retrieve/pii/S2212478014001245.
21. Chatzaraki V, Heimer J, Thali M, Dally A, Schweitzer W. Role of PMCT as a triage tool between external inspection and full autopsy—case series and review. J Forensic Radiol Imaging [Internet]. 2018;15:26–38. https://linkinghub.elsevier.com/retrieve/pii/S2212478018300601.
22. Osborn M, Lowe J, Attanoos R, Gibbs A. Guidelines on autopsy practice. Industrial/occupational-related lung disease deaths including asbestos [Internet]. The Royal College of Pathologists, London; 2017. https://www.rcpath.org/uploads/assets/527983bd-2820-460d-92409b48da8928b1/Industrialoccupational-related-lung-disease-deaths-including-asbestos.pdf.

23. Osborn M, Taylor M, Whibley M, Lawler W, Grieve J, Hamilton S. Guidelines on autopsy practice: autopsy for bodies recovered from water [Internet]. The Royal College of Pathologists, London; 2018. https://www.rcpath.org/uploads/assets/a0eab7db-454b-4556-b9961ecfd8356307/Guidelines-on-autopsy-practice-Autopsy-for-bodies-recovered-from-water.pdf.
24. Christe A, Aghayev E, Jackowski C, Thali MJ, Vock P. Drowning—post-mortem imaging findings by computed tomography. Eur Radiol [Internet]. 2008;18(2):283–90. http://link.springer.com/10.1007/s00330-007-0745-4.
25. Bolliger SA, Ross S, Marino L, Thali MJ, Schweitzer W. Shell fragment aspiration seen at post-mortem computed tomography indicating drowning. J Forensic Radiol Imaging [Internet]. 2015;3(1):87–90. https://linkinghub.elsevier.com/retrieve/pii/S2212478015000027.
26. Raux C, Saval F, Rouge D, Telmon N, Dedouit F. Diagnosis of drowning using post-mortem computed tomography—state of the art. Arch Forensic Med Criminol [Internet]. 2014;2(64):59–75. http://www.termedia.pl/doi/10.5114/amsik.2014.47744.
27. Lo Re G, Vernuccio F, Galfano MC, Picone D, Milone L, La Tona G, et al. Role of virtopsy in the post-mortem diagnosis of drowning. Radiol Med [Internet]. 2015;120(3):304–8. http://link.springer.com/10.1007/s11547-014-0438-4.
28. Mishima S, Suzuki H, Nishitani Y, Fukunaga T. Usefulness and limitation of postmortem computed tomography in bath-related death: four case reports. J Forensic Radiol Imaging [Internet]. 2017;9:51–5. https://linkinghub.elsevier.com/retrieve/pii/S2212478016300557.
29. Leth PM, Madsen BH. Drowning investigated by post mortem computed tomography and autopsy. J Forensic Radiol Imaging [Internet]. 2017;9:28–30. https://linkinghub.elsevier.com/retrieve/pii/S2212478016300739.
30. Lundemose SB, Jacobsen C, Jakobsen LS, Lynnerup N. Exact volumetric determination of fluid in the paranasal sinuses after drowning. J Forensic Radiol Imaging [Internet]. 2015;3(2):111–6. https://linkinghub.elsevier.com/retrieve/pii/S2212478015000155.

8 Post Mortem Computed Tomography of the Heart

Introduction

Cardiovascular disease is the main cause of death in the United Kingdom. Consequently, careful and judicious examination of the heart, including the coronary arteries, is imperative for post mortem computed tomography (PMCT) to be considered a viable alternative to open autopsy in non-suspicious adult deaths. This chapter is presented as an introduction to cardiac PMCT for the general radiologist, considering possible techniques for imaging the heart and a range of findings, from normal variants to potentially critical pathological lesions.

The role of cardiac autopsy in general is to consider the nature of any present cardiac disease, whether it is directly related to death or part of systemic disease [1]. Further considerations are whether the cardiac disease is inherited (important for surviving relatives) or possibly related to non-natural pathology (e.g. illicit drug use).

With regard to imaging, a 'routine', non-contrast PMCT can certainly assess the contents of the pericardial sac, consider coronary, valvular and other cardiac calcifications and in many cases estimate the heart size. However, it cannot assess the lumens of the coronary arteries and is limited in the assessment of myocardium or other soft tissue abnormalities. To enhance arterial visualisation, techniques have been developed for targeted post mortem coronary angiography (in this chapter referred to as PMCTA). PMCT with PMCTA can potentially provide a cause of death in up to 92% of selected cases [2] and may reduce the number of open autopsies needed by up to two-thirds [3]. Despite these promising figures, it is important to understand and appreciate that PMCT assessment of the heart still has limitations.

Clinical cardiac radiology is a specialised field. Indeed, unless the reporter is trained in such techniques of imaging, reporting comparable cardiac PMCT findings and coronary angiography may be challenging. As with the other body tissues in the post mortem setting, PMCT may be confounded by the additional considerations of tissue autolysis and decomposition. However, careful and reasoned

A. Shenton et al., *Post Mortem CT for Non-Suspicious Adult Deaths*,
https://doi.org/10.1007/978-3-030-70829-0_8

consideration of the imaging should still allow the general radiologist, or pathologist, to appreciate the range of cardiac normality and many pathologies.

Cardiac Disease as a Cause of Death

Despite the prevalence of cardiac pathology in the population (principally atheroma, hypertensive cardiac disease and valvular pathologies), proving death is due to cardiac pathology can be less than straightforward. Indeed, one must recognise that many people die with cardiac disease present, but have succumbed from non-cardiac causes. It is too simplistic to attribute death to coronary disease, simply because there is coronary atheromatous calcification. One must consider the history and exclude pathology of a non-cardiac disease group if one desires to define death as reflecting cardiac processes.

It is specifically appreciated that cardiovascular disease is most common in those over 50 years, even when they have no preceding cardiovascular disease symptoms or relevant medical history. Sadly, many cases have cardiac sudden death as the first presentation of their disease. Such deaths can occur during exercise, at rest or even whilst asleep.

The history given may simply be that of sudden death without antecedent symptoms. However, other corroborate data such as shortness of breath, palpitations and/or central angina-like chest pain is useful. Other symptoms may include ‘indigestion’, atypical (neck/abdominal) pain, peripheral oedema and fatigue or symptoms such as these several days earlier.

In the PMCT arena, cases involving a traumatic death may require special consideration, as cardiac pathology may have played a part in events leading up to the death, such as a loss of consciousness or fall, whilst driving/operating machinery, working at a height, etc.

Classic causes of cardiac sudden death (**bold** = most prevalent) include [1]:

- **Occlusive coronary artery disease**
- **Ischaemic heart disease (myocardial infarction, zonal scarring and ventricular dysfunction)**
- **Dissection of the coronary arteries and/or aortic root**
- **Valve disease (stenosis, prolapse, rheumatic scarring, infective and non-infective endocarditis)**
- **Myocardial disease (myocarditis, cardiomyopathies, left ventricular hypertrophy in the context of hypertension, amyloid, connective tissue disease)**
- Congenital arterial anomaly
- Coronary vasculitis
- Coronary spasm
- Structural congenital heart disease (e.g. septal defect, Fallot’s tetralogy, etc.)
- Cardiac tumour (myxoma, sarcoma, etc.)
- Conduction system pathologies (e.g. Brugada syndrome etc.)
- Cardiac trauma

Some of these entities can be demonstrated on PMCT, whereas others will evade radiological confirmation. It is consequently important that the radiologist appreciates the limitations of the PMCT and the possible need for focused open autopsy examination.

Image-guided cardiac biopsy may enhance diagnostic rates by providing histological evidence, with minimal body interaction. This is potentially pertinent to cases of myocardial infarction and myocarditis [4] but is neither widely available nor practiced. When tissue is required, open autopsy focusing on the heart (i.e. chest limited) is probably much easier, with PMCT being used to limit the need for the dissection of other cavities.

Autopsy Examination of the Heart: The Pathologist's Perspective

The open autopsy examination of the heart is generally accomplished at the same time as the examination of the chest, incorporating the lungs, mediastinum and other thoracic contents (see previous chapter). Indeed, without considering the other tissues, it is often difficult to make a value judgement as to any cardiac disease liable to cause death.

When open autopsy of the heart is required after PMCT, our local pathologists tend to favour chest-limited examinations, focusing upon the heart and lungs, often with trans-diaphragm sampling of the liver and one kidney, in order to provide maximum information with minimal tissue dissection/disruption. This approach appears particularly appreciated by families, as minimally invasive.

The heart can be examined in situ by opening the pericardium and directly inspecting the organ and its connections, but is usually removed together with the mediastinum, lungs and related tissues. This may be performed either in isolation, or as grouped tissues with abdominal and/or throat structures.

Whichever dissection solution is applied, the heart is extracted from the pericardium after finger palpation of the opened pulmonary artery has been accomplished (in order to exclude pulmonary embolism). Transection of the aorta and pulmonary artery followed by the pulmonary veins and venae cavae serves to free the heart from the mediastinum.

The heart is considered initially in terms of possible congenital architectural variation by looking closely at the great vessels, the coronary tributary pattern, appendages and chambers. If these are abnormal, it may prompt specialist pathologist referral for congenital or inherited heart disease issues.

If the coronary artery architecture is appropriate, then 3 to 5 mm slices along the length of the coronary arteries are undertaken to exclude thrombosis and to consider the level of atheromatous stenosis (generally graded in 10% increments). The degree of coronary calcification and eccentricity of plaque is also often described as part of the coronary system macroscopic review.

Clearly, devices alter dissection. If there are coronary stents or heavy coronary calcification, then the coronary arteries may require removal en bloc with subsequent decalcification for full assessment. Likewise, calcified valves may require decalcification. Furthermore, the placement of pacemaker wires may require a modification of the dissection protocol. If there are prosthetic valves present, then these should be approached in a schematic way such that the inferior and superior surfaces of the valve tissues are inspected for sepsis, thrombosis or misalignment.

The cardiac chambers are normally considered initially by three transverse slices across the ventricles, ending at a mid-level ventricular slice, thereby showing the arrangement of the right and left ventricles and any scarring, fibrosis or acute infarction. This examination also demonstrates cardiac tissue asymmetry and endocardial thrombosis.

The 'top' part of the heart (i.e. upper part of the ventricles together with the atria) is examined 'along the flow of blood'. In short, the technique starts by opening the right atrium, with incision posteriorly into the right ventricle, exiting along the front of the heart through the pulmonary outflow tract, valve and pulmonary artery. Next, one repeats a similar set of incisions to demonstrate the left atrium, running downwards into the left ventricle. The examination then runs across the front of the heart upwards into the left ventricle outflow tract, across the valve and into the aorta. This is the common standard, although different variants of examination exist which may reflect the pathology under consideration [5].

Consideration of septal defects, calcification of valve tissues, along with stenosis/regurgitant features is normally part of any considered cardiac tissue examination.

As part of the examination, the heart mass can be measured and compared to standard heart weight tables. Furthermore, one can measure items of the internal substructure (valve circumferences, wall thickness, chamber diameter and so on). This may give insight into the status of heart before death.

Sampling for histology is normally guided by the fact that microscopic detail may provide additional information pertinent to the cause of the disease and thereby the death of the individual. Histology sampling is normally targeted, with small numbers of tissue specimens in most cases, through to extensive sampling in those with sudden deaths involving the young. Occasionally, bacterial and virology studies can be simultaneously taken to consider overtly septic processes and the possibility of viral myocarditis, respectively. Deaths involving possible inherited cardiomyopathies normally prompt sampling of the spleen so that appropriate DNA extraction can take place for late considerations [6].

Post Mortem CT of the Heart: Specific Additional Techniques

A familiarity with the range of non-contrast cardiac PMCT appearances is required in all cases, discussed further on in this chapter, as well as an understanding of when further techniques such as coronary calcium scoring, PMCTA or recommendation of open autopsy may be helpful.

In this section, these common techniques for enhancing the imaging assessment of the heart are presented, starting with the consideration of a calcium score (from the non-contrast images) and then targeted coronary angiography. Some centres may choose to apply these techniques routinely to all PMCT cases, whereas others will apply them on a case-by-case basis.

Calcium Scoring of the Coronary Arteries

A non-contrast PMCT may be supplemented with an objective assessment of the burden of coronary calcification by means of calculating a 'calcium score', sometimes referred to the Agatston score (as below) depending on the technique used. This numerical score, as in clinical practice, can be used as a proxy for the presence of coronary atheroma and thereby also for stenosis. Coronary artery calcification is arguably more clearly and easily detected on PMCT, compared to open autopsy [7] (Figs. 8.1 and 8.2).

In the setting of an appropriate clinical history (such as chest pain with sudden collapse/death), a high calcium score can be used to *suggest* a relevant, significant coronary stenosis. Death resulting from a fatal arrhythmia or myocardial infarction is thus inferred on the coronial 'balance of probabilities', assuming the lack of alternate competing fatal pathology or confounding features.

With appropriate software (semi-automated), the score is rapidly calculated and is deemed accurate, given the lack of motion artefacts. However, it is, to some degree, operator dependent, and care must be taken not to include aortic root, valvular, pericardial or mediastinal calcifications. Coronary stents also present a challenge as they can sometimes be difficult to visualise, especially if nestled within calcific plaques, or if there is in-stent calcification. If not recognised, and excluded, they will significantly elevate the score due to their high density. Of particular value,

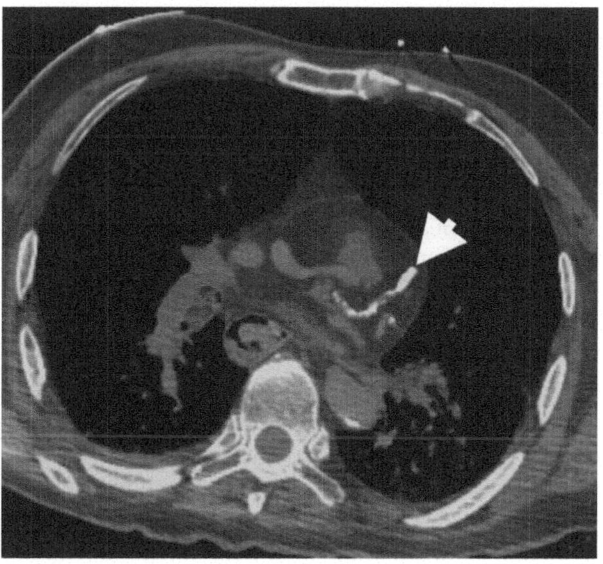

Fig. 8.1 Axial view of the chest on soft tissue windows shows extensive coronary calcification in the left anterior descending coronary artery (arrow), the individual vessel score was 1349

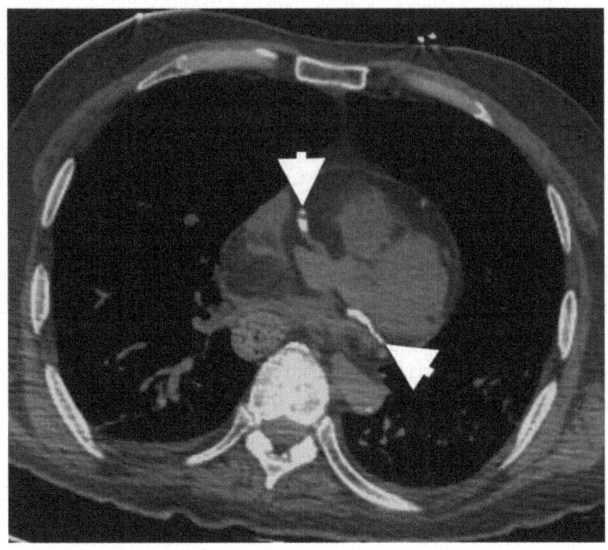

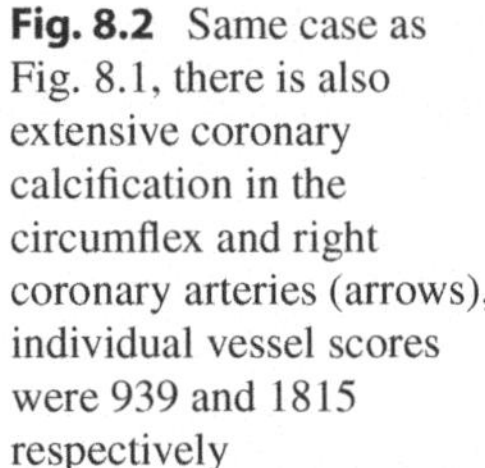

Fig. 8.2 Same case as Fig. 8.1, there is also extensive coronary calcification in the circumflex and right coronary arteries (arrows), individual vessel scores were 939 and 1815 respectively

the calcium score may be calculated even in the presence of moderate decomposition, although the exclusion of other competing and potentially fatal pathologies may not be possible in decomposed bodies.

In the authors' centre, the calcium score is calculated using the Agatston method [8]. Simplified, the score is based on the density of calcification multiplied by its area, taken from a non-contrast axial study at 3-mm slices. It is calculated for each main artery and given as an overall total. The total score, originally derived from those in clinical settings (i.e. the living) can be categorised with regard to the risk of coronary artery disease (CAD) as follows [9]:

0—Very low probability of significant CAD, generally <5%
1–10—Very unlikely probability of significant CAD, <10%
11–100—Mild or minimal coronary stenoses likely
101–400—Non-obstructive CAD highly likely, obstructive disease possible
>400—High likelihood (≥90%) of at least 1 "significant" coronary stenosis

Whilst the categories suggest a score of >400 to be highly significant, for context, scores may occasionally be seen in native vessels (without stents) of more than 3000!

It is to be appreciated that, whilst accurate for calcification, soft plaque is not identified by this method. It has been shown, in the living, that half of the patients undergoing assessment for high coronary risk, atypical symptoms or abnormal stress test who had a normal calcium score actually had non-calcified plaque on coronary angiography. Indeed, it was found that 1.5% of these cases had a severe stenosis! [10]. Thus, a low or even normal calcium score does not exclude a death from high-grade coronary stenosis. Indeed, it is recognised that potentially unstable or vulnerable plaque is often characterised histologically by a high lipid content rather than calcification.

On a practical level, pathologists vary considerably in their threshold for 'significance', modified by the clinical setting and case in front of them but will not usually accept deaths as coronary pathology in those with scores of 400 or less, despite the ante mortem correlates.

In summary, a high calcium score may indicate/support, but does not confirm, a coronary death. Conversely, a low score does not exclude coronary death. For these reasons, careful interpretation of the wider picture, focusing on the circumstances of the death, any reported symptoms and the prior medical history is required. Progression to PMCTA, a limited or full open autopsy may be the appropriate solution.

Post Mortem CT Coronary Artery Angiography

To enhance the information and confidence provided by non-contrast scans, the coronary artery lumens may be directly assessed with PMCT angiography (PMCTA). Whilst the techniques of injecting the contrast may vary to the clinical setting, the results are assessed in much the same way as clinical cardiac CT angiography.

Several methods of coronary PMCTA of varying complexity have been described [2, 4, 11, 12]. The method familiar to the authors involves cannulation of the left carotid artery via a small incision (importantly thus making the examination 'minimally invasive' rather than 'non-invasive') [11]. A 'male length', three-way urinary Foley catheter is passed through to the ascending aorta so that the tip lies above the aortic valve and coronary ostia. The 30 mL catheter balloon is inflated with water (Fig. 8.3) to achieve a seal with the aortic wall. Priming of the catheter with water before inserting may reduce the amount of air introduced and flushing before contrast injection can help dislodge post mortem clot from the aorta. Dilute (5%)

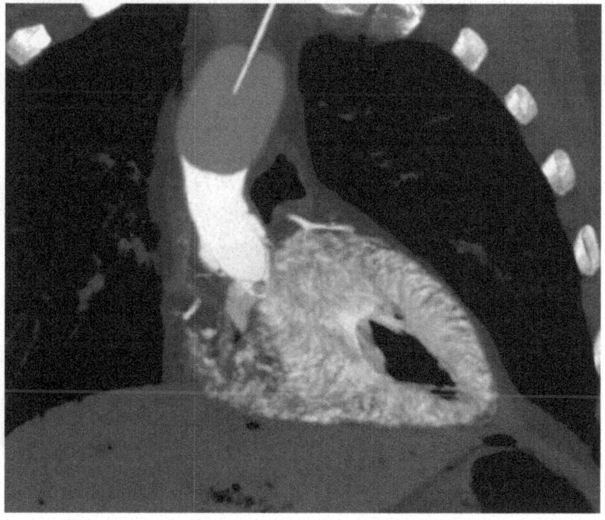

Fig. 8.3 Coronal maximum intensity projection of the chest showing an inflated urinary catheter balloon in the ascending aorta during targeted coronary PMCTA. Contrast is present in the catheter lumen, aortic root, coronary arteries and myocardium

iodinated contrast is injected manually, steadily in volumes of approximately 100–200 mL at a time. Radiological scanning then takes place in a standard manner.

If the aortic valve is competent, then flow of injected contrast material into the left heart is limited, and contrast fills the coronary arteries resulting in a targeted angiogram. However, if there is aortic regurgitation, then the injection pressure may not be sufficient to opacify the full length of each vessel. Contrast should not normally travel into the right side of the heart unless there is a structural defect, reflecting myocardial rupture after infarction, congenital deformity or trauma (Fig. 8.4).

Another potential cause of a non-diagnostic study is the inadvertent protrusion of post mortem clot from the aorta into the coronary arteries [7]. If a coronary artery is not opacified with contrast from its ostium, then 'pseudo-occlusion' by this normal post mortem clot (rather than pathological thrombus) is likely. This is most often seen in relation to the left coronary ostium as, in the conventional supine position, it lies more dependently (Fig. 8.5). Turning the patient prone, or right lateral decubitus, can be helpful in clearing the clot and confirming vessel patency. Non-ostial occlusions are much more likely to be genuine thrombus, as it is rare to find intra-coronary post mortem clot.

Negative contrast (usually air) is sometimes inadvertently injected via the catheter or may already be present due to decomposition, when it is usually found in the non-dependent RCA (Figs. 8.6, 8.7, and 8.8). Some methods of angiography routinely include an air-contrast run [2]. A combination of negative and positive contrast is quite acceptable for manual luminal assessment but can make using vascular analysis software more cumbersome—as the air is not tracked automatically. If necessary, poor opacification or air in the RCA can be overcome by turning the patient prone [11, 12]. However, this adds manual handling issues and time to the examination.

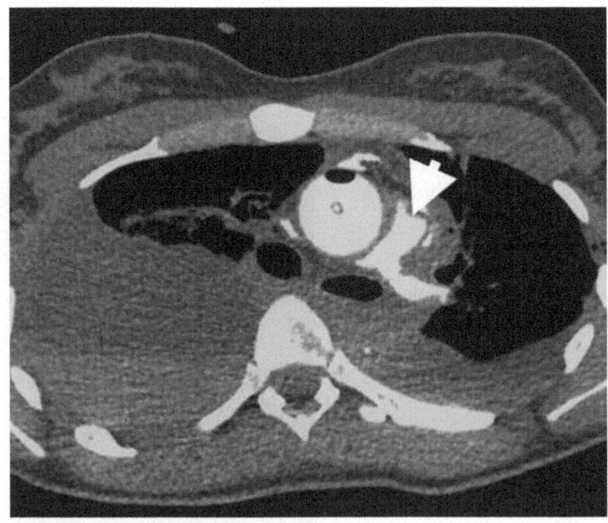

Fig. 8.4 Axial view of the chest during coronary PMCTA after a crush injury. This shows contrast in the pulmonary artery (arrow) which is not a normal finding. Whilst this can arise in the setting of congenital septal defects, in this case open autopsy confirmed a traumatic ventricular septal rupture. Large bilateral traumatic haemothoraces are also evident, yet no rib fractures were seen in this young adult

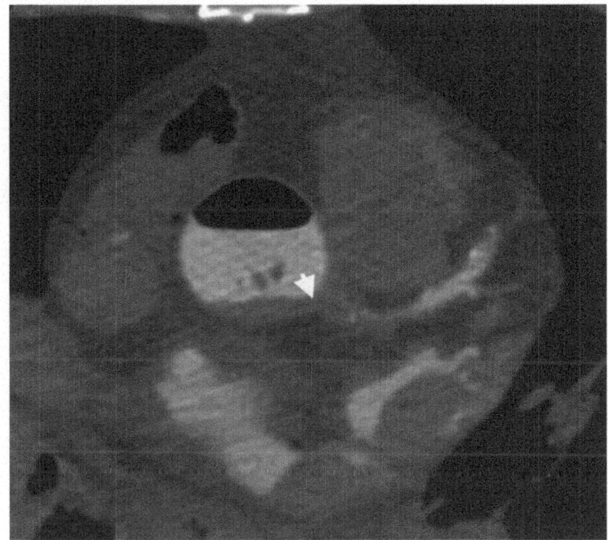

Fig. 8.5 Axial PMCTA view of the heart shows contiguous clot extending from the dependent aorta into the left coronary artery ostium (arrow) and main stem, likely protruded post mortem clot from the aorta—although there is distal vessel contrast implying incomplete 'pseudo-occlusion'

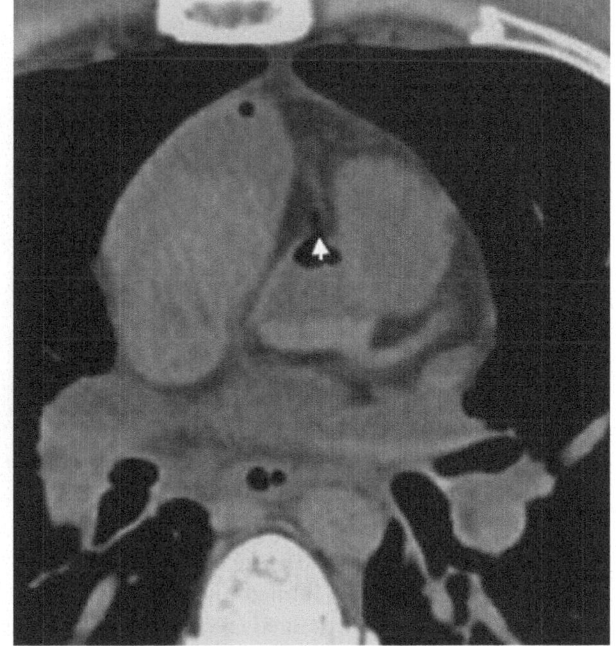

Fig. 8.6 Axial view of the mediastinum on soft tissue windows shows non-dependent air at the right coronary artery origin (arrow). There is also normal blood sedimentation in the aorta and normal positions of the right and left coronary ostia

Once contrast has filled the arteries, a 'myocardial blush' of contrast is sometimes seen, reflecting capillary backfilling and/or interstitial leakage. This may aid in revealing segments of non-perfused, infarcted myocardium (compare Figs. 8.8 and 8.9). However, if excessive, it can also make discrimination of the arteries more difficult.

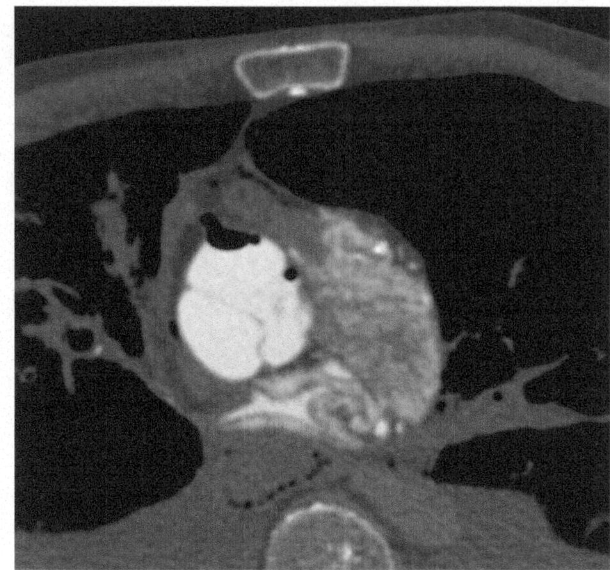

Fig. 8.7 Axial view of the aortic root following PMCTA contrast injection. The normal, anteriorly positioned right coronary origin is filled with air, inadvertently injected. Note is made of a normal tricuspid aortic valve without any calcifications

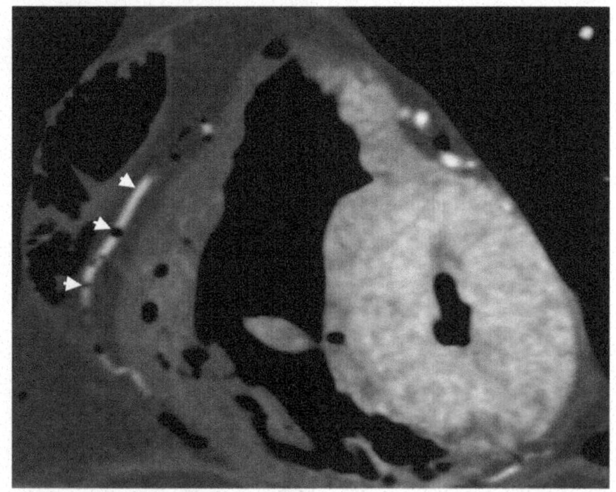

Fig. 8.8 Oblique PMCTA view of the heart to show the right coronary artery (arrows) in the anterior atrioventricular groove. The RCA contains contrast and locules of decomposition gas. There is also gas in the cardiac chambers from decomposition and a left ventricular myocardial blush of contrast

The choice of when to undertake angiography is largely down to local agreement but could, for example, be limited to cases of suspected coronary death, where the Agatston score is below a defined level, such as the clinical calcium score threshold of 400 [13]. This is because, 'on the balance of probabilities', a score of over 400 (in the absence of another cause of death or conflicting history) would support a cause of death due to coronary artery disease, without requiring further investigation such as angiography [13]. In addition, as the coronary calcium score further rises, coronary luminal visualisation becomes more difficult due to calcium blooming artefacts.

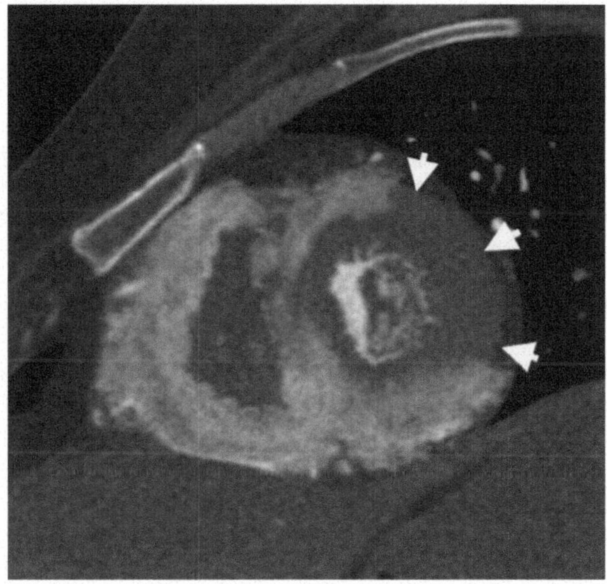

Fig. 8.9 Short axis view of the heart (mid ventricles) following PMCTA shows a well demarcated perfusion defect of the lateral segments of the left ventricle (arrows) suggesting infarct in the distribution of the left circumflex artery. The LCx artery demonstrated occlusive thrombus on PMCTA (not shown in this image) and the setting was sudden death following a few days of heartburn type symptoms and hypertension

One should however be mindful that the pathologist's approach or thresholds for considering PMCTA may differ. If the pathologist is the one sanctioning the test, then he/she may prefer to go straight to open cardiac autopsy review for uncertain cases. Cases where the history clearly suggests another unrelated cause of sudden death (such as suicide or ruptured aortic aneurysm) will not usually need PMCTA. If angiography is undertaken, it is preferable to obtain toxicological sampling in advance to avoid any potential for contamination. Cases with an infection risk may require exclusion from angiographic assessment. As with all specialised tests, it should be appreciated that PMCTA increases the time, cost and invasiveness of the overall post mortem study.

Considering now the potential results, PMCTA can provide diagnostic information about coronary narrowing, which is at least comparable to a standard open autopsy [12]. As with open autopsy, a 70% reduction of intra-luminal diameter is generally taken as a significant stenosis, with 90% considered high grade and usually sufficient (in appropriate circumstances) to assign the cause of death as ischaemic heart disease [1]. Lesser degrees of stenosis (<70%) may be important, but these must be tested against the absence of other pathology [1].

Arterial wall remodelling (a reaction to plaque formation) may be demonstrated and perhaps more easily appreciated on PMCTA, compared to open autopsy macroscopy, but is inferior to histology review. PMCTA also lacks the ability to provide microscopic information about a stenosis (such as intraplaque rupture or haemorrhage), inflammation, evidence of prior vascular dissection and so on. However, it is recognised that this microscopic assessment of atheromatous disease is not routinely performed at open autopsy—making PMCTA a viable alternative solution for many cases.

Normal PMCT Findings

Pericardial Sac

There is often a visible outline or trace of fluid in the pericardial sac, more obvious than on clinical imaging due to the absence of cardiac pulsation artefact. This finding is considered normal (Fig. 8.10). The pericardium should be thin and smooth.

Basic Coronary Anatomy

It is important to be familiar with normal and variant coronary anatomy [14] if one desires to interpret non-contrast scans as well as PMCTA. In the aortic root, there are right and left sinuses of Valsalva from which the coronary arteries arise (Figs. 8.11 and 8.12). There is also a third, 'non-coronary' aortic sinus situated right posterior.

The right coronary artery (RCA) travels anteriorly to the right of the pulmonary artery and along the anterior atrioventricular groove and has branches named acute marginals.

The left coronary artery arises in the form of the left main stem (LMS). It is a short trunk (generally 5–10 mm) that passes between the left atrial appendage and the pulmonary trunk.

The LMS bifurcates into the left anterior descending (LAD) and left circumflex (LCx) arteries. Occasionally, the LAD and LCx arise separately from the left coronary sinus, with this being generally considered to be a normal/benign variant,

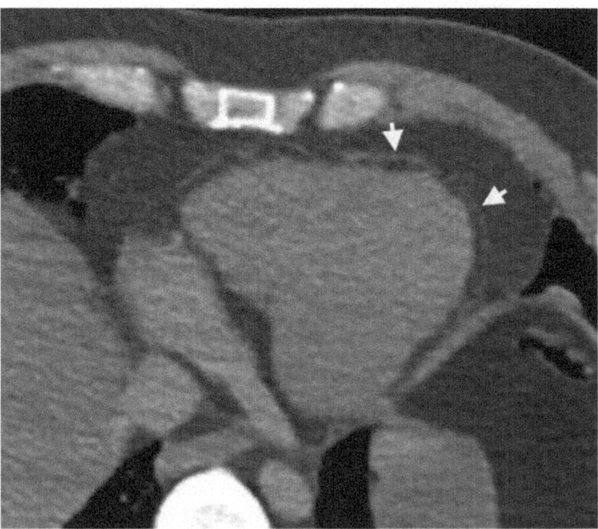

Fig. 8.10 Axial view of the mediastinum on soft tissue windows shows a normal thin pericardium (arrows), outlined by fat

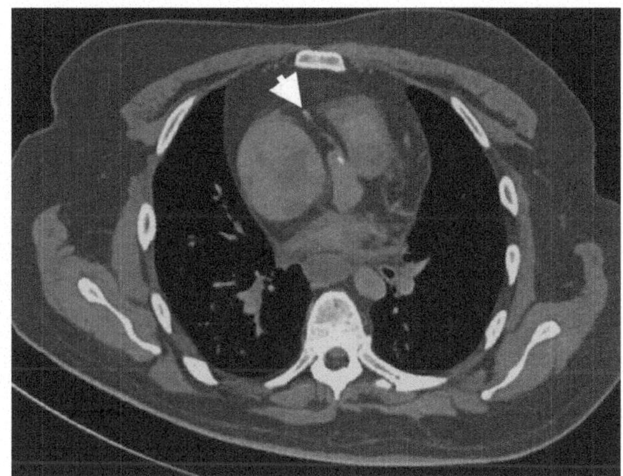

Fig. 8.11 Axial view of the chest on soft tissue windows shows the normal position of the right coronary artery (arrow), arising from a partially collapsed, normal post mortem aorta and travelling anteriorly through the right atrioventricular groove

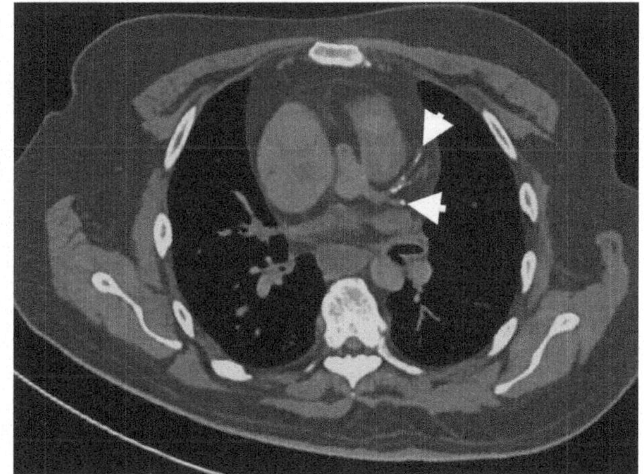

Fig. 8.12 Same case as Fig. 8.11, the normal position of the left main coronary origin is shown with the proximal left anterior descending and circumflex arteries also demonstrated (arrows). Multiple foci of vessel calcification are seen on this non-contrast study

rather than a pathological anomaly. Sometimes the LAD trifurcates with an anomalous artery arising between the LAD and the LCx being called a ramus intermedius.

The LAD travels in the anterior interventricular sulcus, and its branches are called the diagonal arteries. The LCx travels in the posterior atrioventricular groove, and its branches are the obtuse marginals.

'Coronary dominance' is a term which denotes the artery that supplies the distal posterior descending artery (PDA) and the posterolateral branch (PLB), which in turn supply the infero-septal and inferior aspect of the left ventricle. There is right side dominance in 80–85% of adult cases [14], with the other, non-dominant artery expected to be smaller in calibre. All of the coronary vessels should demonstrate a smooth tapering from their origins (Figs. 8.13 and 8.14) if they are normal.

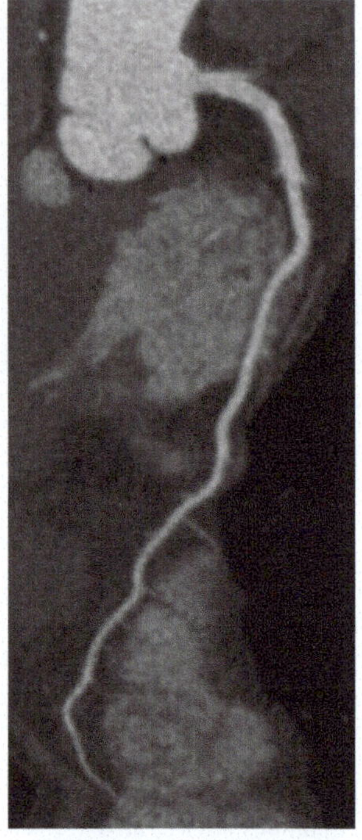

Fig. 8.13 PMCTA curved reconstruction of a normal left anterior descending artery from its origin showing a normal, smooth tapering of the vessel and no stenosis

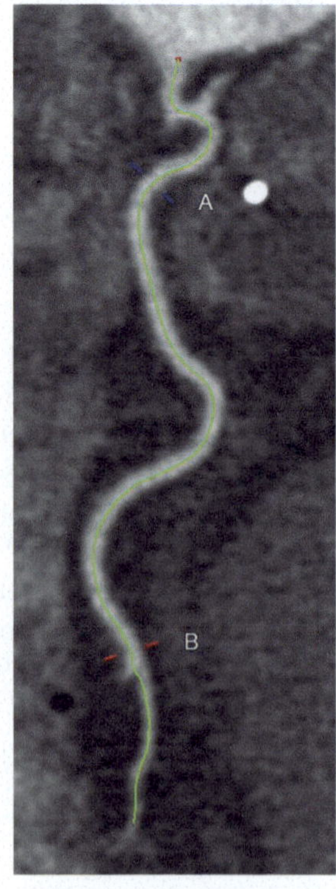

Fig. 8.14 PMCTA curved reconstruction of a normal right coronary artery with vessel tracking software 'centre line' and points of reference (A and B) which allow calculation of relative stenosis between different points

Heart Walls and Contents

Within the heart, there may be a normal fluid–fluid level from the sedimentation of blood, as well as intracardiac gas largely secondary to resuscitation attempts or decomposition. A relative dilatation of the right heart is a common observation on PMCT [15, 16], caused by the pooling of blood on the right side reflecting equalised intravascular pressures when the circulation ceases.

It is difficult to accurately measure myocardial thickness on routine PMCT, since inadvertent inclusion of papillary muscle and epicardial fat can lead to overestimation. The left ventricle is usually the chamber of most pathological interest. Measurement of wall thickness can be made by reconstructing images into a cardiac short-axis view (Fig. 8.9) and then measuring perpendicular to the endocardial surface. Such measurement may be easier when contrast outlines the cardiac chambers (such as when during angiography there is reflux of contrast through the aortic valve).

Once measured, the meaning of the figure obtained needs careful consideration. Bodies scanned very soon after death have the heart walls can appear artefactually thicker on PMCT compared to ante mortem CT due to rigor mortis [17]. The ventricular thickness will also vary depending on the cardiac phase (systole or diastole) at the time of death, further reducing confidence in the measurement. Other factors such as age and 'athleticism' of the deceased may factor into the assessment, and so a 'one-size-fits-all' approach to defining a normal post mortem myocardial thickness is inadvisable.

A method for estimating heart weight from PMCT, based on measuring the left ventricular circumferential area, has been proposed [18], although this is not validated in the presence of decomposition or trauma and is not currently undertaken in our own practice.

As so many factors are at play, it is very difficult to be certain of the value of measuring LV thickness or estimating heart weight at the present time. There is currently more research needed into the application of post mortem CT cardiac measurements, particularly for the post mortem period of several days to weeks after death.

Abnormal PMCT Findings

Pericardial Disease

Pericardial Effusion and Calcification

More than a normal trace of fluid (i.e. a true effusion, Fig. 8.15) may indicate pericardial disease or more likely reflect other systemic disease. If large, the effusion may be linked with poor cardiac function, and flattening of the right ventricle suggests a tamponade effect before death (Fig. 8.16). However, in the post mortem setting one must also consider that flattening of the right ventricle may also be seen due to flaccidity of the heart muscle during decomposition.

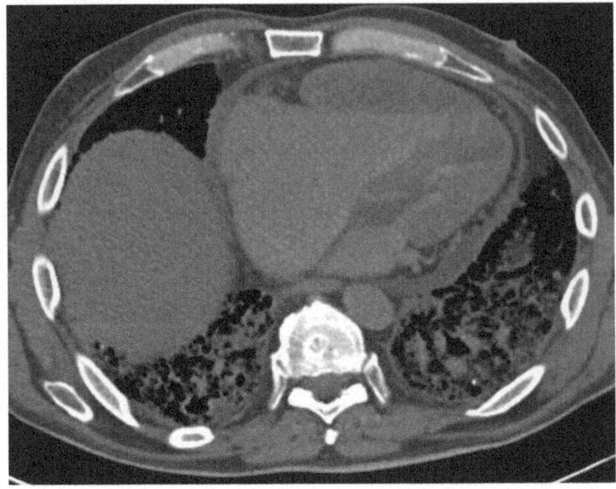

Fig. 8.15 Axial view of the chest on soft tissue windows shows a small pericardial effusion in a case of known pulmonary hypertension and lung fibrosis

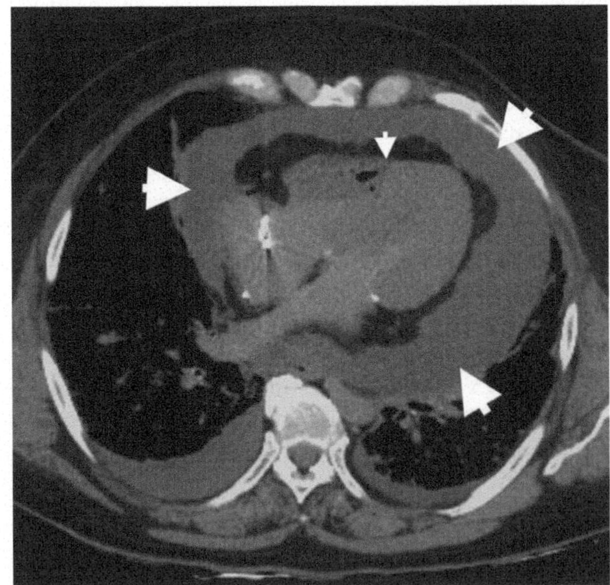

Fig. 8.16 Axial view of the chest on soft tissue windows showing a very large, non-haemorrhagic pericardial effusion (large arrows). There is subtle right ventricular flattening (small arrow), suggesting a degree of tamponade. Note also pacemaker wires with associated artefact, traversing the right atrium

Pericardial calcification is easily identified on PMCT and may be seen at sites of previous infection (viral or tuberculous), inflammation, intervention/surgery or trauma. The significance is higher if it is visibly constrictive or associated with a large effusion.

Haemopericardium

A haemopericardium is seen as a hyperdense pericardial collection. In the absence of external trauma, this is usually from either a ruptured aortic root (reflecting mural dissection) or a ruptured ventricular free wall (following a recent myocardial infarct). Rare causes of this pathology include coronary vasculitis, dissection or injury during intervention.

There are two distinct patterns to a post mortem haemopericardium. First is a horizontal layering of density (Fig. 8.17), similar to that commonly seen when blood products separate in the great vessels during normal hypostasis. Second, and fairly unique to this anatomic location is the 'hyperdense ring' appearance. Here, there is a concentric ring of high-density matrix around the heart (representing clot) in turn surrounded by a ring of low-density serum (Figs. 8.18 and 8.19). It has been suggested that the concentric ring pattern forms when haemorrhage occurs around

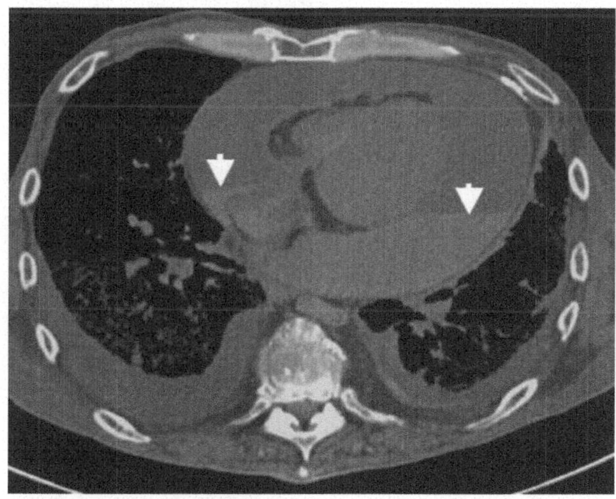

Fig. 8.17 Axial view of the chest on soft tissue windows shows a very large haemopericardium with layered separation of blood (arrows indicate the separation of components yet the whole volume is 'blood'). An intact aortic root (not seen on this image), high coronary calcium score and history of chest pain suggest this to be from a ruptured myocardial infarct

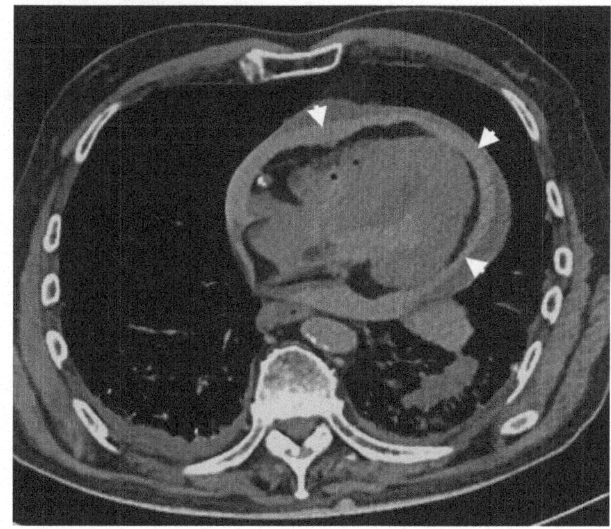

Fig. 8.18 Axial view of the chest on soft tissue windows shows a circumferential ring of high-density clot (arrows) around the heart, surrounded by lower density. This is representative of a haemopericardium. This patient had a high coronary calcium score (2603), neck and shoulder pain followed by sudden collapse, altogether in keeping with ruptured myocardial infarct

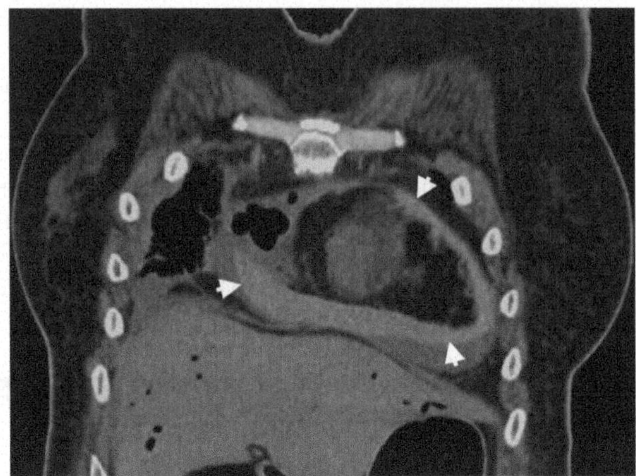

Fig. 8.19 Coronal view of the chest on soft tissue windows, (different case to Fig. 8.18) shows the true circumferential nature of hyperdense clot in this ring pattern of haemopericardium (arrows). This was a known hypertensive patient who suffered chest pain and a sudden collapse

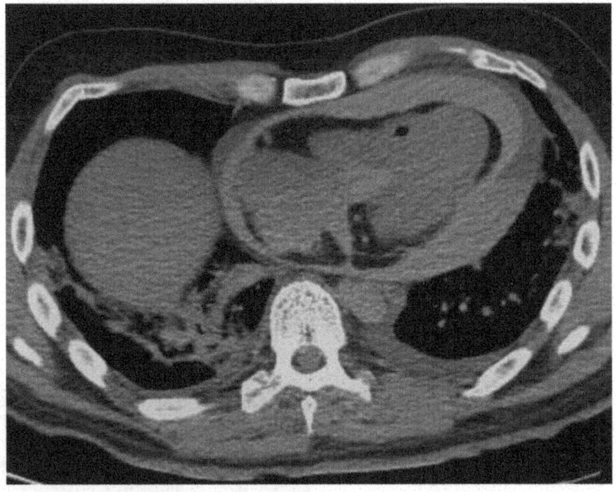

Fig. 8.20 Axial view of the chest on soft tissue windows showing a large haemopericardium with combined patterns; concentric hyperdensity around the heart and also layering of haemorrhage. This suggests a combination of ante mortem and post mortem haemorrhage. Note slight flattening of the right side of the heart anteriorly suggesting tamponade and anterolateral rib fractures from CPR attempts

a beating heart, i.e. blood loss initiated prior to the time of death. The layering pattern more likely forms in the post mortem phase, for example originating from cardiac rupture secondary to chest compressions [19].

The absolute reliability of this categorisation can be debated [20], as there may be other factors to consider. These include the presence of a coagulopathy (pathological or pharmaceutical), continued post mortem oozing from a primary defect and resuscitation injury following a true pathological aortic or ventricular rupture.

Occasionally, both patterns may be seen together (Figs. 8.20 and 8.21), suggesting a combination of both ante mortem and peri/post mortem haemorrhage. The emphasis should be on the ring pattern, as this is considered a vital reaction and therefore relevant to the events leading up to death [19].

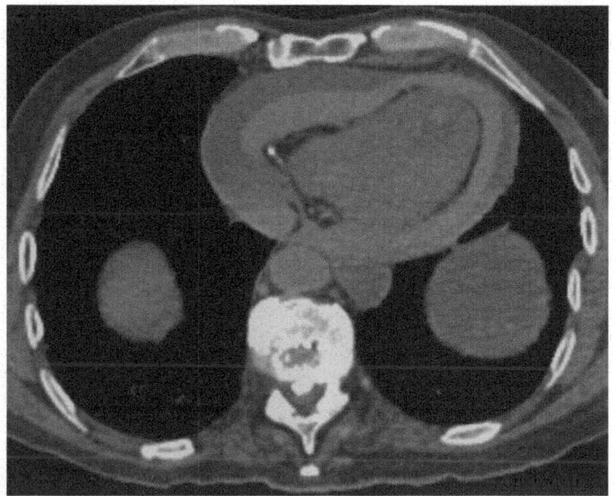

Fig. 8.21 Axial view of the chest on soft tissue windows shows both concentric hyperdensity around the heart and additional layered hyperdensity within the pericardial sac in keeping with a combined pattern haemopericardium. Flattening of the right (anterior) heart suggests tamponade effect

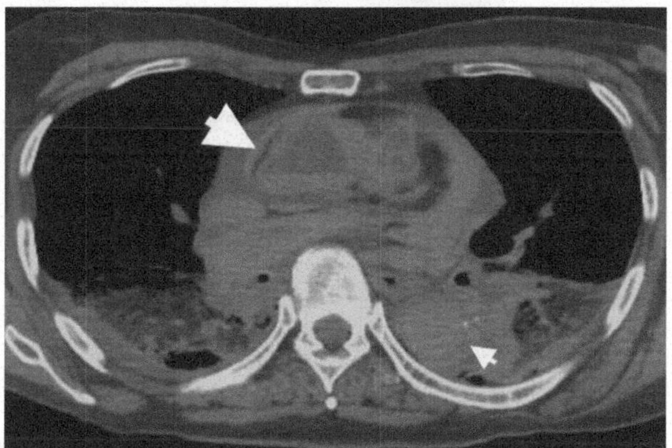

Fig. 8.22 Axial view of the chest on soft tissue windows shows a combined concentric ring and layered pattern of haemopericardium. A ring of hyperdensity extends around the aortic root (large arrow), arch (not seen) and more subtly around the descending aorta (small arrow) in keeping with an aortic dissection which has ruptured into the pericardial space

The origin of a haemopericardium is sometimes directly evident on PMCT. For example, a markedly irregular aortic root with adjacent haematoma is in keeping with aortic rupture or occasionally a dissection plane is evident (Fig. 8.22). By contrast, ventricular wall defects resulting from infarction are often occult unless revealed during angiography (Figs. 8.23 and 8.24). Arguably, in the presence of a normal aortic root, further investigations may not be required as, 'on the balance of probability', myocardial rupture is the most likely cause of tamponade.

Of note, rupture of the left ventricle is most likely to be secondary to infarction. However, whilst a right ventricular rupture may reflect infarction, it may

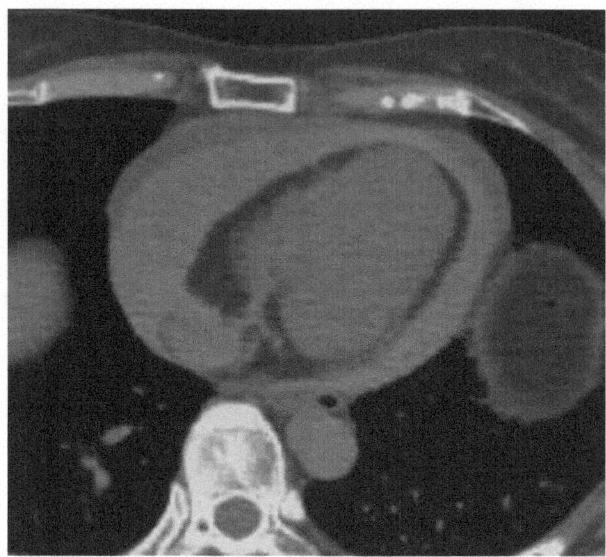

Fig. 8.23 Axial view of the mediastinum on soft tissue windows shows a concentric ring pattern of haemopericardium in a patient who was found deceased in bed with recent history of heartburn symptoms. The aortic root (not shown) appeared normal and the coronary calcium score was low. Coronary angiography was subsequently performed (Fig. 8.24)

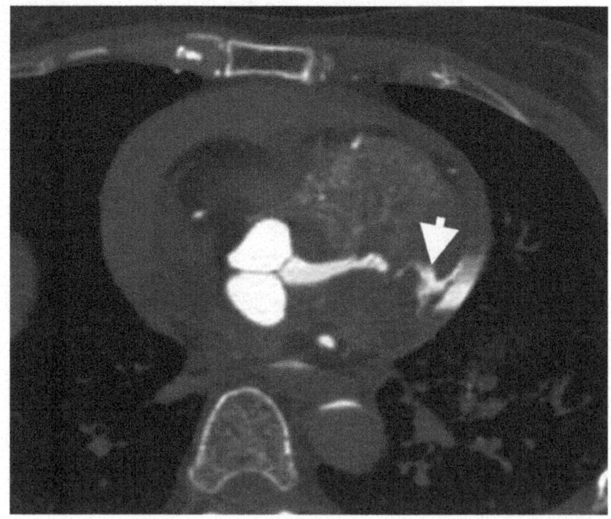

Fig. 8.24 Same patient as Fig. 8.23, a targeted coronary angiogram confirmed an intact aortic root (not shown) and reflux of contrast into the left ventricle demonstrated extravasation into the pericardial sac through a free-wall defect (arrow). This permitted diagnosis of a ruptured myocardial infarct

also be associated with traumatic injury, for example chest compressions during resuscitation. Open autopsy with histology sampling would be required to prove/refute each interpretation yet by careful consideration of the history and imaging, interpretation can usually be made radiologically, again on the balance of probabilities.

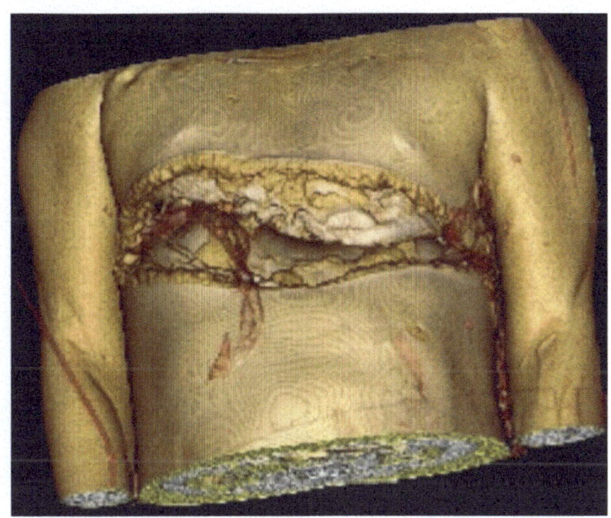

Fig. 8.25 Volume rendered image of the anterior chest wall following a 'clamshell thoracotomy' performed on this penetrating chest trauma patient to evacuate haematoma in the pericardial cavity

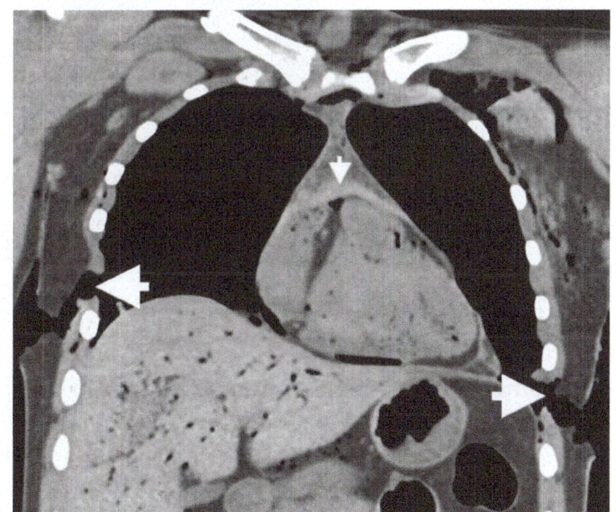

Fig. 8.26 (Same case as Fig. 8.25) Coronal view of the chest on soft tissue windows shows a small volume of residual haemorrhage in the supra-pericardial recess (small arrow) and large soft tissue defects from the clamshell thoracotomy (large arrows). Multiple locules of gas in the soft tissues result either from the primary trauma and/or secondary to the thoracotomy

In the emergency or resuscitation setting, when a haemopericardium with tamponade is suspected (usually due to penetrating thoracic injury, suspected blunt cardiac injury in a shocked patient or identified on bedside ultrasound), then aspiration or drainage may be attempted by means of a thoracotomy (Figs. 8.25, 8.26, and 8.27). Such extensive intervention however results in a scan that is very difficult to subsequently interpret.

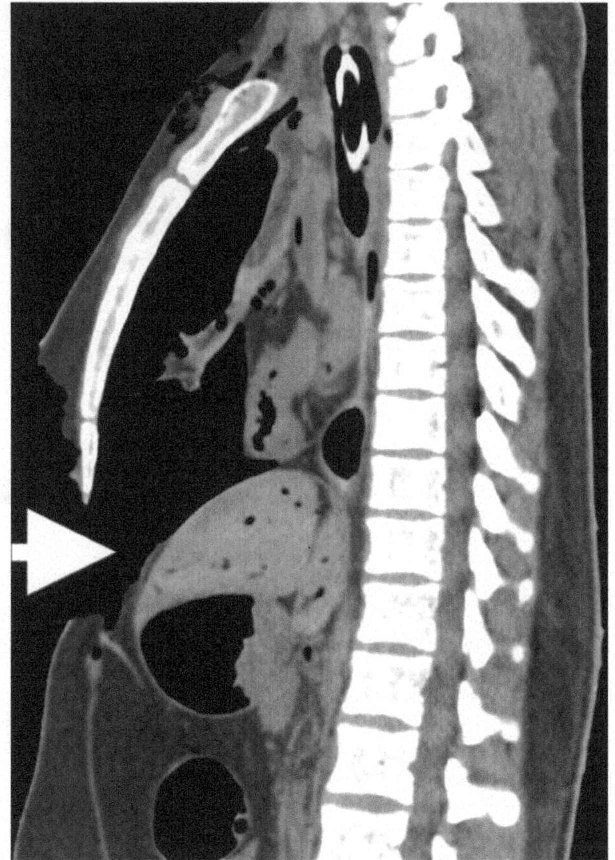

Fig. 8.27 (Same case as Fig. 8.25) Sagittal view of the chest shows the large anterior chest wall defect from clamshell thoracotomy (arrow). Subsequent collapse of the chest tissues/lungs and soft tissue gas make interpretation of the underlying primary injury difficult

Heart Size

Cardiomegaly and the Cardiothoracic Ratio

The assessment of heart size on PMCT is not straightforward. Traditionally, the term 'cardiomegaly' refers to an overall increase in size of the heart and/or the weight of the heart as defined by the pathologist at autopsy. This matter is important, as cardiac hypertrophy may be an important risk factor for sudden death. Thus, it is helpful for the radiologist to give an indication of the heart size, or state when this is not possible, for example in the setting of decomposition or traumatic disruption. One should be aware that the heart was dynamic and may remain in a state of systolic/diastolic contracture after death, akin to rigor mortis.

In clinical practice, the commonly used radiographic assessment of cardiac size is the cardiothoracic ratio (CTR), measured on a postero-anterior (PA) chest radiograph. A normal CTR is 0.5 or less, when the transverse diameter of heart is up to 50% of the inner thoracic cage diameter. The CTR can be measured on PMCT by reconstruction of the image into the coronal plane and performing transverse measurements, as if assessing plain film [21] (Figs. 8.28 and 8.29).

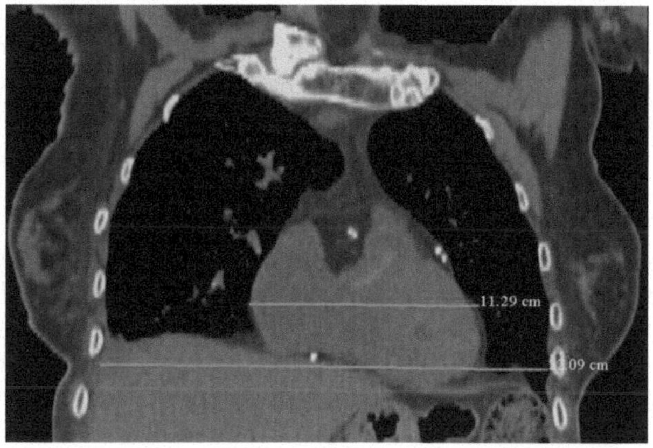

Fig. 8.28 Coronal image of the chest on soft tissue windows showing a simplified example of how to measure the transverse diameters of the heart and thorax in order to calculate the cardiothoracic ratio, in this example the heart size is considered to be normal (11.29/22.09 = 0.51). *Note however that the maximum transverse diameters may not always be in the same coronal plane*

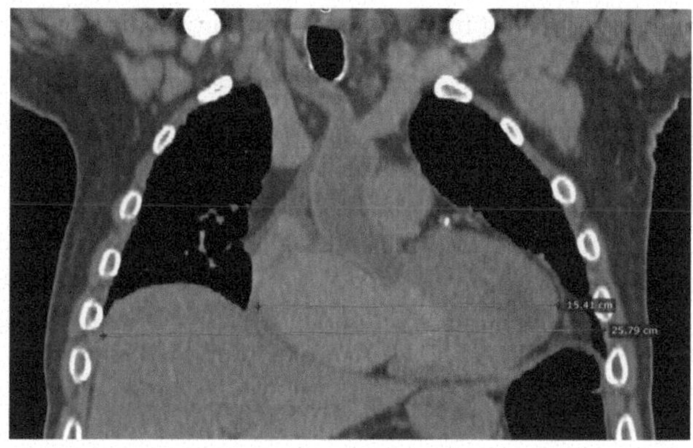

Fig. 8.29 Coronal image of the chest on soft tissue windows showing a simplified example of how to measure the transverse diameters of the heart and thorax in order to calculate the cardiothoracic ratio, in this example cardiomegaly is demonstrated (15.41/25.79 = 0.6)

It has been suggested that a CTR of more than 0.5 (or more than 130 mm cardiac diameter) might indicate cardiomegaly early after death [21]. This has been described with sensitivity/specificity of 89%/71% for the CTR and 89%/93% respectively for heart diameter. However, a body laid supine and in a post mortem state will have some progressive heart 'flattening' with a corresponding potential increase in CTR such that a normal post mortem CTR value has alternatively been judged as 0.54 or more [22]. For a very high specificity (>95%) an even higher CTR threshold of 0.57 may be more appropriate [23, 24], especially if scans are not undertaken within 24h of death. In general, care must be taken not to overcall mild cardiomegaly in the post mortem setting, with CTRs between 0.5 and 0.57 remaining debatable.

Certainly, cardiothoracic ratio may not be an appropriate measurement in cases where there are congenital variations to the thoracic cage, extremes of age or background lung pathologies, such as emphysema [25]. The heart size is difficult to accurately measure and trust if there is visible decomposition (gaseous distension or chamber collapse), pericardial fluid or cardiac injury. Chest wall deformity from trauma (including from chest compressions during resuscitation) may also alter the cardiothoracic diameters and ratio. When these confounding factors exist, it may not be possible to make a confident measurement of heart size on PMCT.

One approach is that measurements (transverse cardiac diameter and CTR) may be calculated from the images and reported in a factual manner that will allow the pathologist to consider the significance in relation to the other findings and scenario. CTR values between 0.5 and 0.57 might be considered 'borderline'. The radiologist should however make it clear when the values are likely to be less reliable owing to the factors highlighted in the previous paragraph. Other attempts to enhance the value of autopsy CTR alone include an adjusted CTR-based score (accounting for body-mass index, age and gender), used to predict cardiac hypertrophy at PMCT, available as an online tool [26], yet this also does not account for the confounding factors mentioned earlier. Reference to any clinical imaging (if available) would be extremely helpful in these borderline circumstances.

Coronary Artery Disease

Coronary Artery Stenosis

There are a variety of pathologies liable to cause coronary lumen narrowing, although one recognises the majority of UK cases reflect atheroma. Stenosis (narrowing) of the coronary arteries may be due to soft plaque, calcific plaque or may be mixed in nature. Any stenosis can be broadly described in terms of location along the vessel (proximal, middle and distal) and to a quantitative degree in terms of the degree of narrowing [27]:

- Minimal stenosis: <25%
- Mild stenosis: 25–49%
- Moderate stenosis: 50–69%
- Severe stenosis: >70%
- Occluded: 100%

A visual aid, originally developed to aid pathologists, may help when becoming familiar with reporting degrees of stenosis [28], although most dedicated angiography software solutions will provide a numeric assessment through vessel reconstructions. Further morphological description of the arteries and stenotic lesions is beyond the scope of this introductory text, and the reader is directed to clinical cardiac radiology and pathology texts and relevant courses [29, 30].

Coronary artery stenosis can result in myocardial ischaemia, with deaths from myocardial infarction or fatal dysrhythmia. Pathological studies have shown that stenoses of more than 85% are linked with a risk of sudden death [31], although, as above, over 70% is referred to as 'severe' [27] and in other sources, 90% is considered 'high-grade' [1]. It is suggested that the degree of significance (enough to attribute cause of death, in the absence of confounding factors) be discussed and agreed between radiologist and pathologist to ensure concordance in interpretations. From the pathologists' perspective, severe stenosis (i.e. over 70–85%) with a fitting history is usually considered sufficient to confirm coronary artery disease as the cause of death. This analysis could be equally extrapolated to radiology (Figs. 8.30, 8.31, and 8.32).

Faced however with a mild-to-moderate stenosis, on the balance of probability, this narrowing being the cause of death is difficult to satisfy, without well-fitting

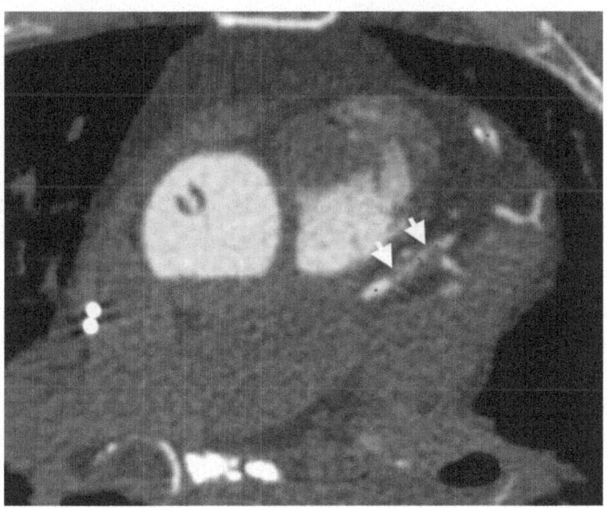

Fig. 8.30 Axial view of the heart following targeted coronary PMCTA, performed to investigate a sudden unexpected death (found deceased). The calcium score was 92 (but all in the LAD). PMCTA reveals severe stenosis of the proximal LAD (arrows). Note the vessel tracking software markers through the stenosis, used to form curved reconstructions of the vessel (Fig. 8.31). The PMCTA catheter tubing is seen in the opacified aortic root and pacemaker wires noted in the SVC

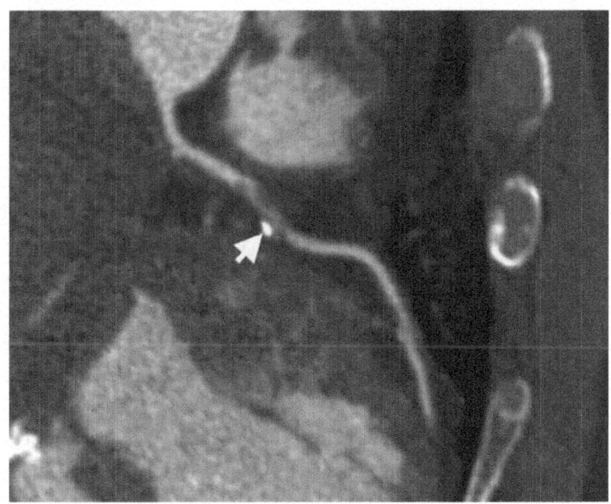

Fig. 8.31 Same case as Fig. 8.30, curved PMCTA reconstruction of the LAD demonstrates the stenosis to be secondary to a mixed density plaque with a calcific focus (arrow). This plaque results in a segment of severe (>85%) luminal stenosis but there is contrast 'run-off' distally (i.e. it is not occlusive)

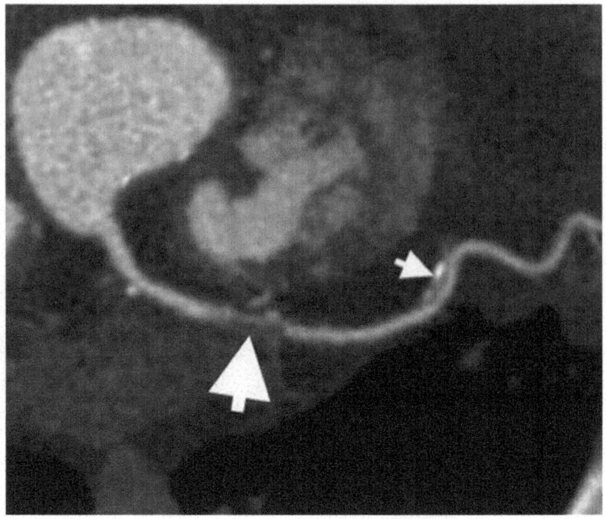

Fig. 8.32 Same case as Figs. 8.30 and 8.31, another curved reconstruction at a different rotation point again demonstrates the severe stenosis of the proximal vessel (large arrow). Note that a further, eccentric mild mixed plaque stenosis is now also seen more distally (small arrow)

circumstances and careful exclusion of alternate pathology. However, it is again emphasised that any even severe coronary disease may be present *but may not be the cause of death.*

It is also worth noting that complete vessel occlusion is not automatically the cause of death, as fully blocked arteries are sometimes seen in autopsies with other (non-cardiac) causes of death. Indeed, individuals may suffer from myocardial infarction from such complete coronary occlusion and yet live on with this cardiac disease. It therefore follows that finding complete occlusion should not be defined automatically as the cause of death, without triangulated ante mortem data and exclusion of alternate causes.

Coronary Artery Bypass Grafting

Targeted coronary angiography will not readily assess cardiac bypass morphology or patency. It is probably not meaningful to perform coronary calcium scores or coronary angiography in patients who have had bypass grafting, as the results cannot reliably be interpreted in the same manner as natural disease. Whole-body angiography, if available, may allow assessment of the bypass vessels [12], but this is rarely performed in the United Kingdom owing to the additional time and financial resource required.

Open autopsy examination of bypass vessels is appreciated as complex to dissect, due to the variable anatomy, fragile nature, local fibrosis and post-surgical scarring. One has to consider whether such assessment (open or radiological) is best for to the overall post mortem examination, if one is assessing a case on the balance of probability. A history of cardiac bypass surgery indicates a significant background risk from heart disease, even with good previous revascularisation outcomes. Again, considering an appropriate history, in the absence of confounding features on external examination and imaging, ischaemic heart disease may be considered the probable cause of death.

Myocardial Bridging

A 'myocardial bridge' is defined as an anomalous course of a major coronary artery, commonly the left anterior descending, where there is overlying myocardium (the 'bridge segment') contrasting with a normal epicardial coronary artery position. The importance of this finding is controversial, as myocardial bridges are common (although prevalence is variably reported) and often asymptomatic [14]. The importance of the finding probably increases with increasing length and depth of the involved segment. In life, relative stenosis of this segment during systolic compression of the "buried" artery can result in pre-stenotic dilatation, retrograde flow and plaque formation at the bridge entrance. Nevertheless, they have been associated with ischaemia, infarction and sudden death.

This finding can be seen on non-contrast PMCT [32], although it is better appreciated following contrast administration [12]. Once seen, the significance of the finding must be interpreted in the context of the clinical history, as it may be entirely incidental (Fig. 8.33).

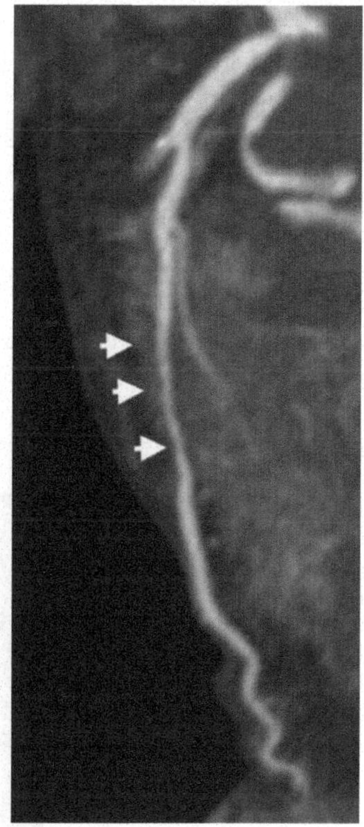

Fig. 8.33 Curved PMCTA reconstruction of the left anterior descending artery demonstrates incidental bridging of the proximal to mid vessel segments through the myocardium (arrows, blushed with contrast) and a resultant underlying mild stenosis

Anomalous Coronary Arteries

Anomalous coronary anatomies are seen in approximately 1% of the general population, with varying degrees of significance. Whilst most clearly demonstrated on PMCTA, it is usually possible to assess the coronary artery origins and the course of the proximal segments on a non-contrast study, as they are usually outlined by fat. Indeed, this could be considered a standard 'review area' in PMCT.

Some anomalous configurations are of doubtful clinical significance, such as a separate origin of the LCx and LAD from the left coronary sinus. This alone would not usually be considered as a cause for sudden cardiac death.

However, if an anomalous coronary artery passes between two arterial structures (commonly the aorta and pulmonary artery, referred to as a 'malignant' inter-arterial course), there is a risk of sudden death (Figs. 8.34 and 8.35). This will usually be associated with exertion but can occur during rest and at any age. Myocardial ischaemia is thought to result from vessel compression during increased demand (hence exacerbated by exercise), leading to infarction or death from arrhythmia.

Examples of such a 'malignant' course include an anomalous right coronary arising from the left aortic sinus and an anomalous left coronary artery arising from the right aortic sinus. Both configurations are recognised to be associated with sudden and exercise-related death [33, 34].

Anomalous origins can also be associated with slit-like ostia, oblique intramural segments and high take-off origins, where the coronary vessel exits the aorta irregularly or at an acute angle to travel a short distance through the aortic wall itself. During exercise, as the aorta expands, it is thought that the ostium is closed like a valve [33].

As with other cardiac findings, it is important to appreciate that anomalous arterial courses may be incidental findings at PMCT [35]. Their presence needs to be considered against the circumstances and other case findings before being suggested to be related to the cause of death.

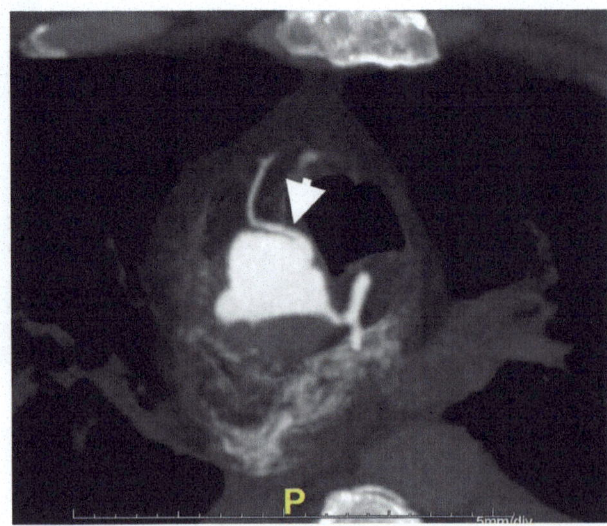

Fig. 8.34 PMCTA oblique axial view at the level of the coronary ostia showing an aberrant right coronary artery origin (arrow) which has acute angulation as it travels between the aorta and (gas filled) pulmonary artery—a so-called malignant course

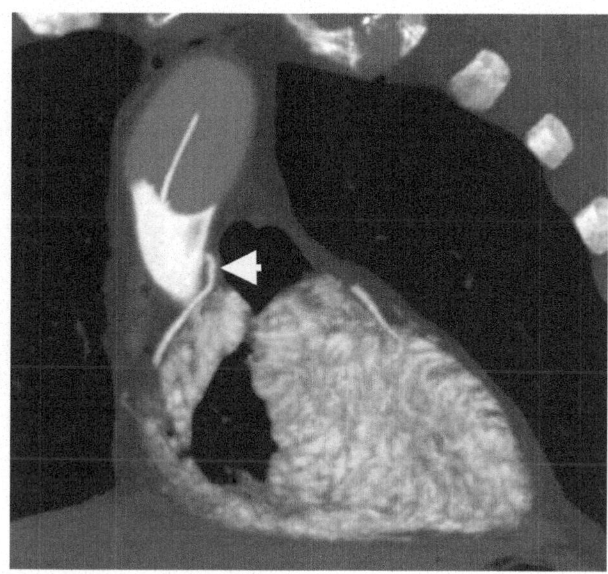

Fig. 8.35 Same case as Fig. 8.34, a coronal MIP view shows the aberrant, mildly compressed right coronary artery winding around the aortic root (arrow)

Myocardial Disease

Myocardial Infarction

It is not possible to directly visualise an acute myocardial infarction on non-enhanced PMCT [36]. The diagnosis of acute myocardial ischaemia or infarction may occasionally be suggested on PMCTA by a geographic perfusion defect corresponding to an arterial territory (Fig. 8.9), along with a stenosis or occlusion of the relevant vessel and appropriate history (perhaps also correlating with ante mortem electrocardiogram/ECG evidence). This complete pattern of findings is rarely seen even in cases of histologically proven infarct [12]. One should be aware that a perfusion abnormality may also be seen as an artefact of PMCTA technique (e.g. ostial post mortem clot or air bubble 'occlusion') or could result from the variables of decomposition.

One should also appreciate that, in sudden coronary occlusion deaths, there may not be enough time for a macroscopic visible myocardial infarct to develop and to be seen at open autopsy. If required, histological sampling from open autopsy may be used to confirm early ischaemia, sometimes using immuno-histology, although this is rarely undertaken in routine deaths.

Old/established infarcts can sometimes be seen on PMCT as regions of fatty replacement, myocardial thinning and calcification (Figs. 8.36 and 8.37). Such previous infarcts and myocardial scars incur a potential arrhythmogenic risk and should be mentioned in the report as they are potentially relevant as a cause of death.

Cardiomyopathy

Cardiomyopathies are an important cause of cardiac death and must always be a differential diagnosis, especially in sudden unexpected deaths of the young or unexplained cardiac failure. Historically, they were considered in terms of primary and

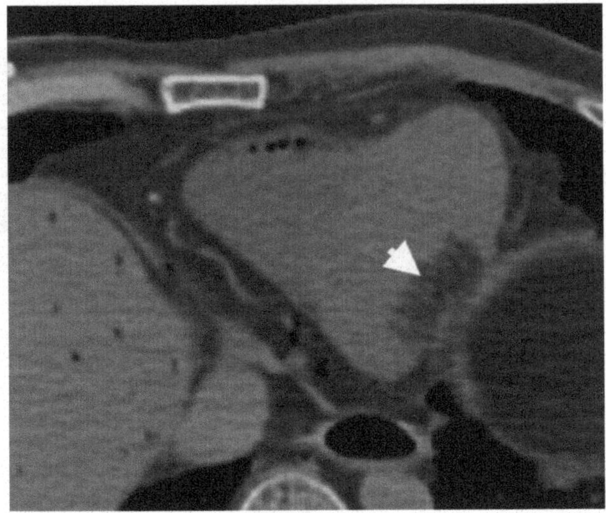

Fig. 8.36 Axial view of the heart on soft tissue windows shows a well demarcated region of fatty replacement in the left ventricular free wall (arrow) in a patient with a known previous myocardial infarct

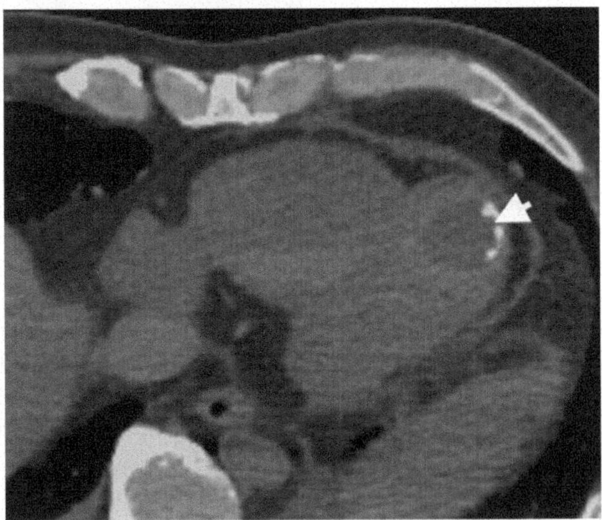

Fig. 8.37 Axial view of the heart on soft tissue windows shows curvilinear calcification of a thinned cardiac apex (arrow) consistent with a known previous myocardial infarct

secondary disorders. It is clear that most of the primary conditions reflect specific gene mutations and often affect the young. This group of cardiomyopathies includes dilated cardiomyopathy (DCM), hypertrophic cardiomyopathy (HCM) and arrhythmogenic (right ventricular) cardiomyopathy (ARVC). Other variants and degenerative cardiomyopathies also exist, and the reader is referred to specialist texts on this matter [37].

By contrast, 'secondary' causes of cardiomyopathy (perhaps better termed as cardiac disease reflecting systemic conditions) include amyloid deposition, hypertension, alcohol misuse, sarcoid and a variety of storage disorders. Their diagnoses may be suggested by the history, but PMCT does have a role in confirming cardiac structural change, features of heart failure and in excluding other pathologies.

Clues for the existence of cardiomyopathy may be apparent, such as profound cardiac enlargement, hence the need to at least consider heart size at PMCT. The thickness of the left ventricle might point to HCM or a storage disorder (such as Fabry disease). Likewise marked fatty change potentially suggests ARVC. A large and dilated heart, seen in cases of DCM, is not specific and can be seen after myocardial infarction, following myocarditis and in a variety of other conditions. Thus, tissue sampling for enzyme assessment, gene/DNA review and histology are all important, making the open autopsy a beneficial and often mandatory protocol in this context.

Given the importance of making this diagnosis, the radiologist should have a low threshold for advising/considering focused invasive autopsy, since the inheritance pattern of these lesions means other family members may be at risk of sudden deaths. This is particularly so as there are an increasing range of genetic subtypes described. The coroner and families are often grateful to have this issue explored by means of open autopsy and potential gene testing.

Valvular Heart Disease

Assessing this mixed group of disorders by routine PMCT has many limitations; in terms of clinical imaging, they would usually be assessed by real-time ultrasound or ECG-gated CT/MRI. More information may be gathered by an experienced cardiac radiologist reporting angiographic images; however, there are findings on the routine non-contrast images that may still be of value.

Valvular calcification is readily apparent on post mortem imaging and provides important information to indicate valve disease. Care should be taken however to separate the valve from aortic root, mitral annular, coronary, myocardial or pericardial calcifications [38, 39].

Aortic valve disease is the most common cardiac valve disease in the Western population, particularly in older age, and the degree of calcification of the valve leaflets correlates with the severity of stenosis. Whilst this can be estimated on PMCT, the true functional significance cannot be assessed. Yet, some understanding of the effects of the valve disease can be inferred from any associated chamber dilatation (e.g. left ventricle in relation to aortic stenosis or left atrium in relation to the mitral valve), mural hypertrophy or aortic root dilatation. These features however may not be measurable/reliable in the post mortem setting and need to be judged by the radiologist for the scan in front of them. There is commonly some post mortem vascular or cardiac collapse that may preclude these estimations (Fig. 8.38). A normal aortic valve has three leaflets, and these cannot usually be seen on routine PMCT but may be evident on PMCTA (Fig. 8.7). The diagnosis of a bicuspid aortic valve would be important, as significant stenosis may be present here, even if the calcific burden is mild.

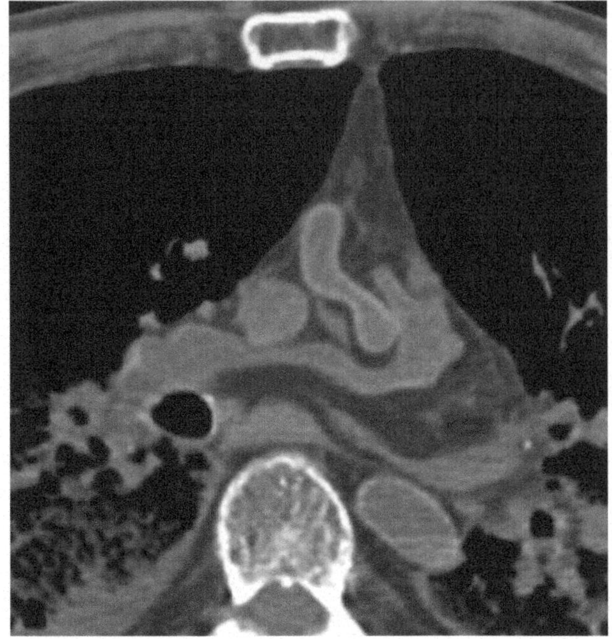

Fig. 8.38 Axial view of the superior mediastinum on soft tissue windows showing normal post mortem vessel collapse—which makes the diagnosis of dilatation difficult/impossible, although the surrounding fat planes are preserved mitigating against rupture

We are aware of the potential clinical use of the Agatston score to objectively calculate the calcific burden of the aortic valve [40], but this is not within our current PMCT practice. For the non-cardiac radiologist, a simpler categorisation, just as that suggested for clinical practice [39], of *'none, mild, moderate and severe'* may be more achievable and appropriate.

Mitral valve leaflet calcification is less common but often seen in the setting of rheumatic disease or advanced renal impairment. It is important to differentiate this from mitral annular calcification (normally seen on the posterior and outer ring of the valve, Fig. 8.39) which is more common, can be extensive, is degenerative in nature and is associated with normal valve function [38].

Non-calcific valvular soft tissue pathology such as mucoid degeneration causing incompetence (floppy mitral valve) and vegetations (infective endocarditis) are unlikely to be identified on PMCT. The replacement of valve by metal prostheses is readily seen on CT, yet with the associated streak artefact it would be difficult/impossible to appreciate whether any thrombus or vegetation is present.

Uncommon Cardiac Conditions

Cardiac Tumours

When there is no ante mortem diagnosis, primary cardiac tumours are rarely seen at PMCT and normally do not feature as autopsy findings, apart from being incidental pathologies. Pragmatically, only the cardiac myxoma and cardiac sarcoma are generally apparent and if identified as abnormalities on imaging, PMCT would have to

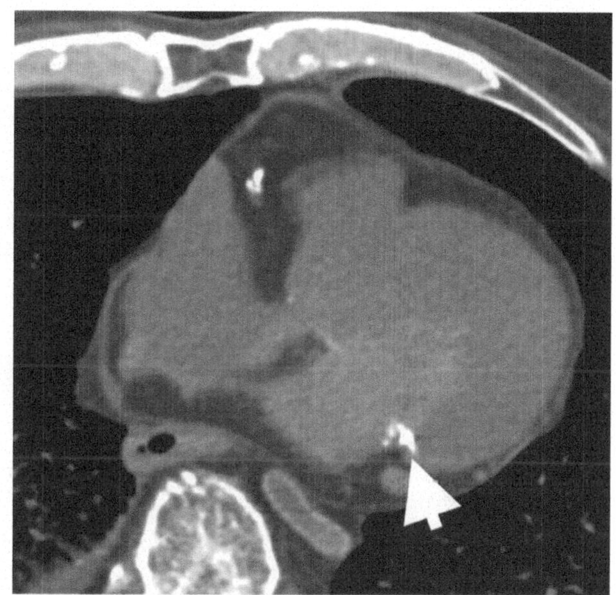

Fig. 8.39 Axial view of the heart on soft tissue windows shows incidental calcification of the mitral annulus (arrow) in an elderly patient

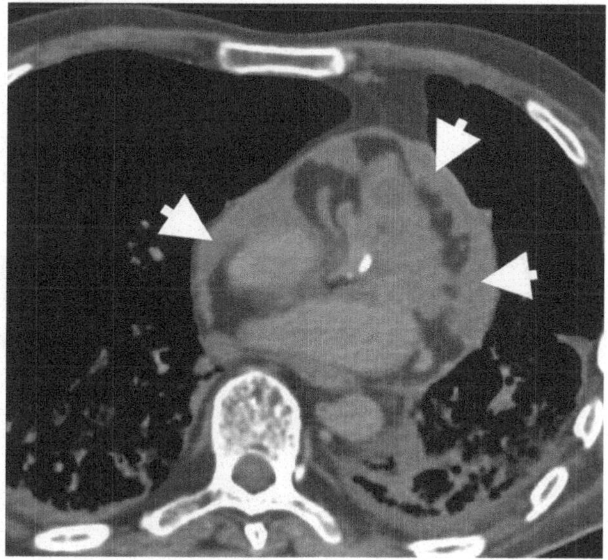

Fig. 8.40 Axial view of the mediastinum on soft tissue windows shows a thickened, lobulated pericardium (arrows) in a case of known disseminated left bronchial malignancy

include a very broad range of differentials. As such, these soft tissue lesions would normally require open autopsy for confirmation.

However, disseminated malignant disease from other sites may terminally involve the pericardium and cardiac tissues with lymphoma, mesothelioma and lung cancer, to name but a few commonly implicated (Fig. 8.40).

Cardiac Trauma

Significant trauma to the heart is usually an unequivocal cause of death, due to induced arrhythmia, haemopericardium with tamponade and/or rapid exsanguination (Figs. 8.41 and 8.42). Mechanisms include both penetrating injuries and blunt force/crush injury to the chest. Large haemorrhagic collections can be seen on non-contrast imaging and may be enough to confirm the traumatic cause of death in the setting of the known trauma history. Coronary angiography can add to the description of the sites of cardiac and vascular disruption if further detail is needed (Figs. 8.4, 8.43, and 8.44).

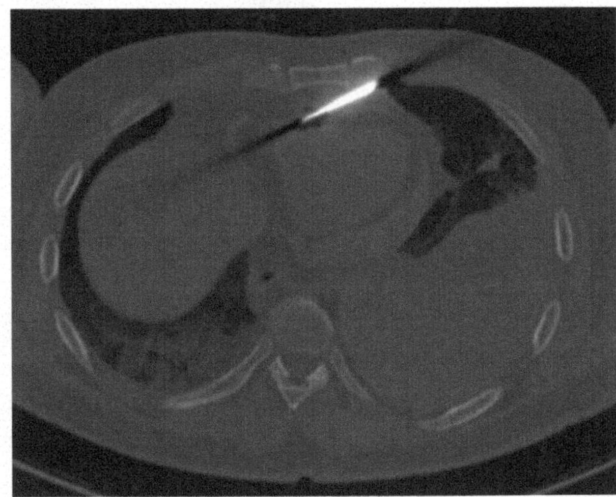

Fig. 8.41 Axial view of the chest on bone windows demonstrates a linear metallic object consistent with a knife blade penetrating the anterior chest wall and pericardium. The tip now lies at the right atrial wall

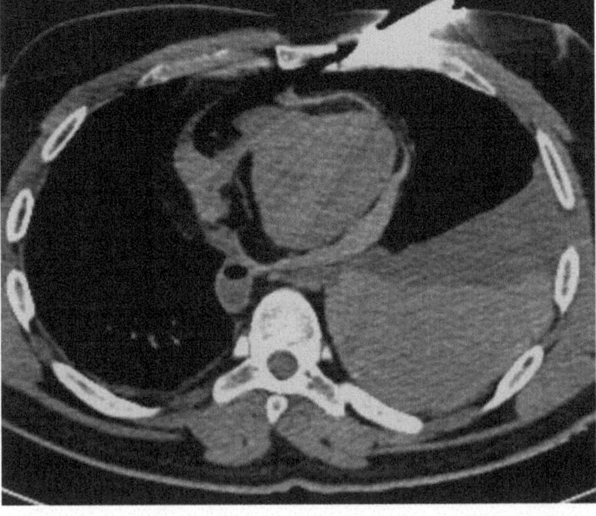

Fig. 8.42 Same case as Fig. 8.41, soft tissue windows at a more cranial level show a hyperdense haemopericardium and massive left haemothorax (with layering of blood products) resulting from fatal penetrating cardiac injury

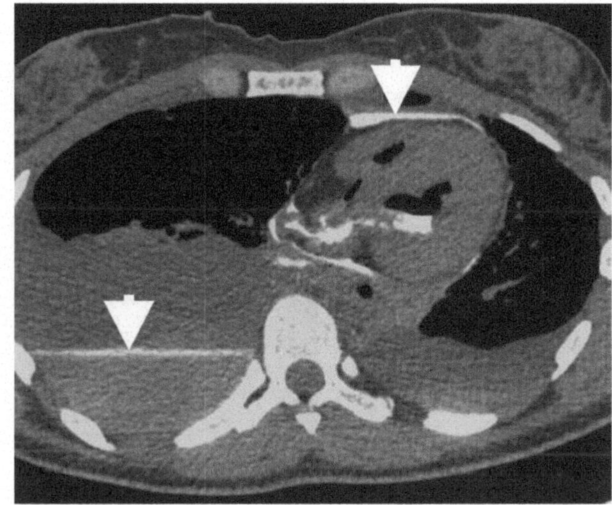

Fig. 8.43 Same case as Fig. 8.4 (PMCTA after chest crush injury with cardiac disruption), shows further leakage of the dense angiographic contrast into the pericardium and right hemithorax (arrows) indicating multiple sites of internal injury

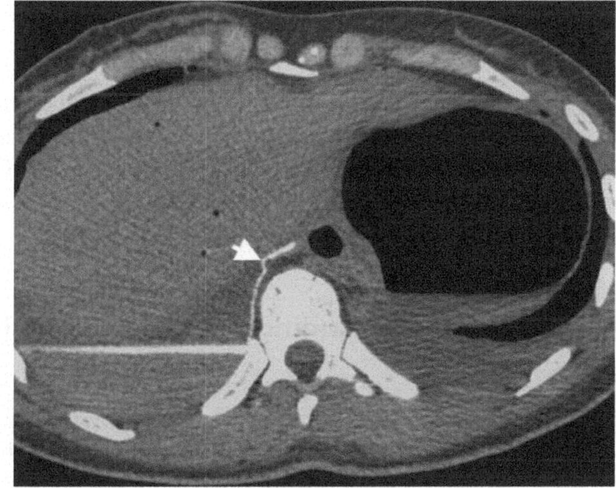

Fig. 8.44 Same case as Fig. 8.4 and 8.43, a more caudal slice shows the exact site of contrast extravasation from the IVC (arrow), indicating a venous tear communicating with the pleural space/large right haemothorax. This was confirmed at open autopsy

Intra-cardiac air embolus should be considered when the history is appropriate, for example after trauma to the body (not necessarily to the heart itself), childbirth or a therapeutic procedure where air may enter the vessels. It is estimated that a volume of 100–250 mL of air is potentially sufficient to cause death [41]. However, in our practice, it is much more common to see air in vascular structures secondary to decomposition or following CPR attempts.

In non-trauma cases, care must be taken not to over-call injury related to cardiopulmonary resuscitation (Fig. 8.45), which can result in multiple rib, sternal and even thoracic spinal fractures, cardiac injury, haemopericardium and haemothoraces. These features are further discussed in Chap. 11.

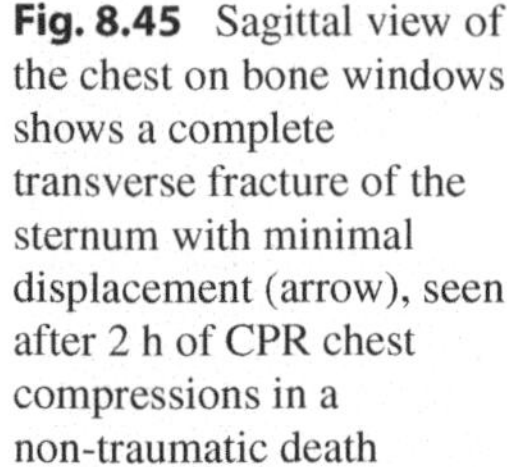

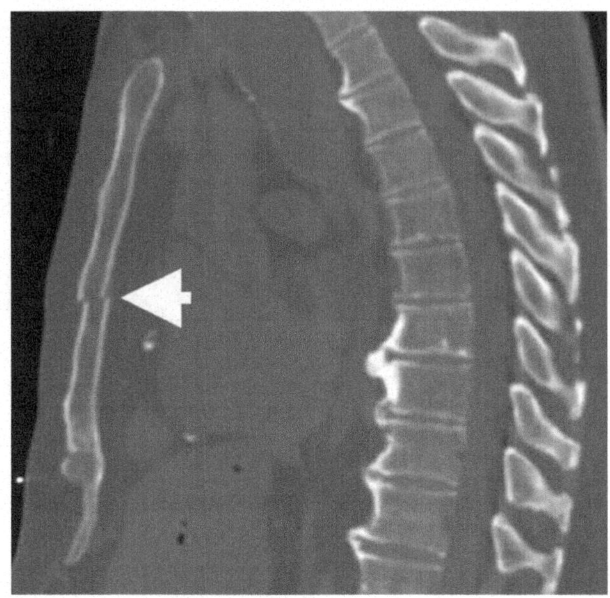

Fig. 8.45 Sagittal view of the chest on bone windows shows a complete transverse fracture of the sternum with minimal displacement (arrow), seen after 2 h of CPR chest compressions in a non-traumatic death

Finally, for interest, one must also be mindful of the issue of 'commotio cordis' in which sudden blunt force applied to the chest is associated with cardiac dysrhythmia and sudden death. Normally, this is the preserve of forensic pathology cases, but could possibly feature as part of the routine PMCT workload. Usually, no cardiac pathology is identified on imaging [34].

Reporting Cardiac Findings: Pearls and Pitfalls

The level of detail to which cardiac findings and their relevance is reported will depend somewhat on whether the reporter undertakes cardiac imaging in the living and their confidence in this subspecialty.

Cardiac PMCT may variably include a non-contrast study, coronary calcification scoring and whole-body or targeted coronary PMCTA as per local agreements or case-by-case assessment.

Any prior cardiac surgery (including valves, stents, bypass grafts, pacemaker or defibrillator devices) should be reported and considered.

An assessment of the features of decomposition should be made in order to inform the confidence of subsequent findings.

The volume/nature of pericardial fluid and presence of pericardial calcification should be made in all cases. An assessment of heart size (transverse measurement or CTR for example) may be made with appropriate caution.

Coronary origins may be assessed for normal or aberrant location, without the need for PMCTA. Valve and/or other cardiac calcifications should be noted.

A calcium score may be calculated, and an interpretation of its significance can be given, remembering that sudden death from coronary artery disease is difficult to diagnose with absolute certainty and reference to the available history should always be made.

The quality of any angiographic study should be noted, for example 'excellent, good, average or poor' [27] and then the findings detailed for each major vessel.

A coronary cause of death is often described with the more global term 'ischaemic heart disease' and usually made on the *balance of probabilities* if a relevant significant coronary stenosis is demonstrated (or inferred from calcium scoring). This highlights that the full implications of reporting stenosis are not fully understood, and this is a research direction needed for adult post mortem imaging [42].

One should note that the terms 'cardiac failure' or 'cardiac arrest' should not feature as a given cause of death as these are 'modes of death'. They require correlation to an underlying pathological mechanism and it is this that the autopsy seeks to describe, such as aortic stenosis.

Example PMCT report phrases:

- The heart is considered to be enlarged with a cardiothoracic ratio of 0.6 (or 60%).
- There is a large haemopericardium with right ventricular flattening, in keeping with tamponade. The aortic root appears normal and given the history a ruptured myocardial infarction is most likely.
- Normal coronary artery origin morphology.
- Coronary stents noted. These have been excluded from the calcium score. The total coronary calcium score is XX; calculated using the Agatston method. This suggests a XX risk of a significant coronary artery stenosis.
- Excellent quality coronary PMCTA with full opacification of all vessels, there is no coronary occlusion or stenosis.
- High-grade (>90%) stenosis of the left anterior descending (or other) artery secondary to mixed plaque.
- Severe aortic valve calcification with associated left ventricular hypertrophy.

References

1. Osborn M, Lowe J. Guidelines on autopsy practice: sudden death with likely cardiac pathology [Internet]. The Royal College of Pathologists, London; 2015. https://www.rcpath.org/uploads/assets/823dfcf4-8eba-40f7-81b7e174675ecdd9/Guidelines-on-autopsy-practice-Sudden-death-with-likely-cardiac-pathology.pdf.

2. Rutty GN, Morgan B, Robinson C, Raj V, Pakkal M, Amoroso J, et al. Diagnostic accuracy of post-mortem CT with targeted coronary angiography versus autopsy for coroner-requested post-mortem investigations: a prospective, masked, comparison study. Lancet [Internet]. 2017;390(10090):145–54. https://linkinghub.elsevier.com/retrieve/pii/S0140673617303331.
3. Roberts ISD, Traill ZC. Minimally invasive autopsy employing post-mortem CT and targeted coronary angiography: evaluation of its application to a routine coronial service. Histopathology [Internet]. 2014;64(2):211–7. http://doi.wiley.com/10.1111/his.12271.
4. Ross SG, Bolliger SA, Ampanozi G, Oesterhelweg L, Thali MJ, Flach PM. Postmortem CT angiography: capabilities and limitations in traumatic and natural causes of death. Radiographics [Internet]. 2014;34(3):830–46. http://pubs.rsna.org/doi/10.1148/rg.343115169.
5. Suvarna SK. National guidelines for adult autopsy cardiac dissection and diagnosis—are they achievable? A personal view. Histopathology [Internet]. 2008;53(1):97–112. http://doi.wiley.com/10.1111/j.1365-2559.2008.02993.x.
6. Suvarna SK. The heart at autopsy, including radiological autopsy of the heart. In: Suvarna S, editor. Cardiac pathology [Internet]. 2nd ed. Cham: Springer International Publishing; 2019. p. 93–126. http://link.springer.com/10.1007/978-3-030-24560-3_5.
7. Michaud K, Grabherr S, Doenz F, Mangin P. Evaluation of postmortem MDCT and MDCT-angiography for the investigation of sudden cardiac death related to atherosclerotic coronary artery disease. Int J Cardiovasc Imaging [Internet]. 2012;28(7):1807–22. http://link.springer.com/10.1007/s10554-012-0012-x.
8. Agatston AS, Janowitz WR, Hildner FJ, Zusmer NR, Viamonte M, Detrano R. Quantification of coronary artery calcium using ultrafast computed tomography. J Am Coll Cardiol [Internet]. 1990;15(4):827–32. http://www.ncbi.nlm.nih.gov/pubmed/2407762.
9. Rumberger JA, Brundage BH, Rader DJ, Kondos G. Electron beam computed tomographic coronary calcium scanning: a review and guidelines for use in asymptomatic persons. Mayo Clin Proc [Internet]. 1999;74(3):243–52. https://linkinghub.elsevier.com/retrieve/pii/S0025619611638603.
10. Kelly JL, Thickman D, Abramson SD, Chen PR, Smazal SF, Fleishman MJ, et al. Coronary CT angiography findings in patients without coronary calcification. Am J Roentgenol [Internet]. 2008;191(1):50–5. http://www.ajronline.org/doi/10.2214/AJR.07.2954.
11. Roberts ISD, Benamore RE, Peebles C, Roobottom C, Traill ZC. Diagnosis of coronary artery disease using minimally invasive autopsy: evaluation of a novel method of post-mortem coronary CT angiography. Clin Radiol [Internet]. 2011;66(7):645–50. https://linkinghub.elsevier.com/retrieve/pii/S0009926011000675.
12. Ross SG, Thali MJ, Bolliger S, Germerott T, Ruder TD, Flach PM. Sudden death after chest pain: feasibility of virtual autopsy with postmortem CT angiography and biopsy. Radiology [Internet]. 2012;264(1):250–9. http://pubs.rsna.org/doi/10.1148/radiol.12092415.
13. Robinson C, Deshpande A, Rutty G, Morgan B. Post-mortem CT: is coronary angiography required in the presence of a high coronary artery calcium score? Clin Radiol [Internet]. 2019;74(12):926–32. https://linkinghub.elsevier.com/retrieve/pii/S0009926019303745.
14. Kini S, Bis KG, Weaver L. Normal and variant coronary arterial and venous anatomy on high-resolution CT angiography. Am J Roentgenol [Internet]. 2007;188(6):1665–74. http://www.ajronline.org/doi/10.2214/AJR.06.1295.
15. Ishida M, Gonoi W, Okuma H, Shirota G, Shintani Y, Abe H, et al. Common postmortem computed tomography findings following atraumatic death: differentiation between normal postmortem changes and pathologic lesions. Korean J Radiol [Internet]. 2015;16(4):798. https://www.kjronline.org/DOIx.php?id=10.3348/kjr.2015.16.4.798.
16. Shiotani S, Kohno M, Ohashi N, Yamazaki K, Nakayama H, Watanabe K, et al. Dilatation of the heart on postmortem computed tomography (PMCT): comparison with live CT. Radiat Med [Internet]. 2003;21(1):29–35. http://www.ncbi.nlm.nih.gov/pubmed/12801141.
17. Okuma H, Gonoi W, Ishida M, Shintani Y, Takazawa Y, Fukayama M, et al. Heart wall is thicker on postmortem computed tomography than on ante mortem computed tomography: the first longitudinal study. PLoS One [Internet]. 2013;8(9):e76026. https://dx.plos.org/10.1371/journal.pone.0076026.

18. Hatch GM, Ampanozi G, Thali MJ, Ruder TD. Validation of left ventricular circumferential area as a surrogate for heart weight on postmortem computed tomography. J Forensic Radiol Imaging [Internet]. 2013;1(3):98–101. https://linkinghub.elsevier.com/retrieve/pii/S2212478013000634.
19. Yamaguchi R, Makino Y, Chiba F, Torimitsu S, Yajima D, Shinozaki T, et al. Fluid-fluid level and pericardial hyperdense ring appearance findings on unenhanced postmortem CT can differentiate between postmortem and antemortem pericardial hemorrhage. Am J Roentgenol [Internet]. 2015;205(6):W568–77. http://www.ajronline.org/doi/10.2214/AJR.15.14808.
20. Mychajlowycz M. The armored heart: differentiating the etiology of hemopericardium on postmortem computed tomography. J Forensic Radiol Imaging [Internet]. 2017;9:6–7. https://linkinghub.elsevier.com/retrieve/pii/S2212478016300685.
21. James P, Morgan B, Rutty GN, Brough A. Cardiothoracic ratio (CTR) measured on postmortem computed tomography (PMCT)—pre- and post-ventilation. J Forensic Radiol Imaging [Internet]. 2016;4:76–80. https://linkinghub.elsevier.com/retrieve/pii/S2212478016300041.
22. Okuma H, Gonoi W, Ishida M, Shirota G, Kanno S, Shintani Y, et al. Comparison of the cardiothoracic ratio between postmortem and antemortem computed tomography. Leg Med [Internet]. 2017;24:86–91. https://linkinghub.elsevier.com/retrieve/pii/S1344622316302267.
23. Winklhofer S, Berger N, Ruder T, Elliott M, Stolzmann P, Thali M, et al. Cardiothoracic ratio in postmortem computed tomography: reliability and threshold for the diagnosis of cardiomegaly. Forensic Sci Med Pathol [Internet]. 2014;10(1):44–9. http://link.springer.com/10.1007/s12024-013-9504-9.
24. Suvarna SK. Teaching and examining for post-mortem CT-scanned autopsies. Diagnostic Histopathol [Internet]. 2020;26(8):343–9. https://linkinghub.elsevier.com/retrieve/pii/S1756231720300815.
25. Screaton N. The cardiothoracic ratio—an inaccurate and outdated measurement: new data from CT. Eur Radiol [Internet]. 2010;20(7):1597–8. http://link.springer.com/10.1007/s00330-010-1721-y.
26. Jotterand M, Faouzi M, Dédouit F, Michaud K. New formula for cardiothoracic ratio for the diagnosis of cardiomegaly on post-mortem CT. Int J Legal Med [Internet]. 2020;134(2):663–7. http://link.springer.com/10.1007/s00414-019-02113-1.
27. Raff GL, Abidov A, Achenbach S, Berman DS, Boxt LM, et al. SCCT guidelines for the interpretation and reporting of coronary computed tomographic angiography. J Cardiovasc Comput Tomogr [Internet]. 2009;3(2):122–36. https://linkinghub.elsevier.com/retrieve/pii/S1934592509000707.
28. Champ CS, Coghill SB. Visual aid for quick assessment of coronary artery stenosis at necropsy. J Clin Pathol [Internet]. 1989;42(8):887–8. http://jcp.bmj.com/cgi/doi/10.1136/jcp.42.8.887.
29. Lim T-H, editor. Practical textbook of cardiac CT and MRI [Internet]. Berlin, Heidelberg: Springer Berlin Heidelberg; 2015. http://link.springer.com/10.1007/978-3-642-36397-9.
30. Michaud K. Ischaemic heart disease. In: Suvarna SK, editor. Cardiac pathology [Internet]. 2nd ed. Cham: Springer International Publishing; 2019. p. 137–51. http://link.springer.com/10.1007/978-3-030-24560-3_7.
31. Davies MJ, Popple A. Sudden unexpected cardiac death? A practical approach to the forensic problem. Histopathology [Internet]. 1979;3(4):255–77. http://doi.wiley.com/10.1111/j.1365-2559.1979.tb03008.x.
32. Ampanozi G, Gascho D, Hatch G, Schulze C, Thali MJ, Ruder TD. What is unsought will go undetected—myocardial bridging on postmortem computed tomography. J Forensic Radiol Imaging [Internet]. 2014;2(1):5–8. https://linkinghub.elsevier.com/retrieve/pii/S2212478013001238.
33. Taylor AJ, Rogan KM, Virmani R. Sudden cardiac death associated with isolated congenital coronary artery anomalies. J Am Coll Cardiol [Internet]. 1992;20(3):640–7. http://www.ncbi.nlm.nih.gov/pubmed/1512344.
34. Suvarna SK. Sudden cardiac death. In: Suvarna SK, editor. Cardiac pathology [Internet]. 2nd ed. Cham: Springer International Publishing; 2019. p. 277–311. http://link.springer.com/10.1007/978-3-030-24560-3_14.

35. Martinez RM, Flach PM, Ebert LC, Bartsch C, Thali MJ, Ampanozi G. Anomalous left coronary artery origin on postmortem imaging in correlation with autopsy. J Forensic Radiol Imaging [Internet]. 2014;2(3):146–8. https://linkinghub.elsevier.com/retrieve/pii/S2212478014000586.
36. Wagensveld IM, Blokker BM, Pezzato A, Wielopolski PA, Renken NS, von der Thüsen JH, et al. Diagnostic accuracy of postmortem computed tomography, magnetic resonance imaging, and computed tomography-guided biopsies for the detection of ischaemic heart disease in a hospital setting. Eur Hear J Cardiovasc Imaging [Internet]. 2018;19(7):739–48. https://academic.oup.com/ehjcimaging/article/19/7/739/4883380.
37. Bunning CR, Suvarna SK. Cardiomyopathies. In: Suvarna SK, editor. Cardiac pathology [Internet]. 2nd ed. Cham: Springer International Publishing; 2019. p. 205–25. http://link.springer.com/10.1007/978-3-030-24560-3_11.
38. Kanza RE, Allard C, Berube M. Cardiac findings on non-gated chest computed tomography: a clinical and pictorial review. Eur J Radiol [Internet]. 2016;85(2):435–51. https://linkinghub.elsevier.com/retrieve/pii/S0720048X15301807.
39. Williams MC, Abbas A, Tirr E, Alam S, Nicol E, Shambrook J, et al. Reporting incidental coronary, aortic valve and cardiac calcification on non-gated thoracic computed tomography, a consensus statement from the BSCI/BSCCT and BSTI. Br J Radiol [Internet]. 2021;94(1117). https://www.birpublications.org/doi/10.1259/bjr.20200894.
40. Pawade T, Clavel M-A, Tribouilloy C, Dreyfus J, Mathieu T, Tastet L, et al. Computed tomography aortic valve calcium scoring in patients with aortic stenosis. Circ Cardiovasc Imaging [Internet]. 2018;11(3). https://www.ahajournals.org/doi/10.1161/CIRCIMAGING.117.007146.
41. Burton J, Rutty G. In: Burton JL, Rutty G, editors. The hospital autopsy [Internet]. 3rd ed. London: CRC Press; 2010. https://www.routledge.com/The-Hospital-Autopsy-A-Manual-of-Fundamental-Autopsy-Practice-Third-Edition/Burton-Rutty/p/book/9780340965146.
42. Morgan B, Adlam D, Robinson C, Pakkal M, Rutty GN. Adult post-mortem imaging in traumatic and cardiorespiratory death and its relation to clinical radiological imaging. Br J Radiol [Internet]. 2014;87(1036):20130662. http://www.birpublications.org/doi/10.1259/bjr.20130662.

Post Mortem Computed Tomography of the Abdomen and Pelvis

9

Introduction

The combined abdominal and pelvic cavities can present a challenge to interpret on post mortem computed tomography (PMCT), as there are many false-positive and false-negative findings to consider [1, 2]. Indeed, there is considerable overlap between the normal (decomposition-related) gas patterns and the findings that indicate true pathology. It is important to appreciate that, as decomposition progresses, the diagnostic potential of the scan also reduces in a progressive manner. This situation can result in decreasing confidence with interpretation and requires a degree of caution and judgement from the reporter. Scanning as early as possible after death is preferred as this will mitigate some of the post mortem effects.

As known from clinical practice, abdominal viscera are difficult to assess without intravenous (IV) contrast. As such, it is important to realise that a number of findings in the abdomen may be difficult to appreciate or even completely overlooked at PMCT. This stands true even without decomposition changes. In addition, if there is paucity of intra-abdominal body fat, the contrast between normal body tissues is reduced and further diminishes visceral definition (Fig. 9.1).

Causes of death in this cavity are however less frequent than those seen in the chest and particularly uncommon with no history of abdominal symptoms. However, when sudden or unexpected, they are often visibly catastrophic and unequivocal, such as a fatal rupture of the abdominal aorta.

Autopsy of the Abdomen: The Pathologist's Perspective

Pathologists tend to work in terms of cavities, often regarding the abdomen and the pelvis as two discrete zones of tissues. The oesophagus clearly falls into the thoracic compartment but may be left intact with the abdominal block. Dissection of all these

A. Shenton et al., *Post Mortem CT for Non-Suspicious Adult Deaths*,
https://doi.org/10.1007/978-3-030-70829-0_9

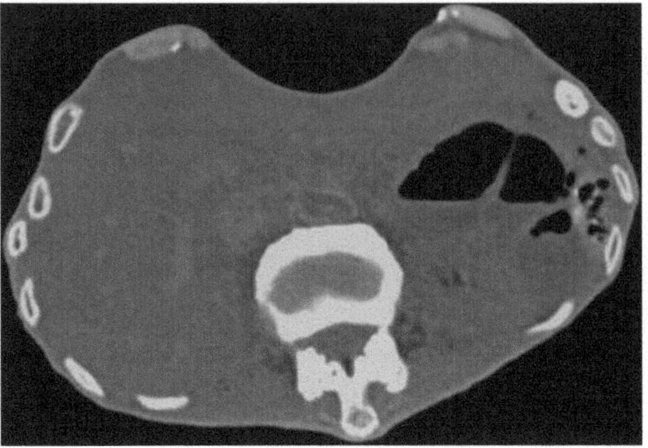

Fig. 9.1 Axial view of the upper abdomen on soft tissue windows showing poor intra-abdominal definition secondary to both the lack of intravenous contrast and intra-abdominal fat. Note the 'scaphoid' cross-sectional profile of the anterior abdominal wall

tissues varies depending on the needs of the case. For example, cases limited to the chest will include the oesophagus but not any of the abdominal viscera.

However, if the abdomen and pelvis do require dissection, then these tissues are removed in one piece along with retroperitoneal compartment elements. Clearly, peritonitis, fluid collections and disseminated cancer (omental cake) should be evident at the point the initial examination is made.

Once the abdomen is open, the jejunum is transected and the bowels are removed progressively by incisions into the fatty mesentery permitting tissue removal en bloc. Visual inspection and palpation are usually all that is required, as tumours with stenosis and diverticular disease are usually quite evident, requiring only localised opening of the bowel lumen. The bowels rarely require complete opening and washout unless the cases involve diffuse mucosal disease.

The remaining tissues can be dealt with in various ways. One could start with the pelvic content after checking the aorta and inferior vena cava. The prostate and bladder (males) or uterus, tubes, ovaries and bladder (females) require direct incision and inspection.

The kidneys are incised along their long axis so that the pelvis can be explored and the ureter traced, if necessary. At this point, the adrenals are normally checked and weighed if significantly large or small.

The upper gastro-intestinal tissues generally are examined initially from the posterior/inferior aspect so that the gall bladder is identified and opened. The common bile duct may be explored in obstruction cases. The spleen is often removed at the time of studying the liver, with consideration of the size and cut surface parenchyma. Any lymphadenopathy should be sampled for histology and may require microbiological testing. Subsequently, the liver can be removed and weighed separately. This allows the stomach (sometimes with the oesophagus still attached) to be opened along the greater curve, through the pylorus into the duodenum. Stomach content may be removed for toxicology analysis at this point. The mucosal content should be considered in terms of haemorrhage and mass lesions. Lifting the stomach upwards and cranially allows the pancreas to be checked and explored, usually by serial transverse slices.

At this point, it should be remembered that the vertebral bone is exposed. Sampling of the marrow compartment is possible by means of sawcut into the vertebral block and removal of a specific section for decalcification and histology.

Histological sampling for the various solid organs and viscera is variably untaken as part of the autopsy, although kidney and liver are common biopsy sites. Photography may be of benefit in some cases as part of the record.

Normal PMCT Findings

Solid Abdominal Viscera

In a body with a reasonable amount of intra-abdominal fat, inherent tissue contrast allows for pragmatic assessment of visceral size and contour (Figs. 9.2, 9.3, and 9.4). This analysis may also demonstrate a surrounding abnormality, such as haemorrhage, inflammatory change or fibrosis. The solid viscera can be recognised for some time post mortem, although they gradually fill with decomposition gas until

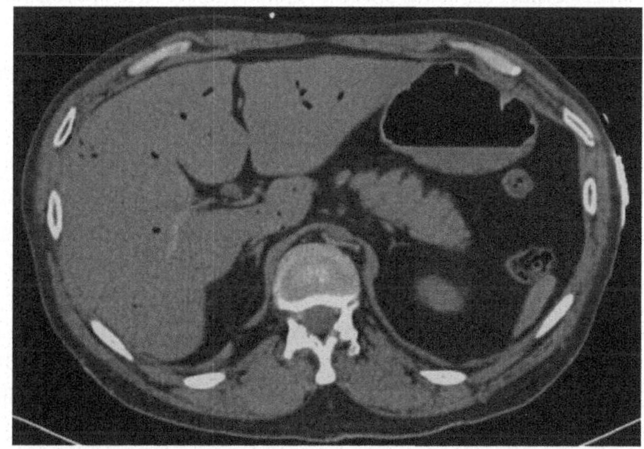

Fig. 9.2 Axial view of the upper abdomen on soft tissue windows shows intra-abdominal fat outlining normal tissues such as the liver, adrenal glands and collapsed aorta

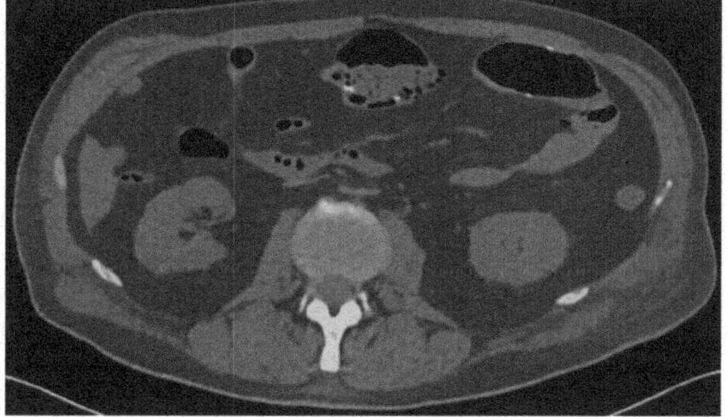

Fig. 9.3 Axial view of the mid-abdomen on soft tissue windows shows intra-abdominal fat outlining normal tissues such as the kidneys and retroperitoneum, collapsed IVC and aorta

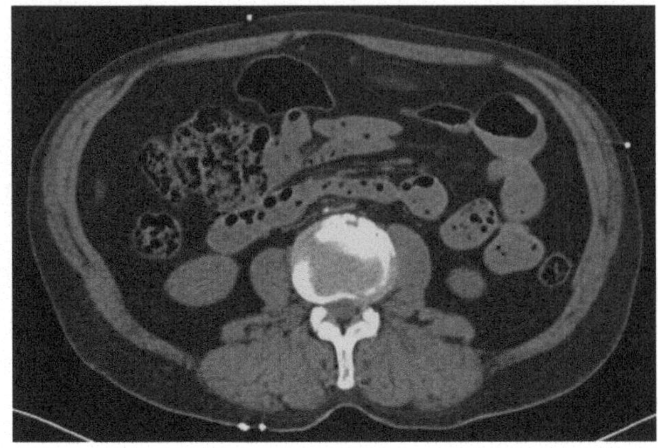

Fig. 9.4 Axial view of the lower abdomen on soft tissue windows shows intra-abdominal fat outlining normal tissues such as large and small bowel loops, abdominal wall muscles, collapsed IVC and aorta

the parenchyma breaks down and becomes one with decomposition fluid. Given that the abdomen and pelvis contain the bacteria-rich bowels, early signs of decomposition in the viscera are common.

It may be helpful to include maximum diameters or length measurements of clearly enlarged or atrophic organs, such as the spleen or kidneys, as a surrogate for organ weight (as might be obtained in open autopsy). Measuring organ density and volume in order to 'estimate' weight is possible with suitable software and may correlate with causes of death such as fatal haemorrhage [3]. However, it is time-consuming, subject to marked variability and probably not reliable enough to be informative in this setting. For example, in one small study it was shown that the liver can decrease in volume by up to 30% by 36 h post mortem, presumably due to passive outflow of blood and compression from the expanding bowels and lungs [4].

Autolysis and Gastromalacia

All tissues autolyse after death. Due to its early autolysis, the pancreas commonly demonstrates a surrounding 'haziness' on PMCT (Fig. 9.5), which may mimic true pancreatitis (Fig. 9.6). The pancreas is rapidly replaced with decomposition gas and soon becomes imperceptible in relation to its surroundings. The adrenals and spleen also undergo early autolysis, although their PMCT appearances remain 'normal' for longer.

Even in life, the stomach can be difficult to assess on contrast-enhanced CT, and the challenge persists in the post mortem setting. One additional post mortem issue is of gastromalacia (decomposition-related 'softening' of the stomach). This can present as stranding around the stomach and appear pathological (Fig. 9.7). Eventually, this causes gastric rupture, resulting in leaked content and a pneumoperitoneum, which is therefore potentially a normal (late) post mortem finding. Gastromalacia may also be the cause of small pleural effusions or pneumothoraces, as the diaphragm is not an absolute boundary, with the pleural space and peritoneum being linked [5].

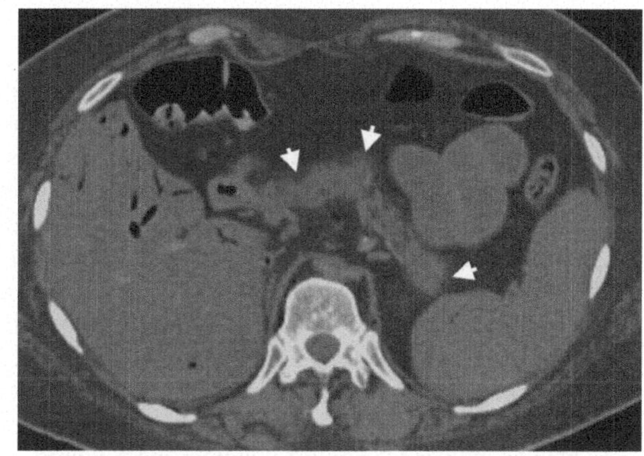

Fig. 9.5 Axial view of the upper abdomen on soft tissue windows shows peri-pancreatic haziness (arrows) secondary to autolysis

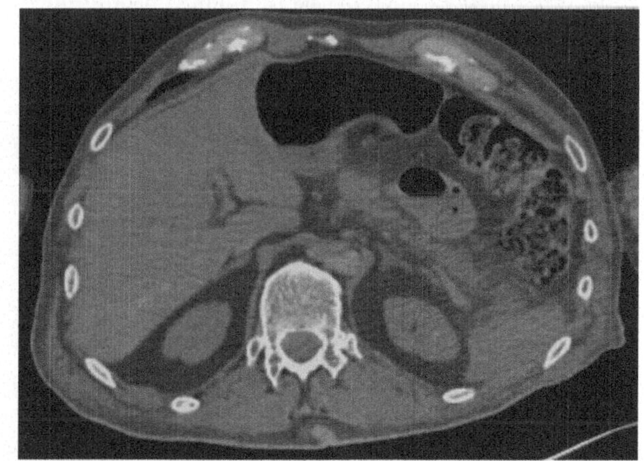

Fig. 9.6 Axial view of the upper abdomen on soft tissue windows showing peri-pancreatic haziness (similar to Fig. 9.5) but instead due to pancreatitis, confirmed at limited abdominal open autopsy

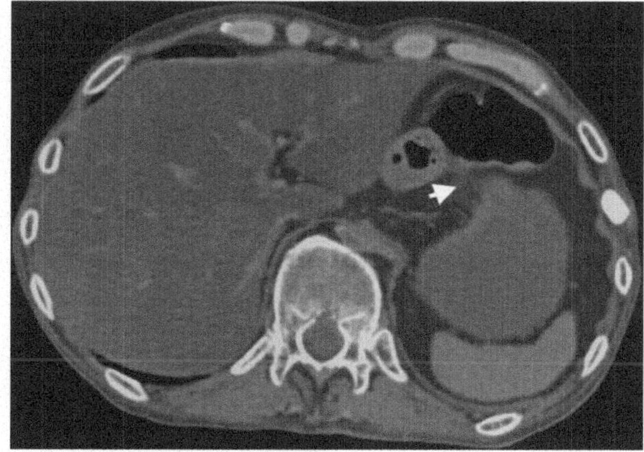

Fig. 9.7 Axial view of the upper abdomen on soft tissue windows shows a low-density (compared to the spleen) fatty liver in a known alcoholic. Normal splenic size and appearances. Faint haziness around the stomach (arrow) is in keeping with autolysis

Pelvic Viscera

In comparison to the upper abdominal viscera, the pelvic tissues (prostate in males, uterus/tubes/ovaries in females) and urinary bladder are often well preserved at PMCT (Fig. 9.8). As with clinical imaging, a basic assessment of size and gross appearances is probably satisfactory to exclude significant (cause of death related) pathology, although an empty bladder is always more difficult to assess. These viscera are rarely implicated a cause of death, unless they are the seat of malignancy—which is usually known from the history.

If a urinary catheter is present it should be noted, although the reporter should consider that its position may have altered post mortem. The presence of a catheter (Fig. 9.9) may well be an incidental observation but could represent a potential infective focus. In the non-catheterised bladder, it is useful to report the approximate bladder volume. Should toxicology be required, it assists the pathologist to know if the bladder is empty as suprapubic aspiration will be futile in this situation.

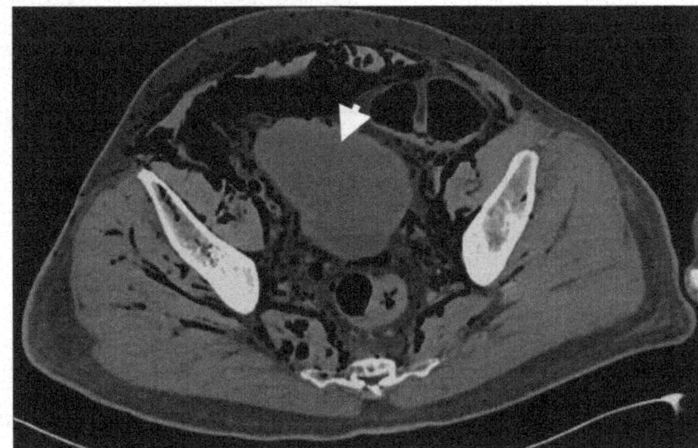

Fig. 9.8 Axial view of the pelvis on soft tissue windows shows the relative preservation of the urinary bladder (arrow) compared to the surrounding soft tissues which contain decomposition related gas

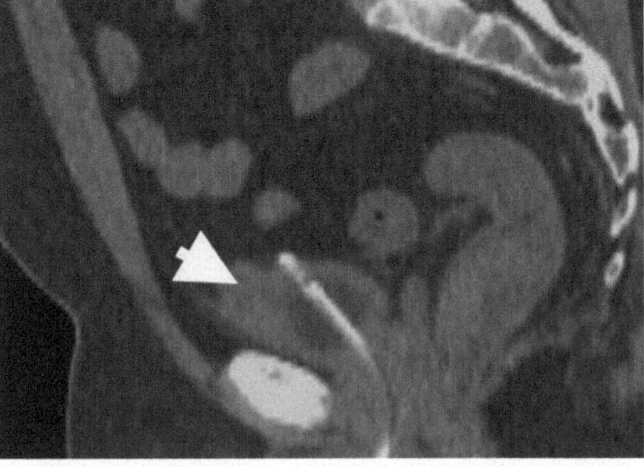

Fig. 9.9 Sagittal view of the pelvis on soft tissue windows showing an empty urinary bladder (arrow) collapsed around a catheter balloon and tube

If aspiration has already occurred, there may be a residual, but sometimes striking, gas track in the anterior abdominal wall (Figs. 9.10, 9.11, and 9.12) not to be confused with unexpected traumatic injury!

The presence of a pregnancy should always merit comment, being both normal and yet potentially relevant to the death of the mother. Fetal measurements may aid as a resource is assessing gestation stage. One should remember that non-pregnancy pathology, such as trauma and suicide, may be the cause of death. Generally, all maternal deaths will require open autopsy.

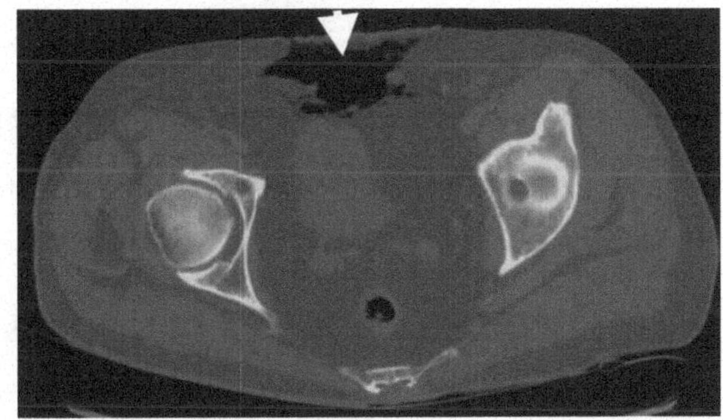

Fig. 9.10 Axial view of the pelvis on bone windows shows a suprapubic, subcutaneous gas collection (arrow) following bladder aspiration for toxicology

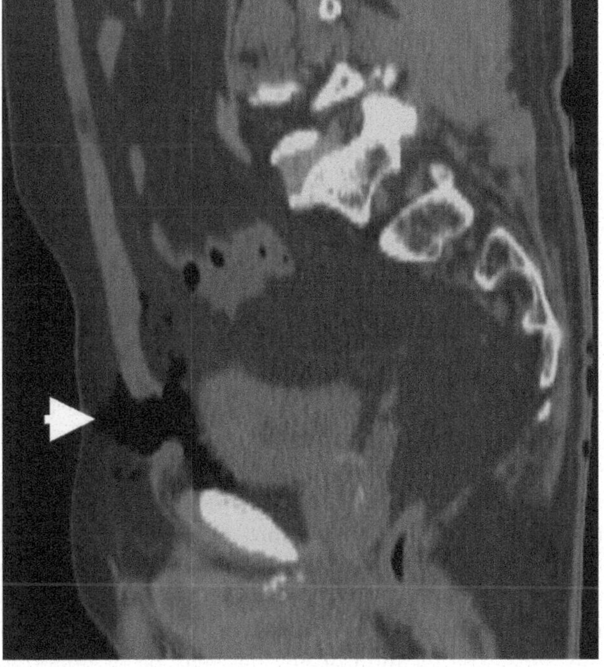

Fig. 9.11 Same case as Fig. 9.10, a sagittal view on soft tissue windows again shows the suprapubic gas (arrow) to track down to the partially collapsed bladder, following aspiration for toxicology

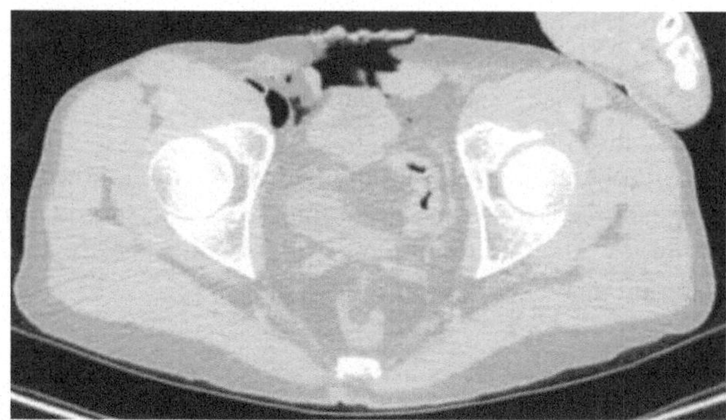

Fig. 9.12 Axial view of the pelvis on lung windows (different case to Figs. 9.10 and 9.11) most clearly demonstrates a suprapubic subcutaneous gas track following bladder aspiration for toxicology with no significant decomposition gas elsewhere

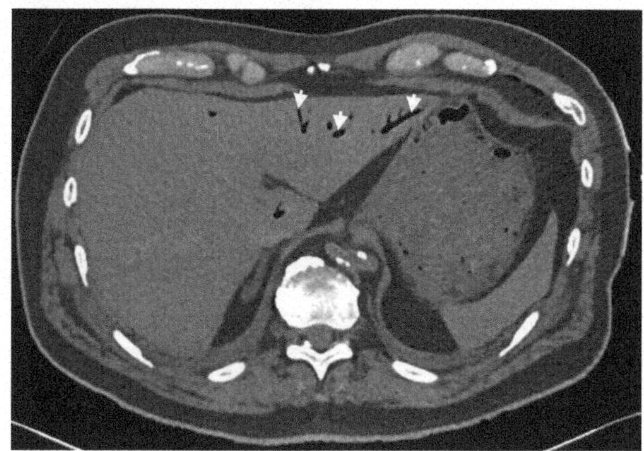

Fig. 9.13 Axial view of the upper abdomen on soft tissue windows shows normal post mortem decomposition gas in the peripheral left lobe of the liver (arrows)

Intra-abdominal Gas Patterns

Due to its high native bacterial load, the abdomen is usually the first location in the body to exhibit changes of putrefaction, such as gas accumulation. At external inspection, early putrefaction may be seen as bloating and a green tinge to the skin, commonly of the right iliac fossa (overlying the caecum), before becoming more generalised. Putrefaction may be rapid in states of infection or sepsis, appearing more prominent than expected for the post mortem interval and environmental conditions (see Chap. 3).

Hepatic gas is a common and normal early decomposition finding on PMCT, seen in the hepatic veins, arteries, portal veins, or a combination of vessels. It is usually seen first in the non-dependent (assuming supine position) left lobe (Fig. 9.13). With smaller volumes it can be difficult to localise, and so gas elsewhere (right heart, main portal vein, systemic veins or arteries) may help confirm location (Fig. 9.14) although, if judged to be due to decomposition or as a consequence of assisted ventilation/resuscitation attempts, its exact location is probably not of significance. The location of any gas may be of importance when pathology is suspected, for example, gastrointestinal distension or traumatic air embolism [6].

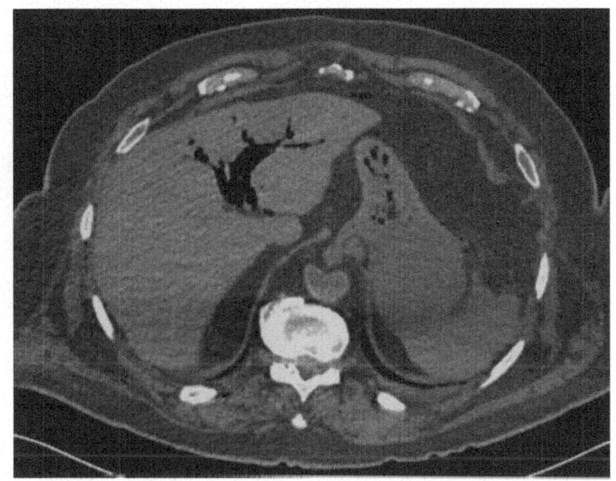

Fig. 9.14 Axial view of the upper abdomen on soft tissue windows shows left portal vein decomposition gas, this could be traced into the main portal vein

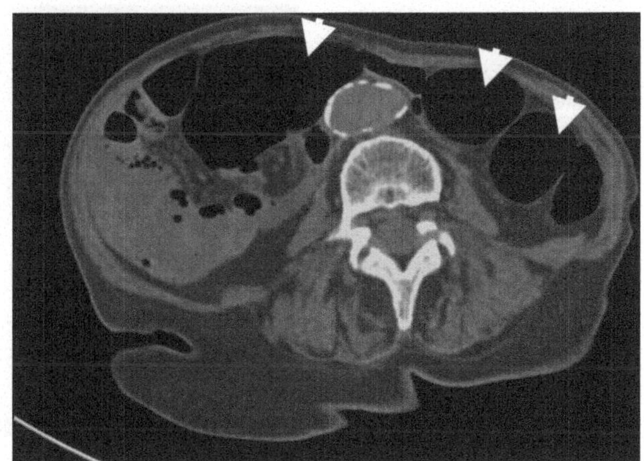

Fig. 9.15 Axial view of the mid abdomen on soft tissue windows shows gaseous distension of the bowel (arrows) due to decomposition. Note also a calcified abdominal aorta, partially 'propped open' by calcification but without evidence of rupture

Gaseous post mortem distension of the bowel is also very common (Fig. 9.15), and the volume of gas here can more than double in the first few days after death [4]. Intramural bowel gas can also be a normal post mortem finding, most likely to be related to decomposition (Fig. 9.16) but may relate to failed cardio-pulmonary resuscitation [2]. If bowel wall gas is present but seems out of proportion to decomposition changes elsewhere and unrelated to the history, the possibility of existing primary pneumatosis intestinalis should be considered although this is considered rare (Fig. 9.17).

Free intra-peritoneal gas is commonly seen with advanced decomposition, although this should always follow obvious visceral and vascular gas accumulation (Figs. 9.18 and 9.19) to avoid mis-interpreting true pathology.

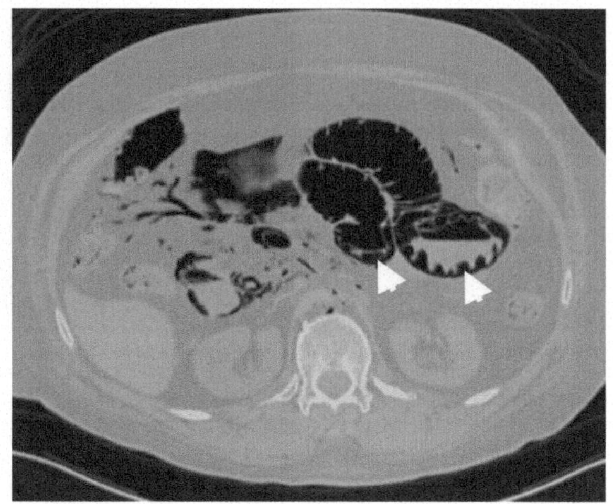

Fig. 9.16 Axial view of the mid abdomen on lung windows shows gas in the bowel wall (arrows) and mesenteric vessels most likely due to decomposition

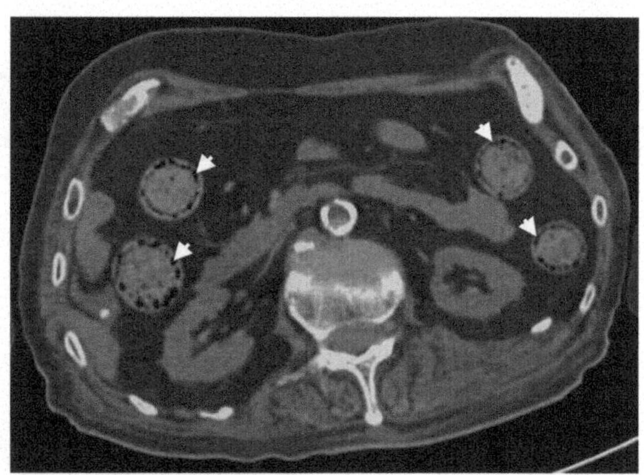

Fig. 9.17 Axial view of the mid abdomen on soft tissue windows shows pneumatosis of the colon (arrows) without significant decomposition gas in the vessels or elsewhere. The cause of death in this case was an unrelated acute pneumonia

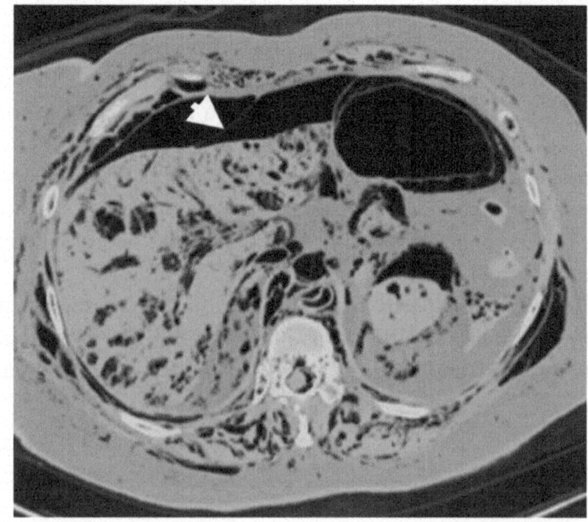

Fig. 9.18 Axial view of the upper abdomen on lung windows shows a moderate-sized pneumoperitoneum outlining the thin falciform ligament (arrow). This is judged secondary to decomposition given the extensive generalised visceral and vascular gas

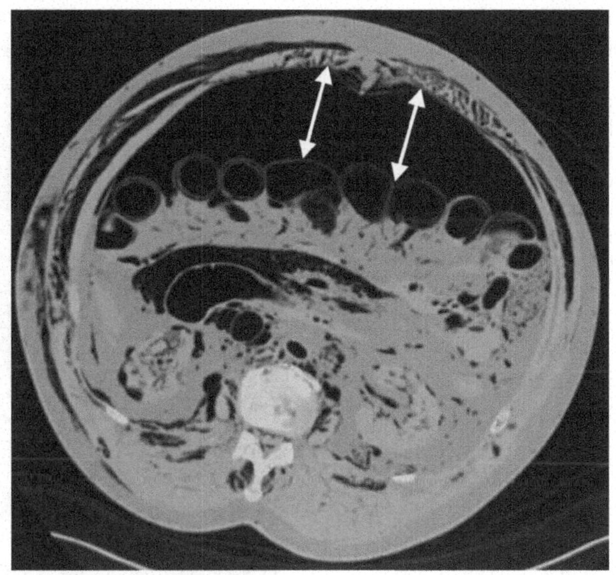

Fig. 9.19 Axial view of the mid abdomen on lung windows shows a large pneumoperitoneum with significant abdominal distension/bloating (arrows), bowel wall, vascular and soft tissue gas all secondary to advanced decomposition

Intra-Abdominal Fluid Patterns

A small volume of intra-abdominal or pelvic free fluid may be physiological (in a young female) or due to progressing decomposition following expected organ autolysis (Fig. 9.20). These post mortem collections should not be misdiagnosed as ascites or haemorrhage [1], with the latter being hyperdense (Fig. 9.21). Fatal intraperitoneal or retroperitoneal haemorrhage is usually extensive and unmistakably identified. Smaller haemorrhagic intra-abdominal collections may result as a consequence of chest compressions (see Chap. 11).

The presence of hyperdense fluid within the gastro-intestinal (GI) tract is notoriously difficult to interpret, as it can be highly variable and non-specific (Fig. 9.22). The bowel content varies in density from multiple factors such as food, medications (Figs. 9.23 and 9.24), previous oral contrast (usually in-hospital deaths) and, of course, haemorrhage [2]. Conversely, when the GI tract fluid is fatty or water dense, another potential artefact arises—the bowel wall can appear abnormally hyperdense. This may be a false-positive finding or, rarely and within appropriate circumstances, indicative of true intramural haemorrhage [2]. As such, much caution should be taken when assessing the bowel wall and its content, especially in the absence of anticipated pathology.

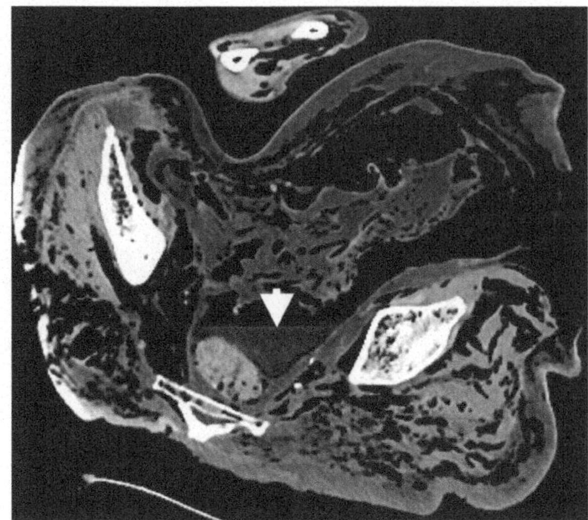

Fig. 9.20 Axial view of the pelvis on soft tissue windows in a moderately decomposed body shows a horizontal fluid level in the pelvis (arrow) due to decomposition, the density of the fluid measured a mean of −97HU i.e. fatty density

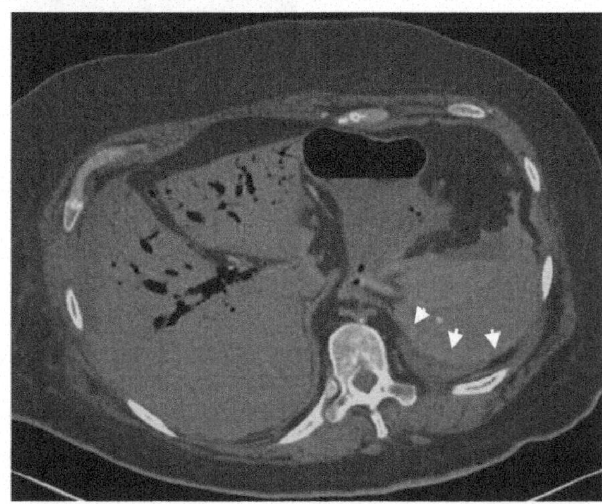

Fig. 9.21 Axial view of the upper abdomen on soft tissue windows showing a small haemoperitoneum, indicated by crescentic hyperdensity on the left (arrows), also note normal decomposition gas anteriorly in the liver. Findings were judged to be secondary to resuscitation attempts

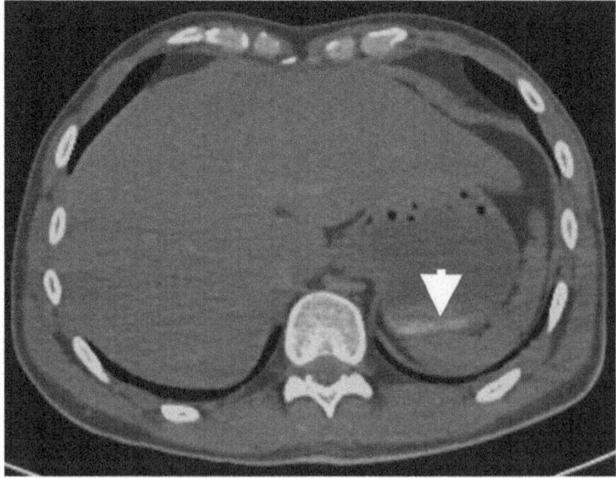

Fig. 9.22 Axial view of the upper abdomen on soft tissue windows shows non-specific hyperdense dependent stomach content (arrow). The given history suggested the possibility of drug intoxication. Findings could indicate partially digested medications but are non-specific, toxicological sampling would usually be required

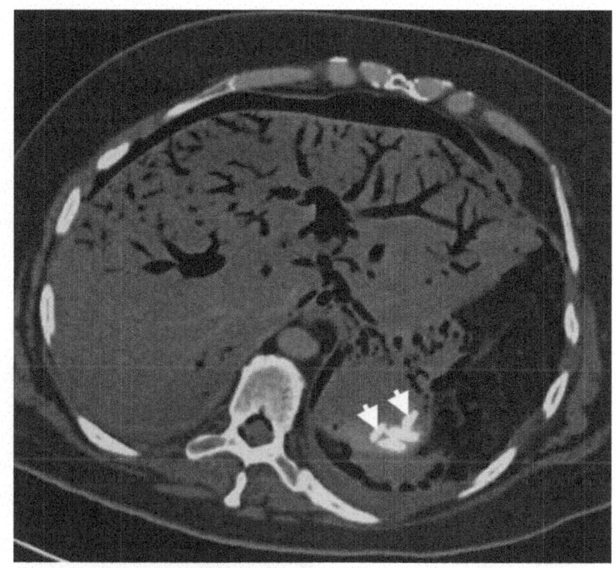

Fig. 9.23 Axial view of the upper abdomen on soft tissue windows shows multiple discrete densities in the stomach (arrows) indicating undigested tablets after an intentional overdose. There is moderate decomposition gas in the liver

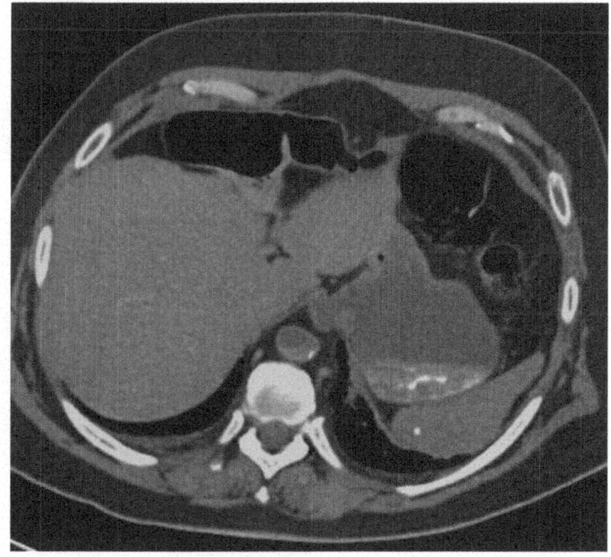

Fig. 9.24 Axial view of the upper abdomen on soft tissue windows shows heterogeneous hyperdensity in the stomach following suicide by overdose of antipsychotic medication. Whilst non-specific this may relate to partially digested medications

It is not defined exactly how the density of blood (which separates due to post mortem hypostasis) and decomposition fluid (due to variable cellular and visceral breakdown) changes over time. Therefore, the reliability of measuring the density of intra-abdominal fluids to accurately determine their nature is somewhat questionable and should be cautiously correlated with the clinical history and circumstances of the body after death.

Abnormal PMCT Findings

Ruptured Abdominal Aortic Aneurysm

This catastrophic cause of sudden death is readily revealed on PMCT. Acute haemorrhage from a ruptured abdominal aorta appears as heterogeneous (but generally high-density) peri-aortic stranding and retro-peritoneal haematoma (Figs. 9.25, 9.26, 9.27, 9.28, and 9.29). Occasionally, there may also be intra-peritoneal (Fig. 9.30) or intra-thoracic extension of the haemorrhage (Fig. 9.31).

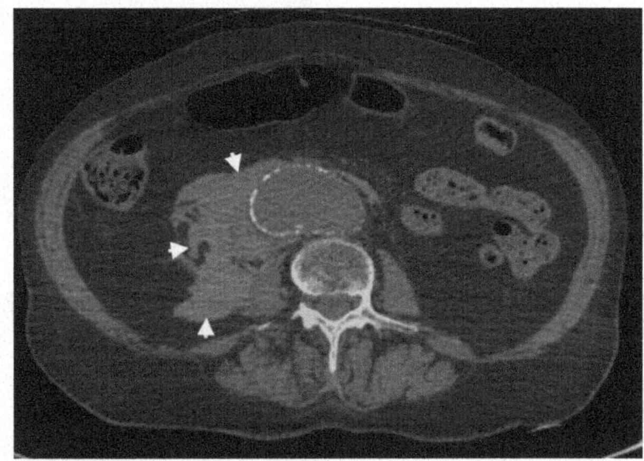

Fig. 9.25 Axial view of the mid abdomen on soft tissue windows shows hyperdense peri-aortic haemorrhagic stranding and right retro-peritoneal haematoma (arrows) from a ruptured abdominal aortic aneurysm. The aorta is outlined by mural calcification

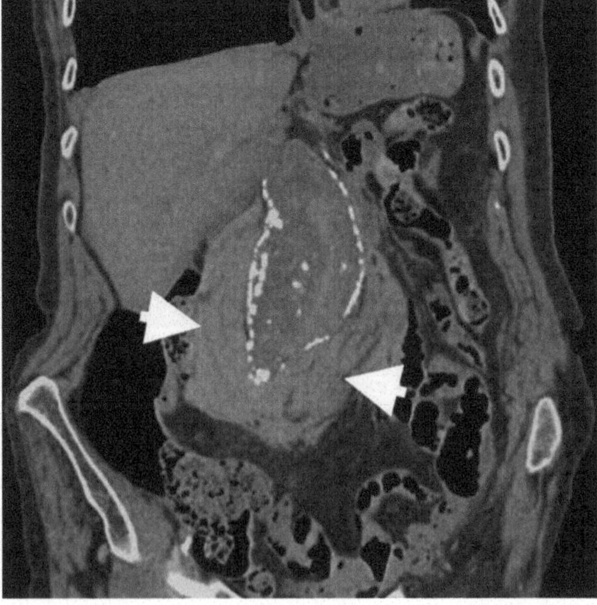

Fig. 9.26 Coronal view of the abdomen on soft tissue windows showing bilateral retro-peritoneal haematoma (arrows) around a heavily calcified, ruptured abdominal aortic aneurysm

The observation that other major vessels are collapsed might also indirectly support a diagnosis of significant haemorrhage, but it must be remembered that on PMCT the vessels, including the aorta are very often at least partially, if not completely, collapsed (Figs. 9.2, 9.3, 9.4, and 9.32). In some cases, vessels and aneurysms partially maintain their shape and size due to the presence of mural calcification (Figs. 9.15, 9.33, and 9.34). The anteroposterior aortic diameter is thus not a reliable measurement to prove an aneurysm in the post mortem setting (as it would be in life), but in the absence of rupture, the exact measurement is of little significance (Fig. 9.33). An incidental aneurysm, highlighted by calcium and thrombus or fibrous tissue, should not be taken as fatally ruptured without very obvious secondary signs.

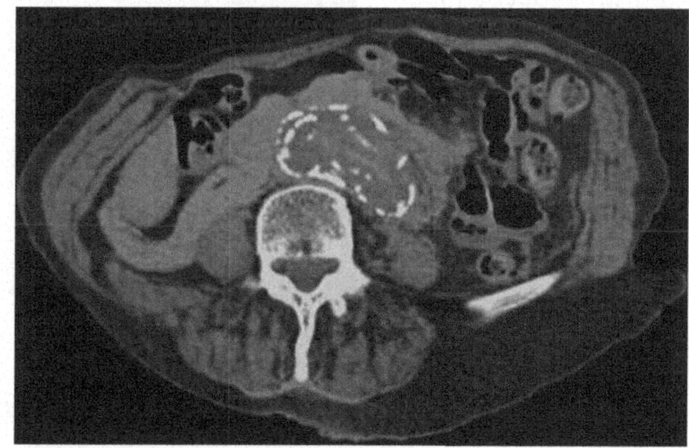

Fig. 9.27 Axial view of the mid abdomen on soft tissue windows shows hyperdense peri-aortic and right retro-peritoneal haematoma around a partly collapsed, calcified aortic aneurysm

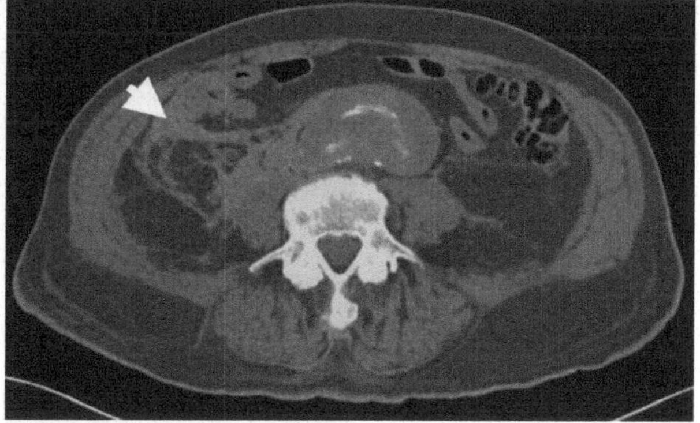

Fig. 9.28 Axial view of the mid abdomen on soft tissue windows showing a ruptured abdominal aortic aneurysm with extension of haemorrhage posterior to the ascending colon (arrow)

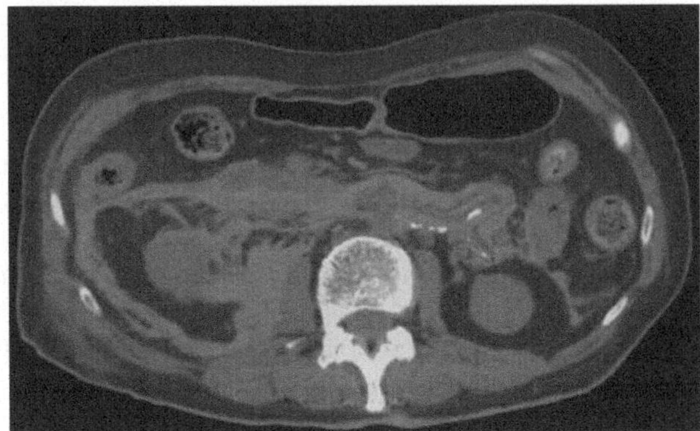

Fig. 9.29 Axial view of the mid abdomen on soft tissue windows shows extensive retroperitoneal haemorrhage extending through peri-renal and para-renal spaces, secondary to rupture of a now collapsed, crumpled aortic aneurysm

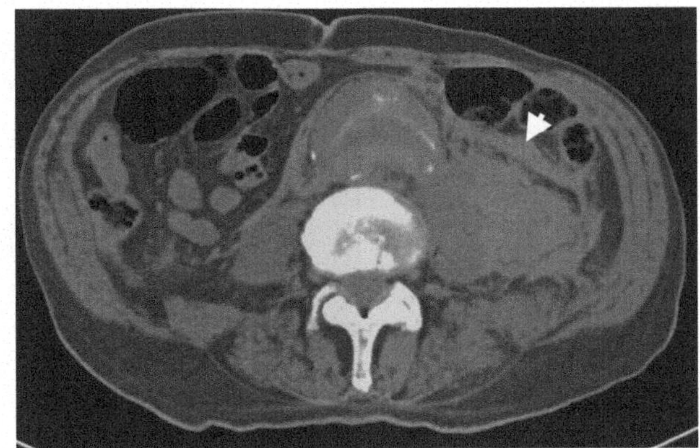

Fig. 9.30 Axial view of the mid abdomen on soft tissue windows shows a large left retro-peritoneal haematoma with intra-peritoneal extension resulting from a ruptured abdominal aortic aneurysm

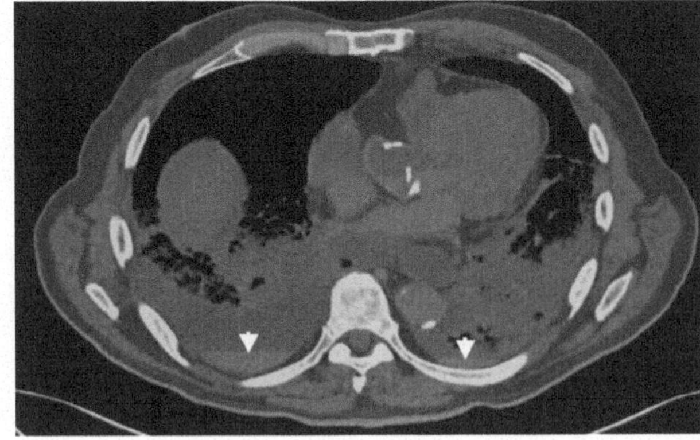

Fig. 9.31 Axial view of the chest on soft tissue windows shows bilateral, dependent haemothoraces with layered separation (arrows), following ruptured abdominal aortic aneurysm (not seen on this slice)

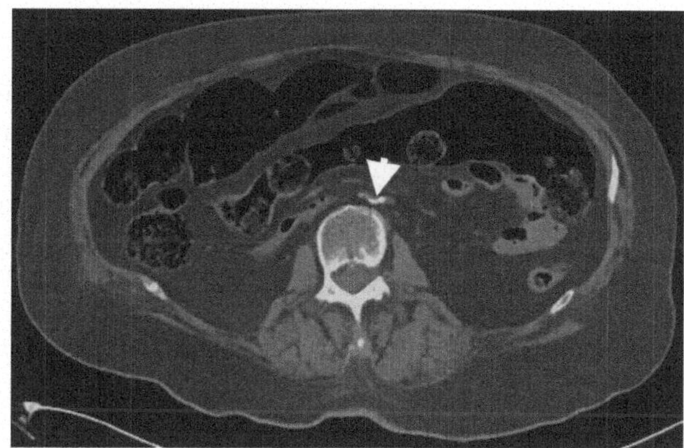

Fig. 9.32 Axial view of the mid abdomen on soft tissue windows shows a collapsed abdominal aorta (arrow), there is a small focus of mural calcification but no aneurysm or evidence of rupture

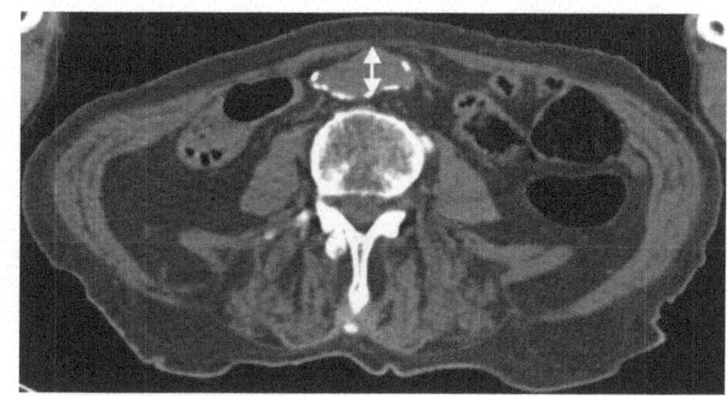

Fig. 9.33 Axial view of the mid abdomen on soft tissue windows shows a partially collapsed abdominal aortic aneurysm, diagnosed in life as measuring 44 mm anteroposterior. Post mortem the measurements were 22 mm anteroposterior (arrows) and 45 mm transverse

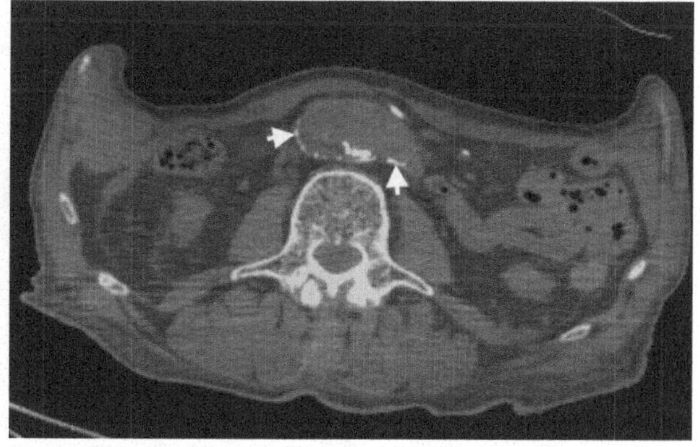

Fig. 9.34 Axial view of the mid abdomen on soft tissue windows showing a partially collapsed abdominal aortic aneurysm with multiple mural foci of calcification (arrows)

Hepato-Biliary Pathology

On PMCT, as for clinical non-contrast studies, the densities of the solid viscera are usually similar to each other. This is a recognised limitation in defining various pathologies.

Fatty infiltration of the liver, simple or hyperdense cysts and haemorrhage may still be appreciated (Figs. 9.35 and 9.36). More unusually, a diffuse increase in liver attenuation may be seen due to amiodarone use (Fig. 9.37), glycogen storage disease or mineral deposition (e.g. haemochromatosis).

Established liver cirrhosis is normally evident as a shrunken and irregular organ. Gallstones may also be visible on PMCT, with thickened gallbladder wall and surrounding inflammatory stranding suggesting cholecystitis. Rarely, resuscitation-related trauma can be seen with liver tears and local haemorrhage.

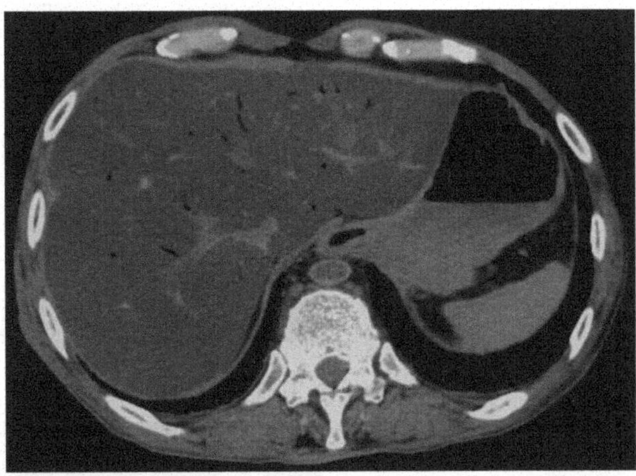

Fig. 9.35 Axial view of the upper abdomen on soft tissue windows showing generalised low density of the liver parenchyma (compared to the spleen), indicating fatty infiltration/hepatic steatosis in a known alcoholic

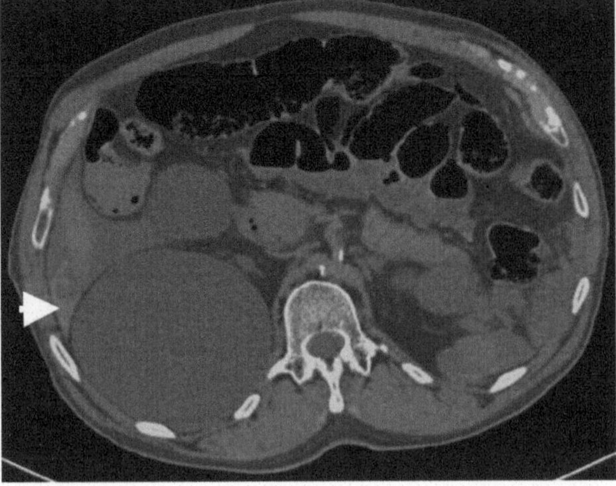

Fig. 9.36 Axial view of the mid abdomen on soft tissue windows shows a large simple cyst arising from the right kidney (kidney not seen on this slice) and adjacent small volume of right para-colic gutter haemorrhage (arrow) judged to have resulted from resuscitation attempts

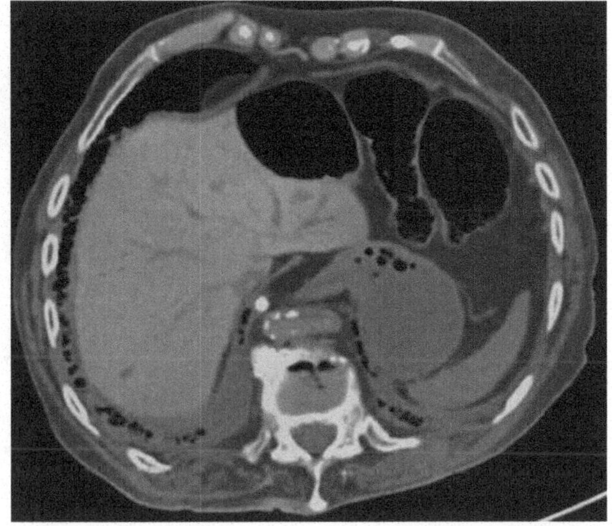

Fig. 9.37 Axial view of the upper abdomen on soft tissue windows showing generalised high density of the liver due to amiodarone use, correlated with the drug history

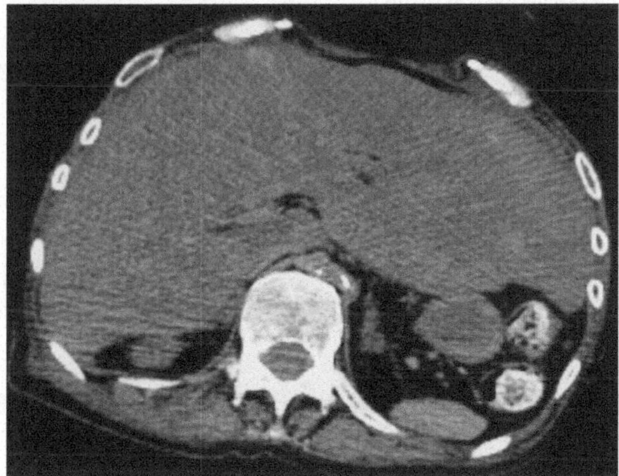

Fig. 9.38 Axial view of the upper abdomen on soft tissue windows showing an enlarged, subtly heterogeneous liver suggestive of multiple metastases (given that there was also a small volume of ascites and a suspected bowel primary). The patient had refused investigations in life

Unfortunately, pathology such as biliary dilatation, vascular thromboses, visceral infarcts, tumours or metastases may remain undetectable, unless extensive or sizeable (Figs. 9.38, 9.39, and 9.40). This should be kept in mind if such pathology is anticipated from the clinical scenario and the limitations of the study in excluding such pathology should be communicated in these circumstances.

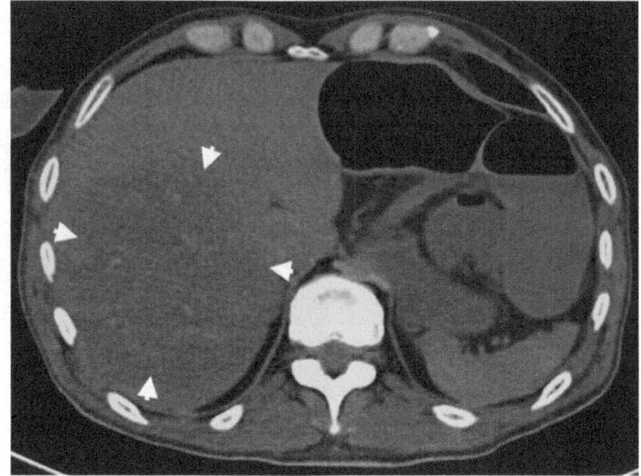

Fig. 9.39 Axial view of the upper abdomen on soft tissue windows shows a large slightly hypoattenuating known metastatic lesion in the right lobe of liver (arrows) in a case with a known rectal primary

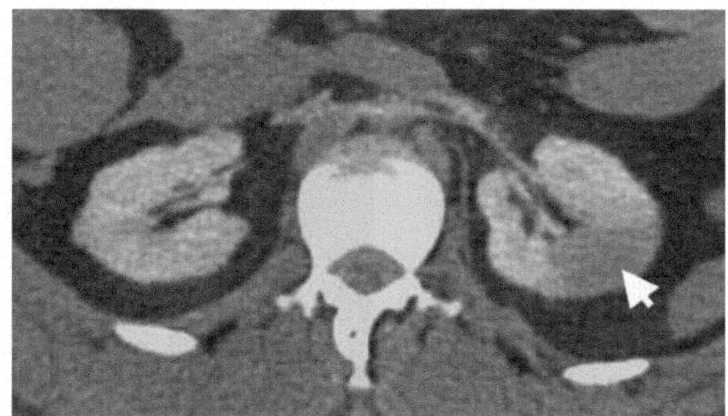

Fig. 9.40 Axial view of the kidneys on soft tissue windows shows a left renal infarct (arrow), clearly identified due to the presence of iodinated contrast enhancing the normal renal parenchyma. Contrast had been administered just before death, during emergency radiological intervention for aortic trauma

Intra-abdominal Inflammatory Change and Infection

In a body with a reasonable volume of fat outlining tissues and no significant confounding decomposition changes, the secondary findings that suggest inflammation and infection include visceral oedema (Fig. 9.41), peri-visceral fat stranding, fascial thickening, causative calculi (Figs. 9.42, 9.43, and 9.44) and frank abscess (Fig. 9.45).

As with any imaging though, infection may be apparent but clearly a causative organism cannot be defined without obtaining supportive microbiological evidence, or preceding in vivo cultures. With such findings, if there is an appropriate clinical history to support (or at the very least not contradict) an infective pathology, one may only infer 'infection' and/or 'sepsis' as the cause of death without detailing the specific responsible organism.

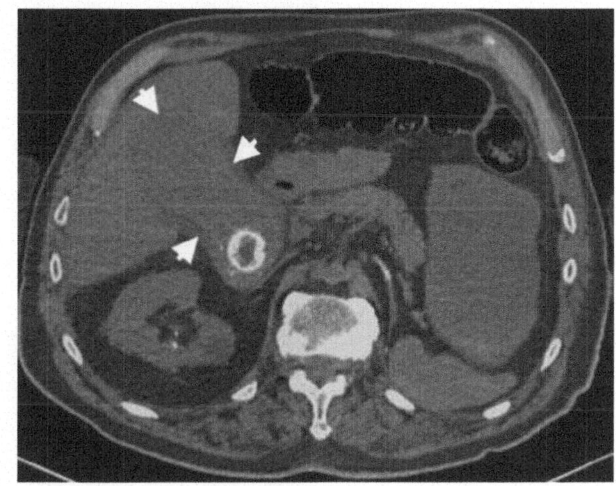

Fig. 9.41 Axial view of the upper abdomen on soft tissue windows shows a thickened gallbladder wall (arrows), in keeping with cholecystitis. There is a calcified gallstone in the gallbladder neck

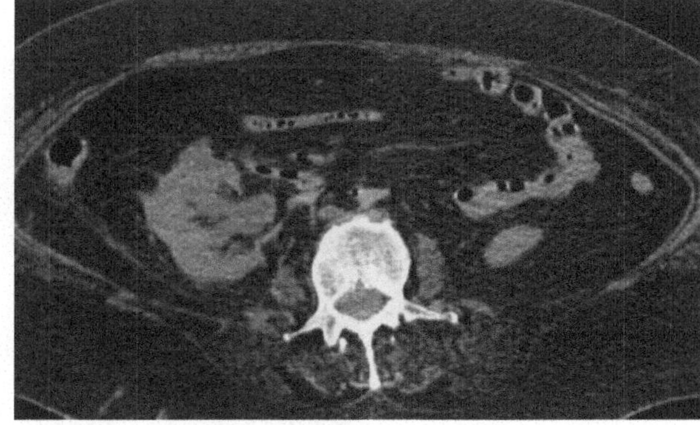

Fig. 9.42 Axial view of the mid abdomen on soft tissue windows shows right-side perinephric inflammatory stranding and mild hydronephrosis. The patient had abdominal pain and a rapid deterioration

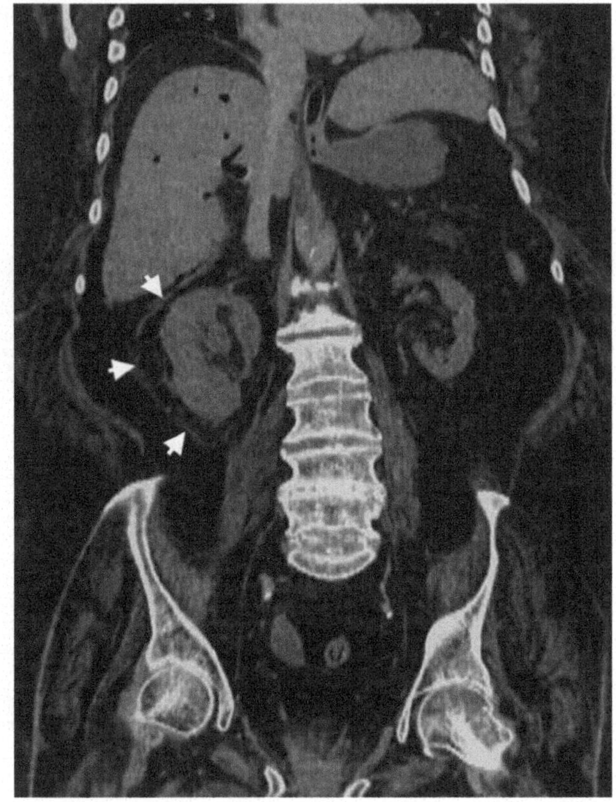

Fig. 9.43 Same case as Fig. 9.42, a coronal view of the abdomen and pelvis shows a swollen right kidney with perinephric inflammatory stranding and thickening of the fascia (arrows) compared to the left

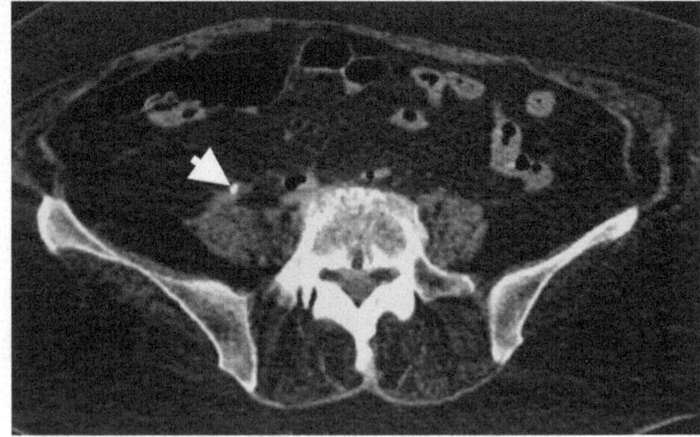

Fig. 9.44 Same case as Figs. 9.42 and 9.43, axial view of the lower abdomen demonstrates a right-side ureteric calculus (arrow) as the cause of obstruction and likely secondary infection. At limited open PM the right kidney was full of pus. Cause of death was therefore sepsis from pyelonephritis, secondary to obstructing renal calculus

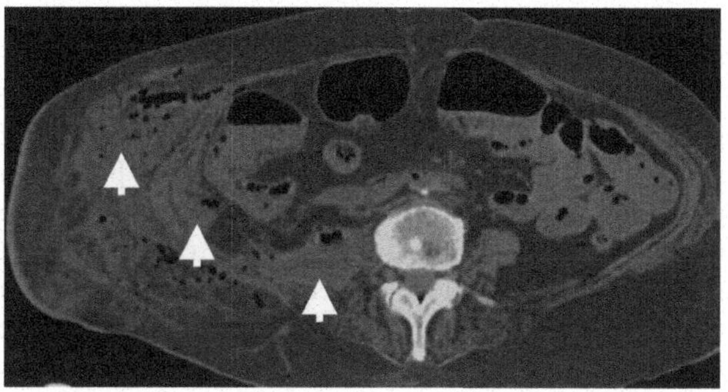

Fig. 9.45 Axial view of the mid abdomen on soft tissue windows shows a right retroperitoneal, abdominal wall and subcutaneous mixed fluid and gas collection (arrows) in keeping with extensive abscess. The exact origin was not identified on PMCT

Abdominal Neoplasia

In our experience, it is rare to come across unknown malignancies as a cause of sudden or unexpected death, and so this is an unusual diagnosis to make on PMCT without further investigations (Fig. 9.38). Bowel malignancy may present acutely with an obstructing mass lesion or perforation. Mesenteric and omental thickening is variably identified by PMCT as a marker for disseminated malignancy in the abdomen. This may be supported by a large mass within the pancreas, stomach or ovary as common primary sources. The presence of a large fluid collection would also support the diagnosis diagnosis of malignancy or hepatic dysfunction. Other findings in widespread malignancy may include liver deposits (Fig. 9.39) from lung, breast, bowel or pancreatic primaries, adrenal metastases, commonly from the lung and adenopathy (suggesting lymphoma or secondary cancers).

Correlation against the medical history is invaluable. Limited sampling (fluid aspiration, needle core biopsy or focused small autopsy incision and biopsy) serves to assist the final diagnosis.

The Pancreas

Given its rapid autolysis (Fig. 9.5), there is often minimal data derived from assessment of this tissue on PMCT, and it is important to be aware that normal changes can mimic acute pancreatitis (Fig. 9.6). However, benign and malignant tumours can persist for longer periods to allow consideration. Chronic damage (e.g. alcohol-mediated calcifications) may support background clinical data and tie in with cirrhosis in those misusing alcohol. The identification of cysts and pseudocysts may be variably confirmed, depending on their size and the post mortem interval.

Bowel Volvulus and Perforation

Bowel volvulus (e.g. small bowel, sigmoid or caecal) can be difficult to clinically diagnose, reflecting the variable presentations and yet can be rapidly fatal [7]. The supporting clinical history may be rather vague, equally applied to the post mortem setting and especially for community deaths. In the setting of suspected bowel pathology such as volvulus, free fluid suggests 'transmigration peritonitis', which in turn may have resulted in sepsis and death.

Bowel imaging in the post mortem setting is generally challenging, but, when present, the PMCT features of volvulus are helpfully specific and similar to clinical imaging. There is distension of the affected bowel segment (localised and more prominent than due to decomposition) possibly with associated 'coffee bean', 'beak' or 'whorl' imaging signs (Fig. 9.46). There may be associated rupture, leading to free fluid and pneumoperitoneum (Figs. 9.47, 9.48, and 9.49), although in such cases the distended bowel may decompress making the exact diagnosis difficult. Free air and free fluid are readily visualised on PMCT but are non-specific.

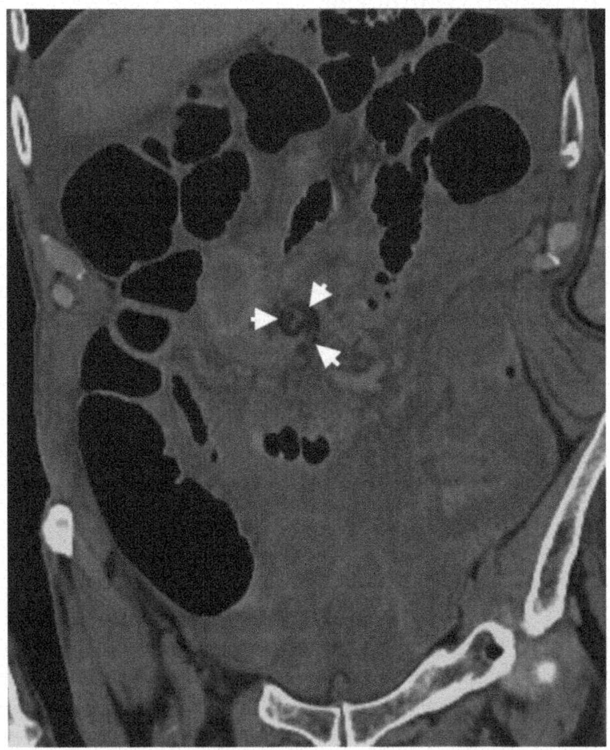

Fig. 9.46 Coronal view of the abdomen on soft tissue windows shows mildly distended bowel loops, free fluid and a central 'whorled' mesenteric root (arrows) in a patient who presented with acute abdominal symptoms. Imaging findings are in keeping with ruptured small bowel volvulus

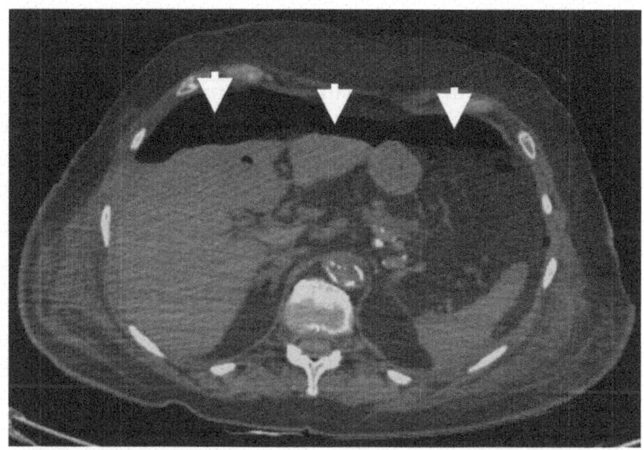

Fig. 9.47 Axial view of the upper abdomen on soft tissue windows shows an anterior pneumoperitoneum. The lack of decomposition gas accumulation elsewhere suggests this to be secondary to a pathological perforation

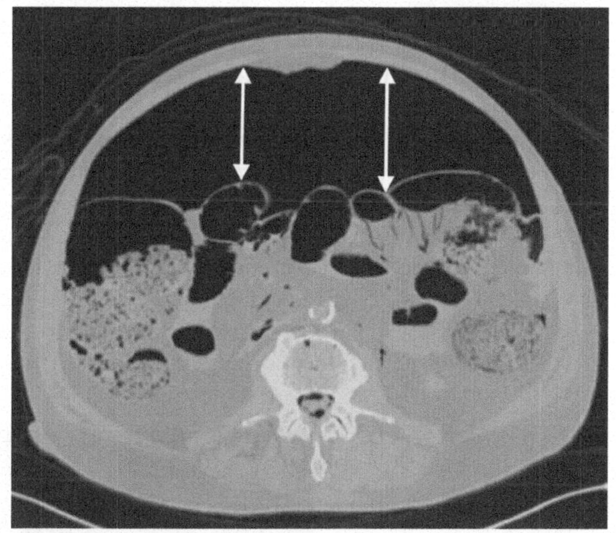

Fig. 9.48 Axial view of the mid abdomen on lung windows shows a pathological large pneumoperitoneum, distending the abdomen (arrows), with minimal features of decomposition in the surrounding tissues (compare to Fig. 9.19 which shows a decomposition related pneumoperitoneum)

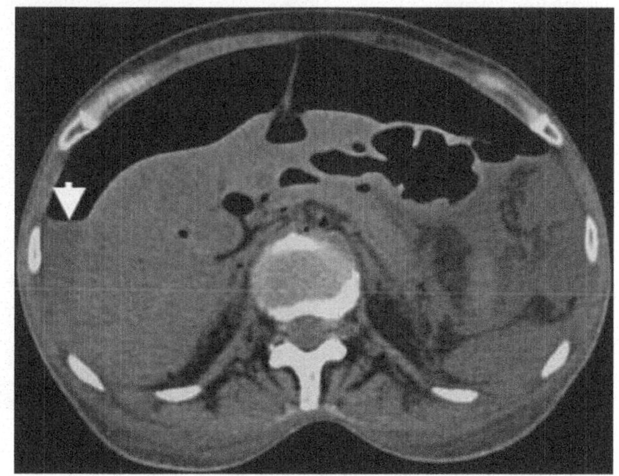

Fig. 9.49 Axial view of the upper abdomen on soft tissue windows shows a pathological pneumoperitoneum with the falciform ligament outlined anteriorly. Moderate volume of free fluid lateral to the liver (arrow) also suggests true perforated viscus rather than decomposition

Bowel Ischaemia

In clinical imaging, intra-venous contrast can be used to demonstrate bowel vitality, with abnormal, non-enhancing loops clearly seen. On PMCT, without such contrast, it is difficult (if not impossible) to appreciate bowel ischaemia unless there are secondary signs and/or a very high clinical suspicion.

Mural oedema and bowel dilatation seen in a defined vascular territory (e.g. superior mesenteric artery) and/or associated pathological gas pattern (bowel wall gas, portal gas and eventually pneumoperitoneum) may support this interpretation. Yet, these clinical hallmarks of bowel ischaemia significantly overlap with the normal and more common changes in decomposition. Consequently, making this diagnosis with confidence is difficult on PMCT alone. Without compelling history *and* imaging, a limited abdominal compartment invasive autopsy may remain necessary to confirm the diagnosis.

Gastrointestinal Tract Haemorrhage

Massive gastro-intestinal (GI) tract haemorrhage, seen as extensive hyperdense haematoma potentially with separation of blood products due to hypostasis (Figs. 9.50, 9.51, and 9.52), may lead to sudden death from exsanguination or precipitate an acute cardiac event from hypotension. Sites of origin include peptic ulcers, varices, tumours, aorto-oesophageal or aorto-enteric fistulae and may be suggested by the past medical history (dyspepsia, alcohol, medications) or presenting features (such as haematemesis or melaena). Consideration of any available clinical data and the distribution of visualised haemorrhage may allow a broad suggestion of the site of

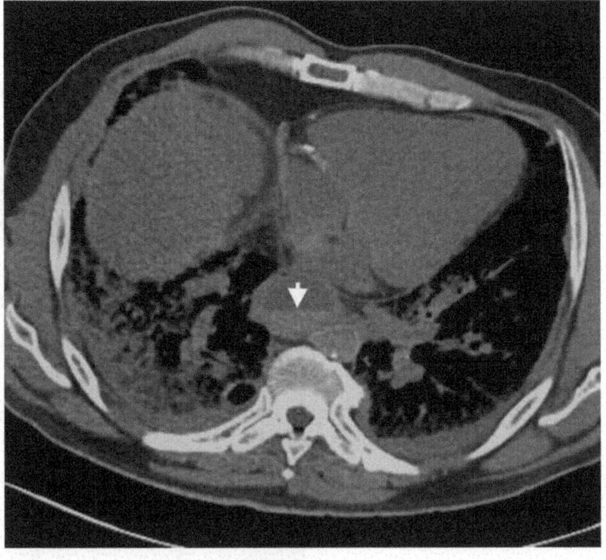

Fig. 9.50 Axial view of the lower chest on soft tissue windows shows haemorrhagic layering in the mildly distended oesophagus (arrow), confirmed haemorrhage at open autopsy

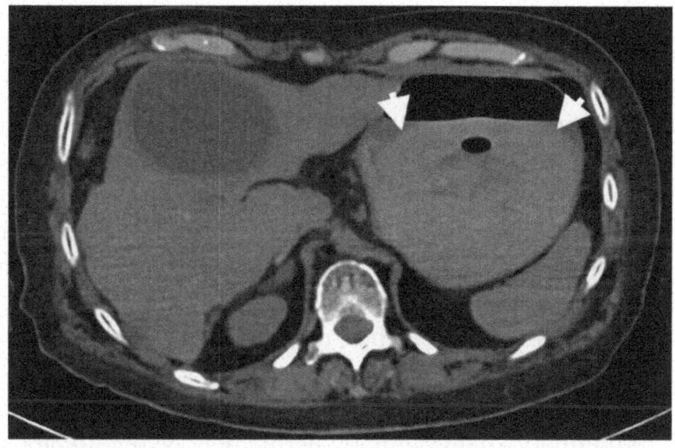

Fig. 9.51 Axial view of the upper abdomen on soft tissue windows shows a large volume of irregular, solid hyperdense gastric content in keeping with haematoma (arrows). This was confirmed at open autopsy. An incidental large simple liver cyst is noted

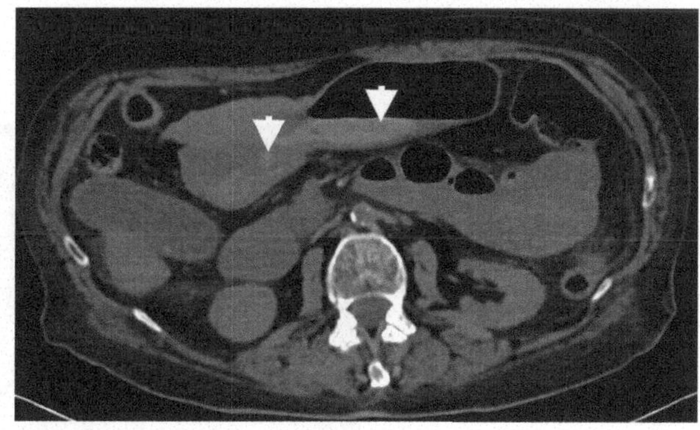

Fig. 9.52 Same case as Fig. 9.51, axial view of the mid abdomen shows further irregular haematoma in the distal stomach (arrows)

origin (gastric, duodenal etc.), *on the balance of probabilities*, although the exact site of haemorrhage may not be demonstrated on routine PMCT. A limited abdominal invasive autopsy may proceed although, even then, it is not always possible to identify the point of haemorrhage.

Abdominal Trauma

Compared to clinical imaging with contrast, PMCT generally has a low sensitivity for detecting intrinsic solid organ injury such as contusions. Significant/large injuries are detected with higher sensitivity and specificity (due to anatomic distortion, associated gas tracks and haemorrhage). Most life-threatening liver injuries, supported by the history and external features, can be detected by PMCT [8] making it, overall, a suitable technique for the post mortem examination of trauma.

Early post mortem scanning is helpful to avoid the confusion of traumatic gas patterns with normal changes in decomposition (Fig. 9.53). For interpretation of trauma cases, it is also worth noting that putrefactive decomposition occurs more rapidly at sites where bacteria have been introduced into the body by an injury.

Abdominal trauma, including that sustained during cardiopulmonary resuscitation, (see Chap. 11) may result in injuries of the liver (owing to its size) followed by injuries of the spleen, kidneys and other viscera (Figs. 9.54, 9.55, 9.56, and 9.57). Lacerations appear as linear low attenuation defects with, or without, visceral contour disruption, gas tracks or haemorrhage (which may be minimal in cases of external exsanguination).

Renal injuries often lead to retroperitoneal haematoma, which can tamponade, given the limited anatomic space. By contrast, hepatic and splenic injury can haemorrhage freely into the much larger intraperitoneal space with subsequent internal exsanguination. Pelvic fractures raise the possibility of bladder and iliac vessel ruptures.

Abdominal organ positions are usually well demonstrated within body fat, and so a traumatic diaphragmatic hernia may be readily appreciated. However, this may be more difficult to confirm if there is basal lung collapse, pleural effusion or haemothorax, especially on the right where liver density may match congested lungs and is not outlined by fat as the spleen or stomach may be [9].

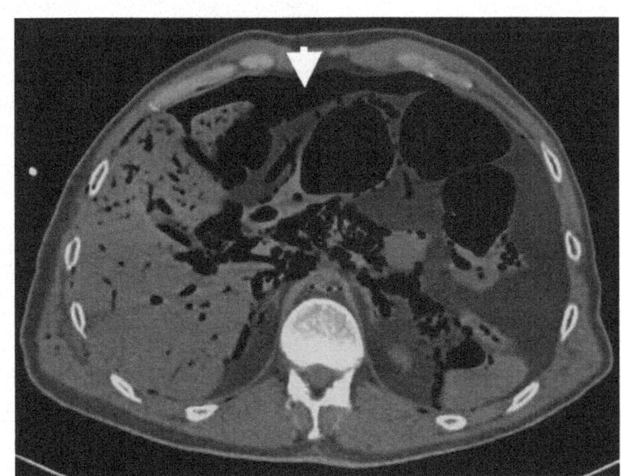

Fig. 9.53 Axial view of the abdomen on soft tissue windows shows a small pneumoperitoneum (arrow) following a road traffic collision. This was however judged most likely due to decomposition given the gas presence elsewhere (scanned 12 days post mortem)

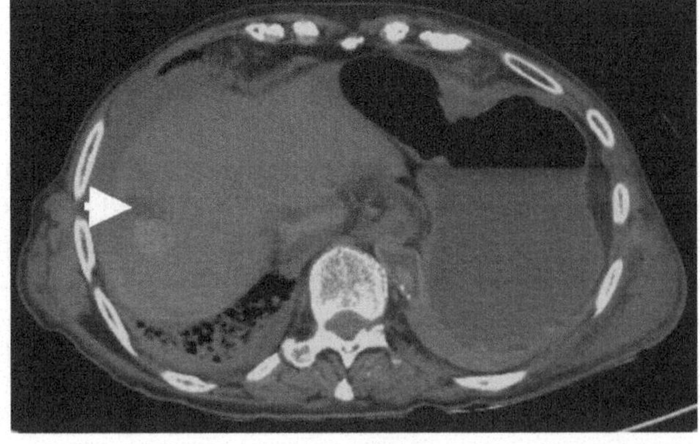

Fig. 9.54 Axial view of the upper abdomen on soft tissue windows shows a haemoperitoneum secondary to large traumatic liver laceration (arrow)

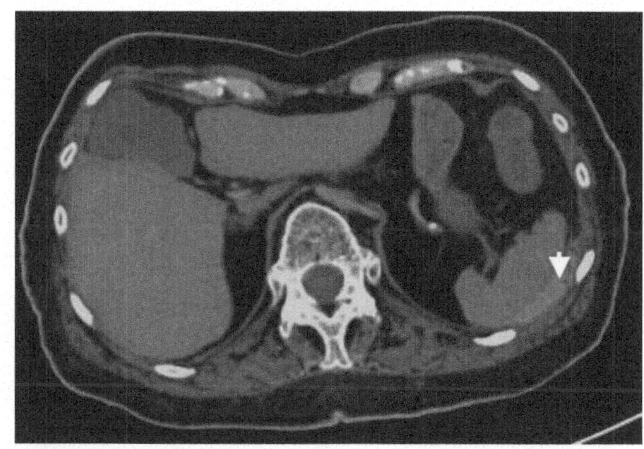

Fig. 9.55 Axial view of the upper abdomen on soft tissue windows showing small peri-splenic haematoma (arrow). This resulted from cardiopulmonary resuscitation with multiple rib fractures sustained (not illustrated). The cause of death was acute pulmonary embolus

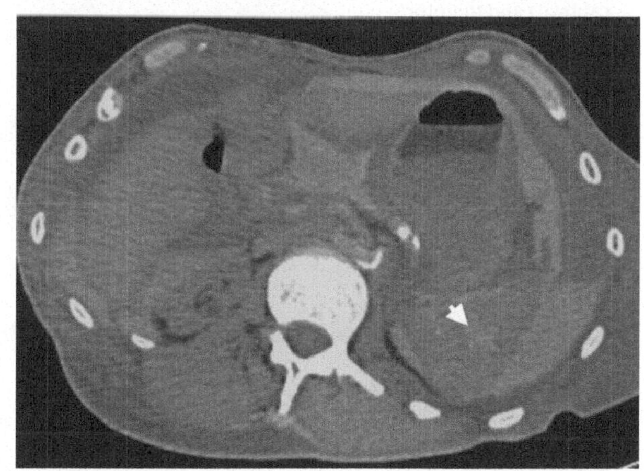

Fig. 9.56 Axial view of the upper abdomen windowed to show an extensive layered haemoperitoneum which also outlines a splenic laceration (arrow)

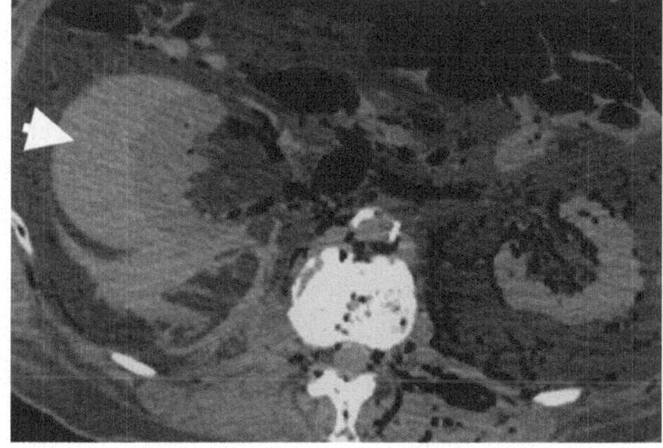

Fig. 9.57 Axial view of the kidneys on soft tissue windows showing a right perinephric haematoma (arrow). There was a presumed history of unwitnessed trauma in this anticoagulated alcoholic. Moderate background decomposition gas noted

Bilateral Adrenal Haemorrhage

This is a rare pathology which has a variable and often non-specific clinical presentation [10]. It is associated with states of sepsis, anticoagulation, antiphospholipid syndrome, trauma and surgery. Imaging findings are usually straightforward with hyperdense, swollen adrenal glands (Fig. 9.58), but the finding needs to be correlated with the medical history to form clear conclusions.

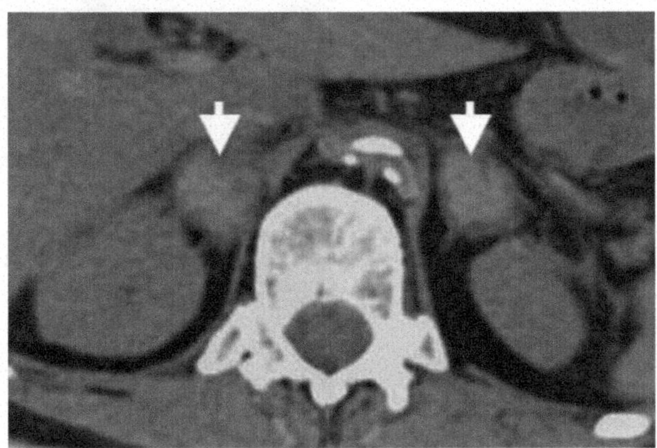

Fig. 9.58 Axial view of the adrenal glands on soft tissue windows shows bilateral hyperdense adrenal haemorrhages (arrows) in a patient who also had acute pneumonia (not shown) and therefore likely sepsis

Reporting Abdominal and Pelvic Findings: Pearls and Pitfalls

An initial assessment of the quality and reliability of the imaging, in relation to body fat and decomposition factors, defines the degree of confidence with which subsequent findings can be held.

There is significant overlap between normal decomposition-related gas patterns and those representing true pathology.

When the scan is adequate, fatal events such as aortic rupture, significant traumatic injury or pathological bowel perforation should clearly be evident.

Subtle findings, of both the viscera and bowel, can often be difficult to confirm to clinical standards and require careful correlation with all available data. Remember that causes of sudden or unexpected death in this cavity are unusual, compared to the chest.

Example PMCT report phrases:

- There is a small volume of retroperitoneal haemorrhage. In the absence of a history of trauma, this most likely relates to the attempted cardiopulmonary resuscitation.
- Peri-pancreatic stranding is noted, in keeping with autolysis.

- Generalised moderate gaseous bowel distension is seen, related to decomposition. No focal mass or transition point to indicate obstruction.
- Small pneumoperitoneum, small volume of fluid in the pelvis, visceral and vascular gas are all in keeping with decomposition.
- There is a moderate pneumoperitoneum, more than expected for decomposition, given the relative lack of gas accumulation elsewhere and therefore judged to be pathological.
- There is advanced decomposition with extensive intra-abdominal soft tissue gas largely replacing the viscera. There is no gross diagnostic feature in relation to the solid viscera or bowel, but no significant haemorrhage or osseous trauma is present.
- There is extensive retroperitoneal haematoma surrounding a partially collapsed, partially calcified abdominal aortic aneurysm. Findings are in keeping with a fatal aortic rupture.
- Generalised omental thickening and ascites, in keeping with the known history of disseminated malignancy.

References

1. Charlier P, Carlier R, Roffi F, Ezra J, Chaillot PF, Duchat F, et al. Postmortem abdominal CT: assessing normal cadaveric modifications and pathological processes. Eur J Radiol [Internet]. 2012;81(4):639–47. https://linkinghub.elsevier.com/retrieve/pii/S0720048X11000830.
2. Ishida M, Gonoi W, Okuma H, Shirota G, Shintani Y, Abe H, et al. Common postmortem computed tomography findings following atraumatic death: differentiation between normal postmortem changes and pathologic lesions. Korean J Radiol [Internet]. 2015;16(4):798. https://www.kjronline.org/DOIx.php?id=10.3348/kjr.2015.16.4.798.
3. Chatzaraki V, Verster J, Tappero C, Thali MJ, Schweitzer W, Ampanozi G. Spleen measurements with reference to cause of death and spleen weight estimation: a study on postmortem computed tomography. J Forensic Radiol Imaging [Internet]. 2019;18:24–31. https://linkinghub.elsevier.com/retrieve/pii/S2212478019300024.
4. Klein WM, Kunz T, Hermans K, Bayat AR, Koopmanschap DHJLM. The common pattern of postmortem changes on whole body CT scans. J Forensic Radiol Imaging [Internet]. 2016;4:47–52. https://linkinghub.elsevier.com/retrieve/pii/S2212478015300289.
5. Bolster F, Ali Z, Daly B. Postmortem gastromalacia. J Forensic Radiol Imaging [Internet]. 2016;5:70. https://linkinghub.elsevier.com/retrieve/pii/S2212478015000386.
6. Jackowski C, Sonnenschein M, Thali MJ, Aghayev E, Yen K, Dirnhofer R, et al. Intrahepatic gas at postmortem computed tomography: forensic experience as a potential guide for in vivo trauma imaging. J Trauma Inj Infect Crit Care [Internet]. 2007;62(4):979–88. https://insights.ovid.com/crossref?an=00005373-200704000-00025.
7. Baumeister R, Gauthier S, Bolliger SA, Thali MJ, Ross SG. Forensic imaging in an unusual postmortem case of sigmoid volvulus. J Forensic Radiol Imaging [Internet]. 2015;3(3):186–8. https://linkinghub.elsevier.com/retrieve/pii/S2212478015000519.
8. Christe A, Ross S, Oesterhelweg L, Spendlove D, Bolliger S, Vock P, et al. Abdominal trauma—sensitivity and specificity of postmortem noncontrast imaging findings compared with autopsy findings. J Trauma Inj Infect Crit Care [Internet]. 2009;66(5):1302–7. https://insights.ovid.com/crossref?an=00005373-200905000-00006.

9. Panda A, Kumar A, Gamanagatti S, Mishra B. Virtopsy computed tomography in trauma: normal postmortem changes and pathologic Spectrum of findings. Curr Probl Diagn Radiol [Internet]. 2015;44(5):391–406. https://linkinghub.elsevier.com/retrieve/pii/S0363018815000420.
10. Fatima Z, Tariq U, Khan A, Sohail MS, Sheikh AB, Bhatti SI, et al. A rare case of bilateral adrenal hemorrhage. Cureus [Internet]. 2018. https://www.cureus.com/articles/13145-a-rare-case-of-bilateral-adrenal-hemorrhage.

Post Mortem Computed Tomography of the Bones and Soft Tissues

10

Introduction

This chapter considers the skeleton and its related soft tissues in more depth, rather than as part of a body cavity. One should differentiate this group of tissues as the skeleton or osseous tissue (axial/appendicular) and the soft tissues of the limbs (mainly muscle, but not forgetting the skin and subcutis, nerves and vessels), considering each and also their relation to the body as a whole.

Post mortem computed tomography (PMCT) has the advantage of incorporating a complete body assessment of the bones, joints and soft tissues. This gives significant insight into the range and extent of related pathology, traumatic or other, in addition to the previously discussed body cavity assessment.

Causes of death relating to these tissues are commonly traumatic. Although trauma is considered 'unnatural' in relation to death, it can be 'non-suspicious'. It will therefore be commonly encountered as part of the investigation in a coronial/medico-legal setting. Examples include a witnessed accidental fall, suicide or a medical event with collapse that results in subsequent injury. If the deaths are not witnessed, one might reasonably initially regard such cases as suspicious (i.e. potentially needing forensic input) until proven otherwise.

It is important to have broad familiarity with assessment of the musculoskeletal system, as in contrast to most clinical CT ranges, the post mortem study usually includes from vertex to toes. Even without a history of trauma, the imaged skeleton and extremities should be examined. There may be unexpected findings that alter the evaluation of the case, for example those relating to trauma, but also infection or neoplasia.

Thin slices and multiplanar reconstructions are especially important, particularly when the body is not scanned in a perfect orthogonal plane (Fig. 10.1), although most bodies can be reasonably aligned in the scanner without issue. Reconstruction software will allow for manipulation of images to confirm bone integrity and alignment—particularly important for the spine (Fig. 10.2).

A. Shenton et al., *Post Mortem CT for Non-Suspicious Adult Deaths*,
https://doi.org/10.1007/978-3-030-70829-0_10

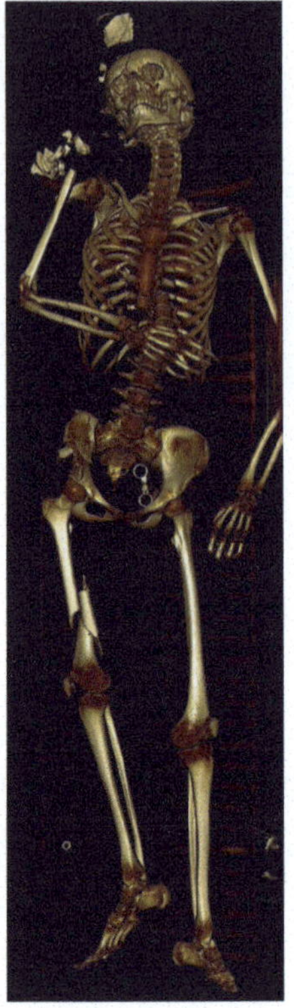

Fig. 10.1 Volume-rendered image of the whole skeleton demonstrating multiple fractures following major trauma. This gives an overview of how the body is positioned within the body bag at the time of scanning

The musculoskeletal and soft tissues are only assessed to a basic level in a routine open autopsy (as highlighted in the following section), as more detailed review requires time-consuming and potentially disfiguring dissection. Often, such investigations have a low yield of significant pathology to justify this.

PMCT may be sufficient to allow the omission of subsequent skeletal or limb dissection. Alternatively, when such autopsy is planned, it may provide a complimentary assessment or indeed guide the dissection.

Autopsy of the Bone and Soft Tissues: The Pathologist's Perspective

The osseous, muscular and soft tissue compartments are evaluated at open autopsy to a minor extent, when considering the standard autopsy technique which focuses on the main organ tissues (see previous chapters). Opening the body, by the standard incisions, requires the anterior rib plate to be removed by saw/shear cuts along with some of the chest musculature, in association with a longitudinal incision into the abdominal wall. This allows a macroscopic review of the alignment of the vertebral

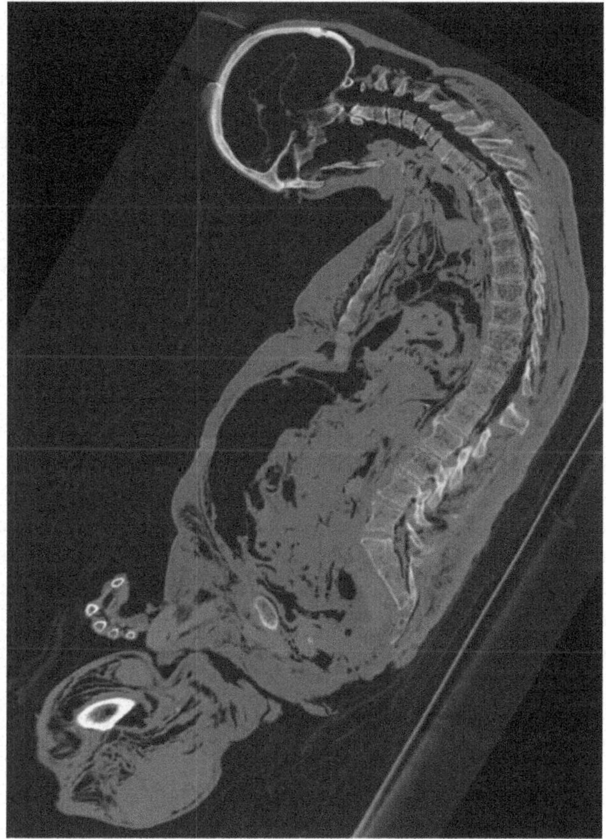

Fig. 10.2 Reconstructed view along the long axis of the vertebral column, on bone windows. This reconstruction allows easy assessment of vertebral body heights and alignment, even in cases of decomposition with abnormal positioning such as here

column, once organs from the chest and abdomen have been removed—and is normally all that is required in terms of bone assessment.

The ribs can be inspected individually by slicing through the musculature and soft tissue between them, thereby looking for fractures, haemorrhage and/or distortion of tissues (Paget's disease, tumours, etc.). Consideration of the marrow compartment, since most cases involve adults and the elderly, tends to focus on the vertebrae. This compartment is opened by means of bone chisel excavating through the coronal plane of the vertebral bodies, producing a vertebral bone strip.

It is uncommon to need to interact with bone fractures or undertake widespread skeletal dissection, unless there is a particular clinical issue to be addressed. An example might be a fractured neck of femur, with possible sepsis or poor fixation of a prosthetic device, prompting resection of the upper femur and the artificial hip joint in one piece. One should always be mindful of the issues of reconstruction in cases where body viewing after post mortem will take place. External fixators need to be removed during autopsy.

Some other devices with regard to bones also require removal. These include certain orthopaedic implants that have explosive potential during body cremation. There are similar considerations as to the removal of pacemakers, nerve stimulator units and other electronic devices, which also have a small explosion risk in crematoria (see Chap. 4). One, often forgotten, benefit of modern prosthetic devices is the unique device serial number and identification code, potentially permitting identification of a very decomposed body.

Small fragments of bone and marrow can be taken and subject to fixation, decalcification and histology, for example in cases of metabolic bone disease. However, since most cases of bone pathology revolve around standard osteoporosis and malignancy, this is rarely an issue. One should also be mindful of potential distal effects of bone injuries requiring special histology (e.g. stains on snap-frozen lung tissue to look for fat embolism).

The soft tissues (skin and musculature) are rarely considered beyond macroscopy, unless there is a specific issue that merits attention. Such cases may have atypical ulceration in the extremities, superficial injuries or possible neoplasia. In addition, one may incise the calf and thigh veins in order to consider if there are residual deep vein thrombotic elements in cases of pulmonary embolism.

Ultimately, each case deserves individual attention and consideration with the clear understanding that, unlike for imaging, returning to the body is rarely possible, one should always try to achieve all necessary tests during the autopsy.

Normal PMCT Findings

The Skin, Subcutaneous Tissues and Muscles

Although directly observable to a viewing pathologist, the radiologist may forget that the skin and subcutis are relevant soft tissues, which should be considered at the same time as the bone and muscle. Hypostasis is a normal early post mortem change that can be seen in the body and limbs on PMCT as dependent skin thickening and subcutaneous oedema (Figs. 10.3 and 10.4). Generally, such changes are symmetrical. As decomposition progresses, the skin can subsequently blister (Fig. 10.5) and eventually slip off, see also Chap. 3.

Sometimes, drawing attention, these decomposition changes may be asymmetric if one side of the body has been more exposed in the open or nearer a heat source (Figs. 10.6 and 10.7). A close review to exclude potential unilateral pathology (such as infection, malignancy or venous thrombosis) should be made, as well as consideration of the environment, before judging such findings.

The muscles may be broadly assessed for a normal bulk and symmetry, usually straightforward when there is sufficient body fat to outline them. Atrophy, hypertrophy, traumatic or mass lesions may be noted and correlated with the clinical history. Significant limb asymmetry may be commonly explained by a known dense hemiplegia, congenital abnormalities or unilateral degenerative changes.

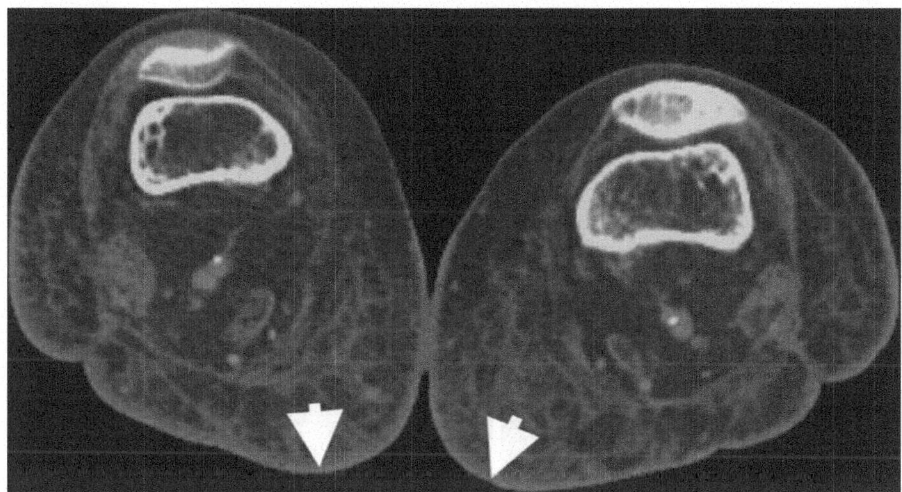

Fig. 10.3 Axial view at the level of the distal femurs, on soft tissue windows, showing dependent thickening of the skin (arrows) and subcutaneous oedema, in keeping with normal post mortem hypostasis

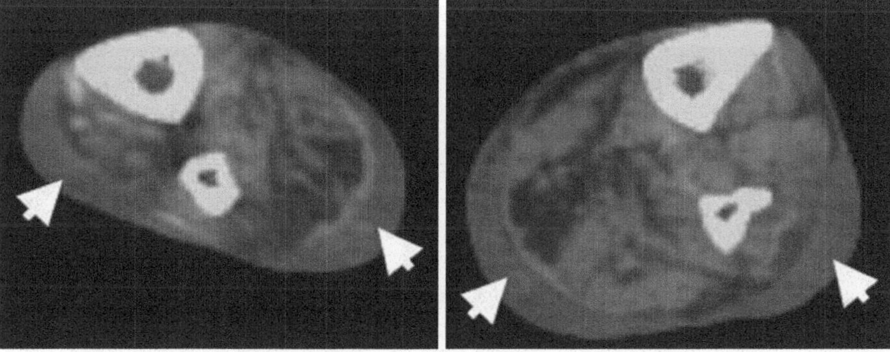

Fig. 10.4 Axial view of the lower legs on soft tissue windows shows dependent subcutaneous fluid accumulation with early blistering of the skin (arrows), due to decomposition. The legs are not seen at exactly the same level due to asymmetric post mortem positioning

The Skeleton

Unlike soft tissues, the skeleton remains generally unaltered for some years after death. Initially, decomposition causes gas to accumulate in the intraosseous vessels and marrow (Figs. 10.8 and 10.9), and this is not to be confused with fractures. The mineralized structure of the bones otherwise remains intact such that they can be assessed for pathologies akin to the clinical setting (Fig. 10.10).

There may be orthopaedic implants relating to joint replacements or fixation of previous fractures, unrelated to the cause of death but which should be mentioned

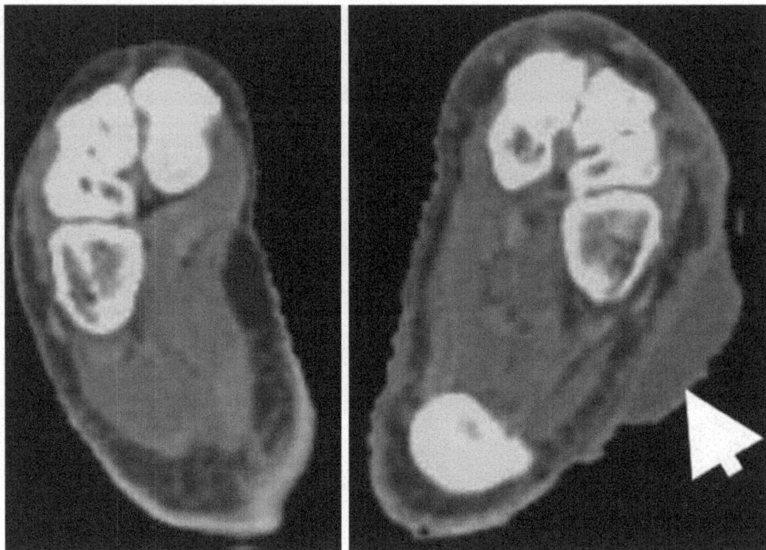

Fig. 10.5 Axial view of both feet on soft tissue windows shows thickened dependent skin due to hypostasis with additional left-side skin blistering due to decomposition (arrow)

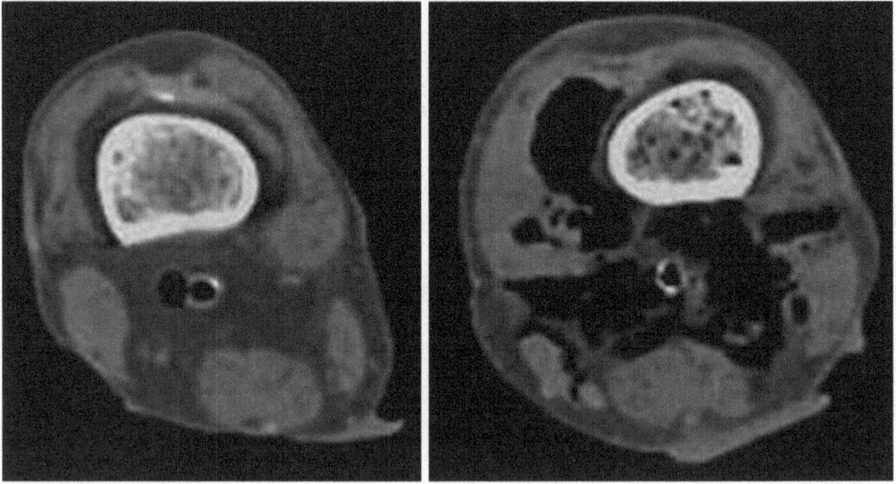

Fig. 10.6 Axial view of the thighs on soft tissue windows shows asymmetric decomposition, more prominent in the left leg where there is more soft tissue and bone marrow gas resulting in swelling of the limb

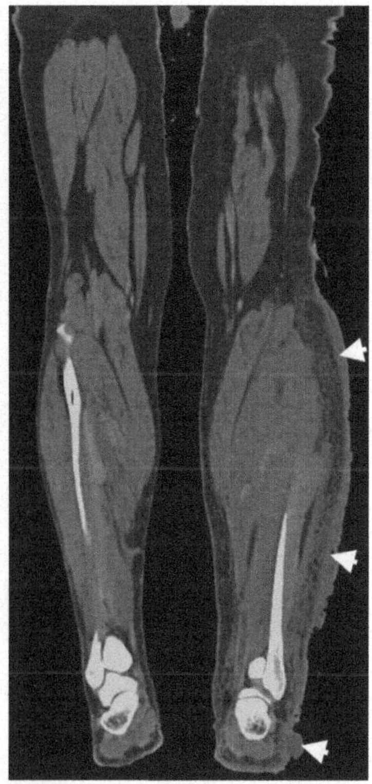

Fig. 10.7 Coronal view of the legs on soft tissue windows shows swelling, subcutaneous oedema and extensive skin blistering of the lateral left leg (arrows) due to asymmetric decomposition (the left side was nearer to a heat source)

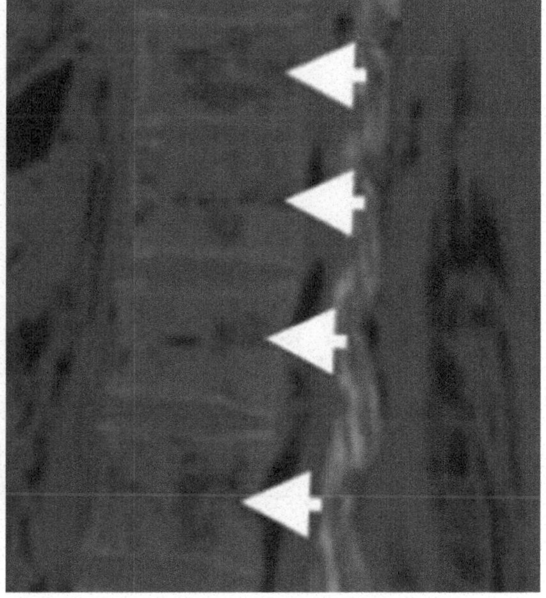

Fig. 10.8 Sagittal view of the spine on bone windows showing gas in the vertebral vessels and marrow (arrows), potentially simulating fracture/s. Decomposition gas in the surrounding tissues is also present

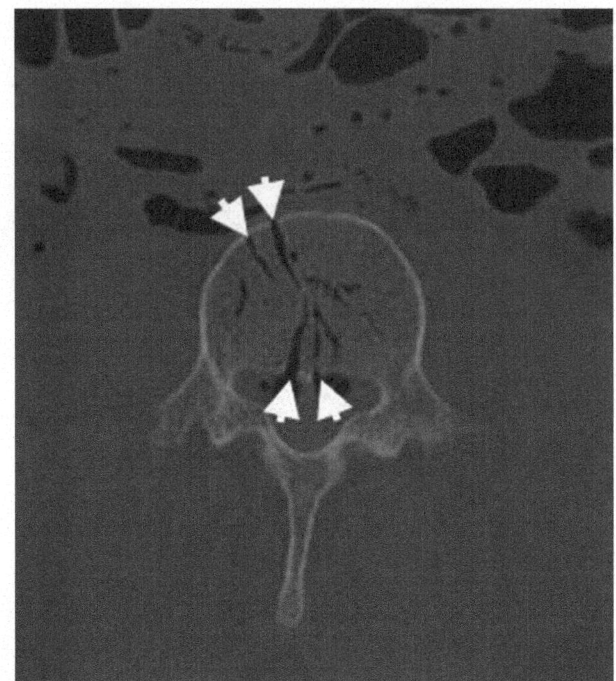

Fig. 10.9 Axial view of a vertebral body on bone windows shows linear decomposition gas in the vertebral venous plexus and marrow vessels (arrows), potentially mimicking fracture in the setting of trauma

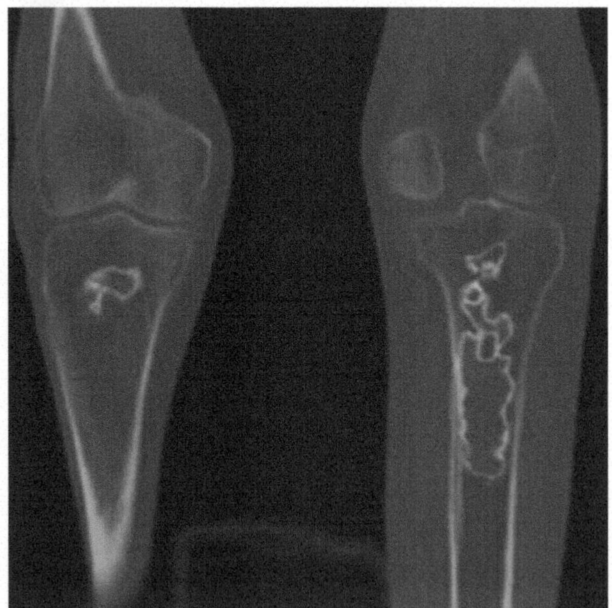

Fig. 10.10 Coronal view of the proximal tibias on bone windows showing incidental, bilateral bone infarcts of doubtful acute significance

for completeness and correlation (Fig. 10.11). Other commonly encountered skeletal devices left in place following attempted cardiopulmonary resuscitation (CPR) are intra-osseous needles placed for emergency vascular access (Fig. 10.12). For more detail regarding implanted devices see Chap. 4.

Over time, the soft tissues surrounding the bones will decay (Fig. 10.13), eventually resulting in 'skeletonisation'. Furthermore, as the ligaments decompose there will be a variable physical disarticulation at the joints (Fig. 10.14), not to be assumed traumatic. The process and significant variability of decomposition are discussed in Chap. 3.

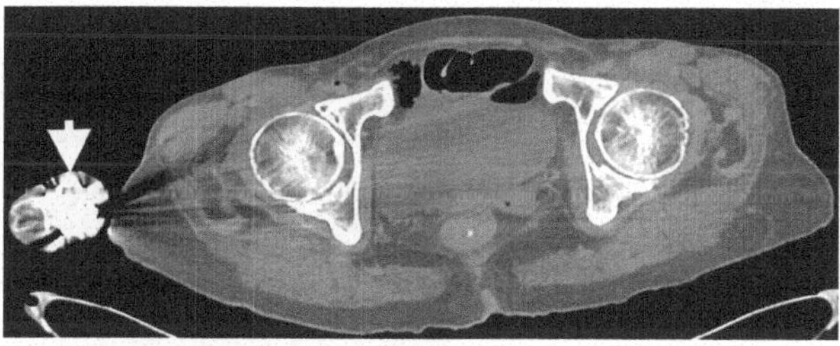

Fig. 10.11 Axial view at the level of the pelvis on soft tissue windows. The body has been scanned with its 'arms by side'. There is streak artefact from a distal radial fracture fixation plate (arrow), unrelated to the cause of death and not severely detrimental to image assessment of the pelvis. When the artefact is more significant, a further 'arms up' acquisition may be made if necessary to clear this artefact

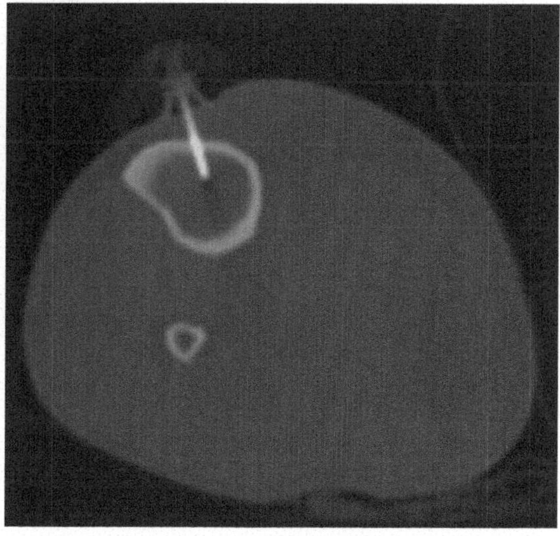

Fig. 10.12 Axial view of the right proximal tibia showing an intra-osseous needle, placed during resuscitation attempts, its tip is in the marrow cavity

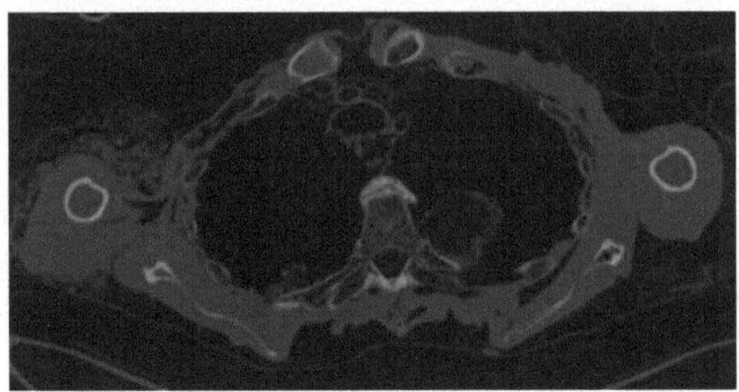

Fig. 10.13 Axial view of the chest on bone windows shows decomposition related loss of soft tissue around a preserved skeletal structure

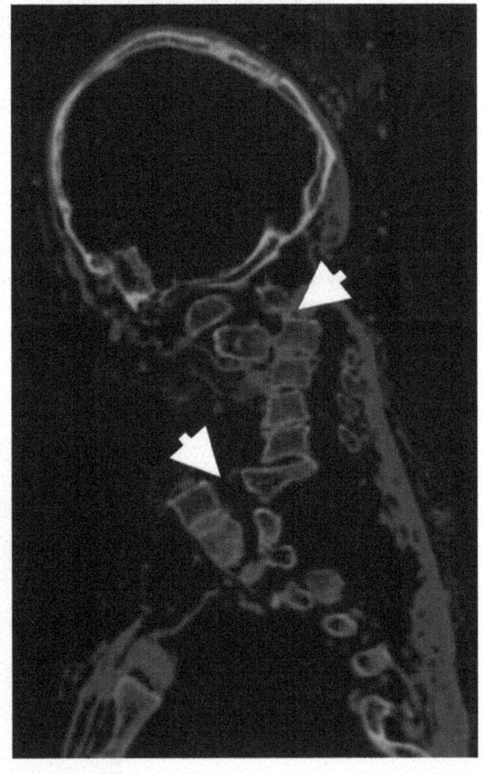

Fig. 10.14 Oblique sagittal view (due to body positioning) on bone windows shows advanced decomposition, almost skeletonisation, with multiple spinal disarticulations (arrows). There was no history/suspicion of trauma

Abnormal PMCT Findings

Degenerative Changes and Arthritis

While arguably 'normal' for aging populations, degenerative osseous findings and also those associated with the various arthritides are commonly seen on imaging, often with no relevance to the events surrounding death. PMCT is effective in showing established joint changes. Significant joint pathology should be documented, as occasionally it may have a relationship with systemic disease (e.g. rheumatoid arthritis and cardiac pathology) and prior trauma (Figs. 10.15 and 10.16).

Gas is sometimes seen clinically in degenerative intervertebral discs and is also seen on PMCT (Fig. 10.17). On PMCT, however, such gas should be considered alongside the gas pattern elsewhere to exclude decomposition. In the setting of trauma, if gas is seen in a single disc, without evidence of degeneration or decomposition elsewhere, it may also reflect a traumatic disruption.

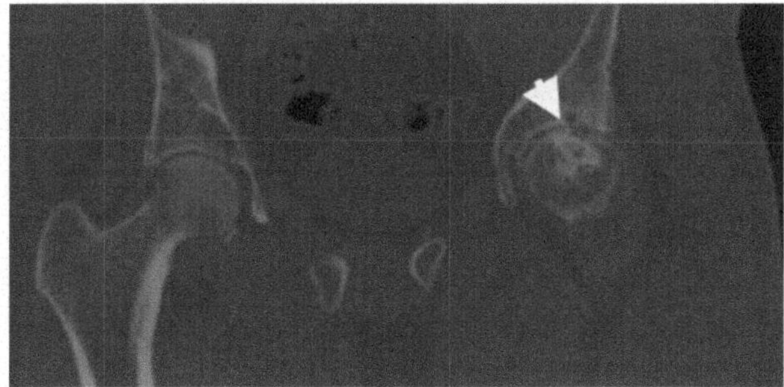

Fig. 10.15 Coronal view of the pelvis on bone windows showing left-side hip joint degeneration (arrow). The left proximal femur is not fully seen as there was flexion at the left hip joint taking the bone out of plane. Note the normal right hip joint appearances

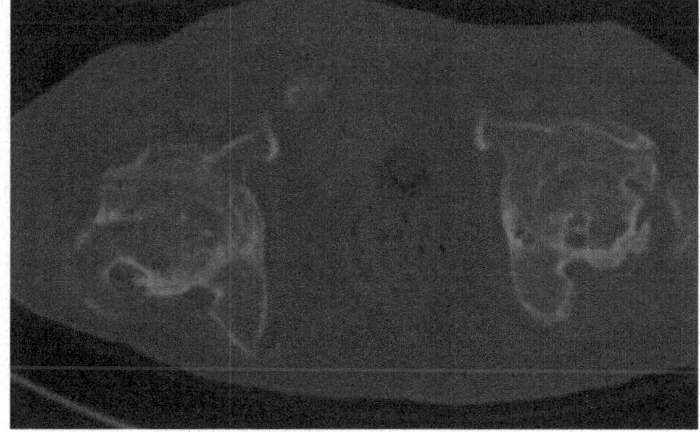

Fig. 10.16 Axial view of the pelvis on bone windows shows severe bilateral hip joint degeneration with loss of joint space, subchondral cystic and sclerotic changes, marked osteophytosis and bony remodelling

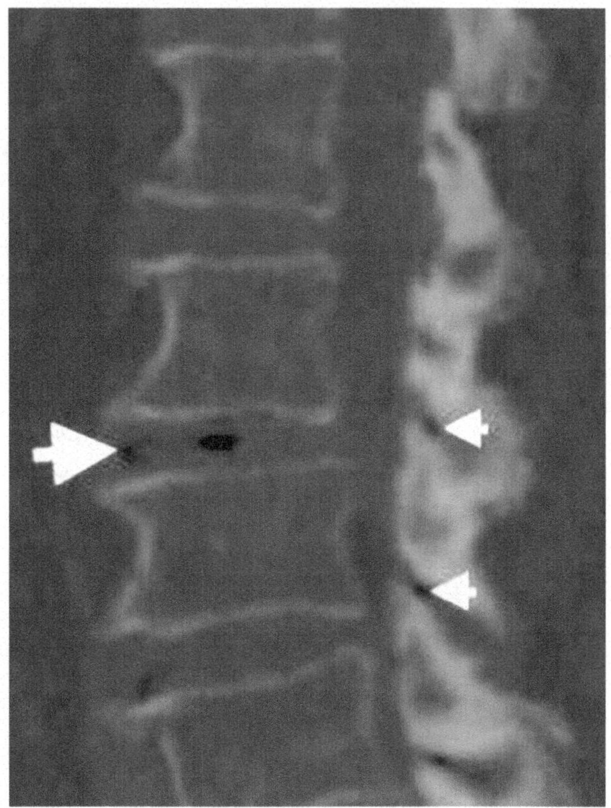

Fig. 10.17 Sagittal partial view of the thoracolumbar spine on bone windows shows small foci of gas in a disc (large arrow) and also facet joints (small arrows), consistent with degenerative changes

Appendicular Fractures

Any fracture should be documented in terms of bone involved, position of the fragments, and extent of soft tissue injury. Fractures of the proximal femur (Figs. 10.18 and 10.19) may particularly compromise mobility and certainly have associated morbidity and mortality.

Long bone fractures (Fig. 10.20) may also cause significant pain and haemorrhage but are unlikely to be fatal in isolation. Even relatively minor fractures (Fig. 10.21) may have had an impact on mobility and morbidity and highlight the value of the 'whole-body' approach to the post mortem assessment.

Even when not fatal by itself, the radiologist should bear in mind that a fracture may be an indirect cause of death. The blood loss may be sufficient, in those with significant cardiovascular disease, to precipitate an acute cardiac ischaemia and/or dysrhythmias. The possibility of fat embolism is also often overlooked as a cause of death in the first 2 days after long bone injury, especially in those fractures which are surgically treated. Alternatively, resultant immobility may precipitate deep vein thrombosis and pulmonary embolism.

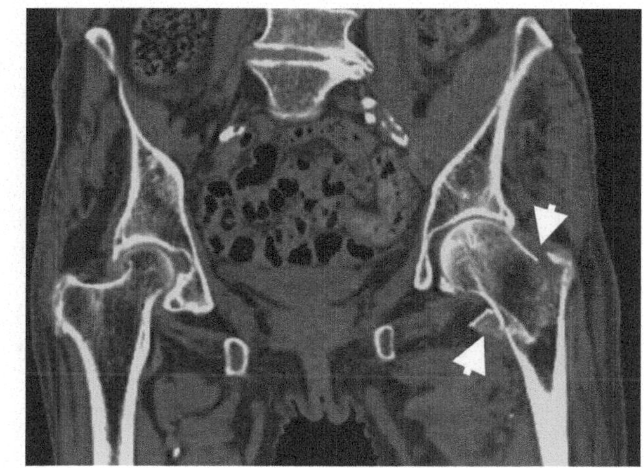

Fig. 10.18 Coronal view of the pelvis on soft tissue windows shows an unexpected comminuted, intertrochanteric fracture of the left proximal femur (arrows) with minimal surrounding haematoma

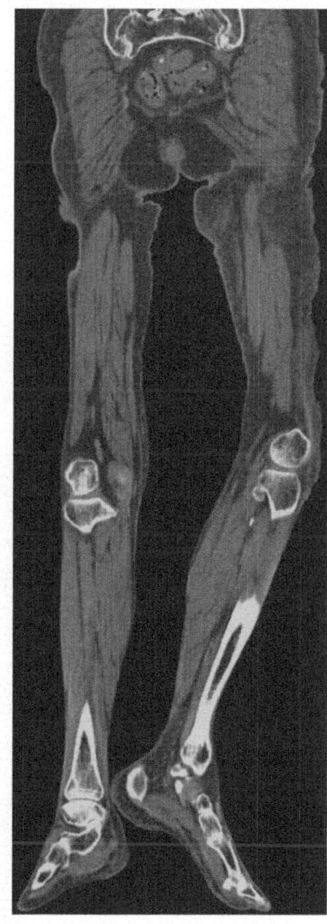

Fig. 10.19 Same case as Fig. 10.18, a coronal view of both legs shows the left leg to be shortened and externally rotated secondary to the hip fracture

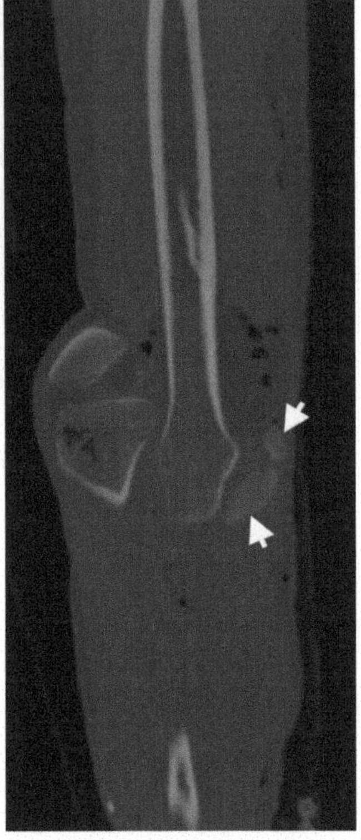

Fig. 10.20 Sagittal view of the knee showing a severe fracture-dislocation with shortening, following a road traffic collision. Large fragments of the femoral condyles are seen in the popliteal region (arrows)

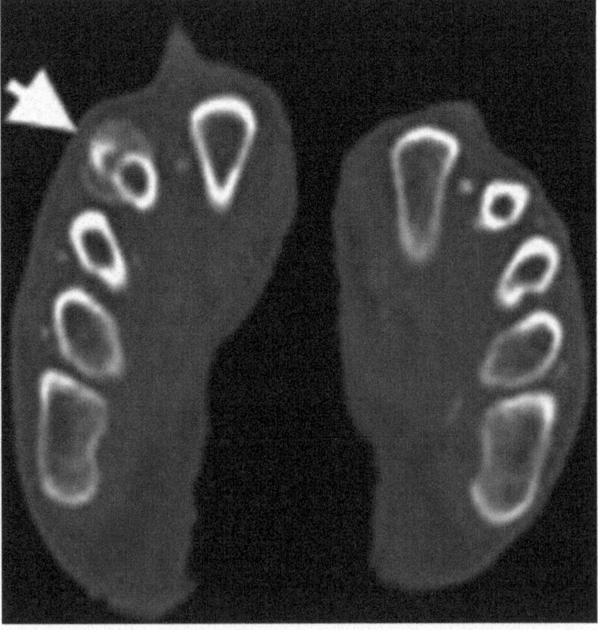

Fig. 10.21 Axial view of both feet on bone windows shows a healing fracture of the right second metatarsal with callus (arrow), seen at the very lower limits of the study range

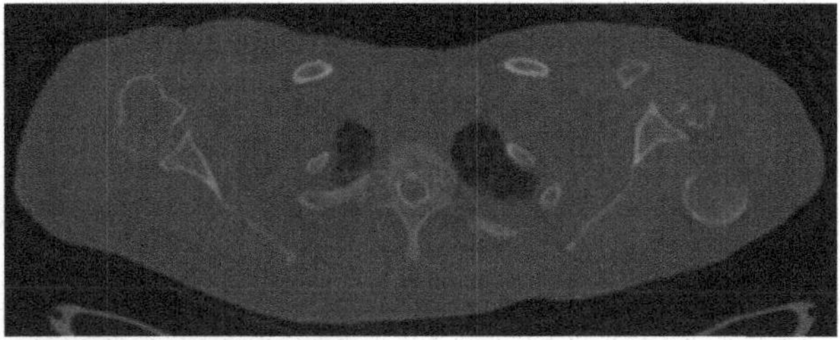

Fig. 10.22 Axial view at the level of the gleno-humeral joints shows an incidental left humeral head fracture dislocation of unknown/unexplained cause (presumed to have been sustained around the time of death) in a case of intra-abdominal sepsis. A congruent right gleno-humeral joint is noted

One should also be open to the possibility of a fatal medical event resulting in a collapse, which might result in peri mortem, incidental fracture/s or even that perhaps injury has been sustained during the post mortem handing of the body (Fig. 10.22).

Vertebral Fractures

Fractures of the spine usually directly involve bones (Figs. 10.23 and 10.24) but can also relate to discs and/or ligaments with variable disruption to vertebral alignment. One should be aware that vertebral collapses of an osteoporotic origin/pattern are a common finding in the elderly and rarely of significance, despite there often being considerable symptoms in life.

By contrast, fractures of the high cervical spine, or those with vertebral separation, are much more likely to be relevant to the cause of death, owing to potential associated brainstem or cord injury. Signs of vertebral separation include straightforward widening (Fig. 10.25), yet one should be aware that fractures can re-align. The position of the bones at the time of scanning may be significantly different to the bony alignment at the time of death. More subtle misalignment, spur/teardrop fracture configuration, visible haematoma and intervertebral gas are also relevant signs and yet can be missed on CT if not meticulous in assessment. Furthermore, fractures through the disco-ligamentous complex without associated bony injury may remain occult [1–3] yet have associated cord injuries [4].

A higher suspicion for subtle or occult injuries should be held when assessing a 'rigid' spine (e.g. in the setting of diffuse idiopathic skeletal hyperostosis (DISH) or ankylosing spondylitis, Fig. 10.26). In these conditions, the discs become the relative points of weakness. Disc heights should be compared to adjacent levels to avoid missing subtle widening. If there is no history of trauma, one should bear in mind that a rigid or fragile spine may more readily incur post mortem injury during the process of body handling/transport [5] or following attempted cardiopulmonary resuscitation (Fig. 10.27).

As with clinical CT, it can be difficult/impossible to age vertebral fractures, especially endplate collapse or wedge/compression types (Fig. 10.28). Previous imaging and/or reports can aid in PMCT assessment, although these are not always available.

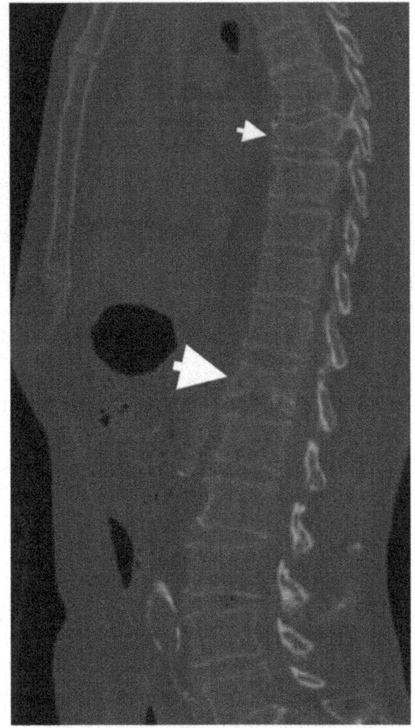

Fig. 10.23 Sagittal view of the thoracolumbar spine on bone windows shows a comminuted acute fracture of T12 vertebral body (large arrow) with lucent fracture lines. There is no posterior loss of height or retropulsion. An anterior wedge compression fracture at T7 (small arrow), is considered indeterminate in age

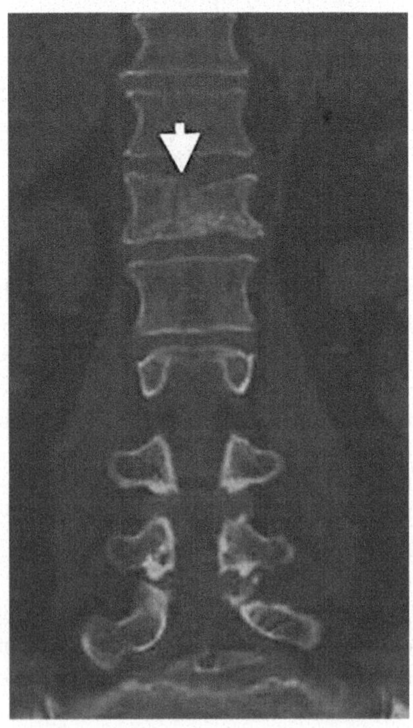

Fig. 10.24 Coronal view of the acute T12 fracture seen in Fig. 10.23 shows a vertical fracture line and upper endplate depression (arrow)

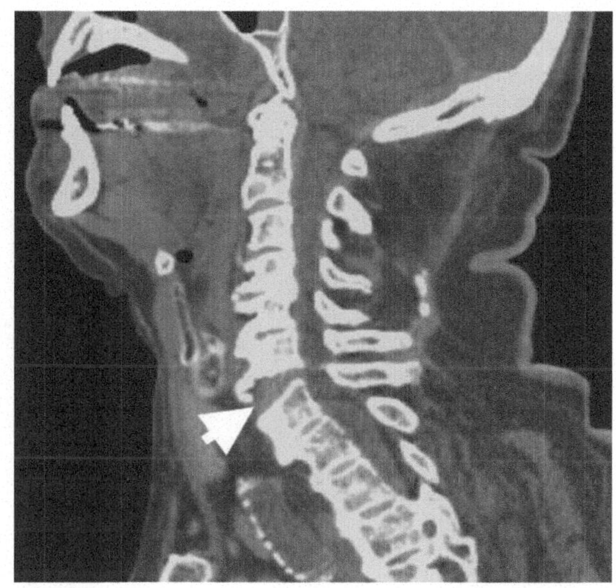

Fig. 10.25 Sagittal view of the cervical spine on soft tissue windows showing fracture through the C6–7 disc with residual anterior widening/ separation (arrow)

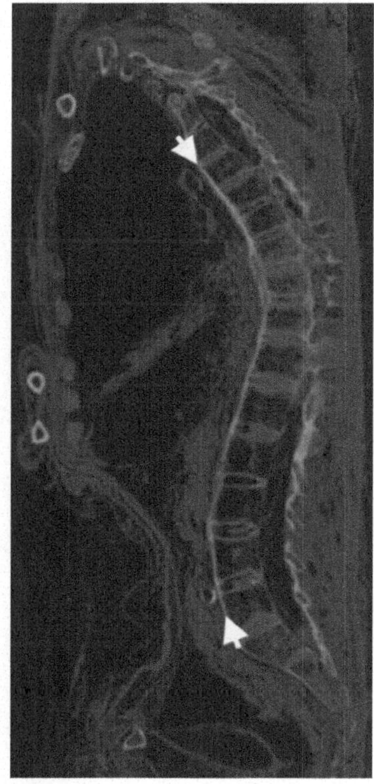

Fig. 10.26 Sagittal view of the thoracolumbar spine on bone windows shows intact, flowing ossification of the anterior longitudinal ligament (arrows) resulting in a rigid spine. The body is otherwise in a severely decomposed state

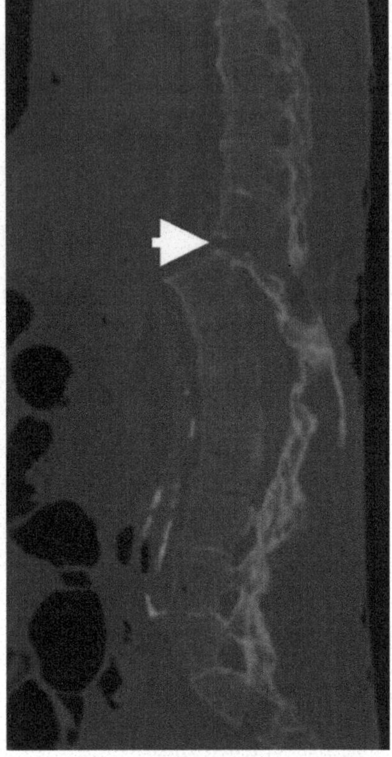

Fig. 10.27 Sagittal view of the thoracolumbar spine on bone windows showing a displaced fracture through the T10–11 disc space (arrow) in a person with known ankylosing spondylitis. This was judged to be secondary to chest compressions during CPR, as there was no other history of trauma

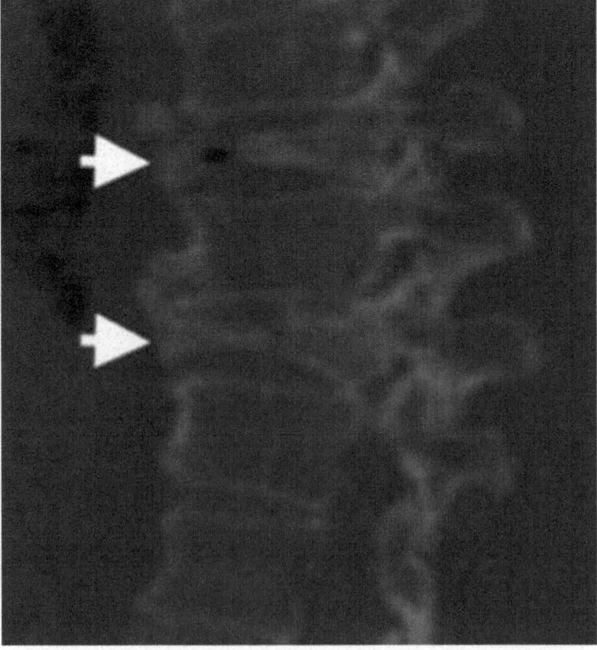

Fig. 10.28 Sagittal view of the thoracolumbar junction on bone windows showing multiple severe wedge compression fractures (arrows)

The presence of haematoma or swollen para-spinal musculature suggests that injury occurred shortly before/about the time of death. Such soft tissue findings are more easily considered at open autopsy, which has the potential benefit of histology sampling to aid assessment but are found to varying extent (including not at all) on PMCT [2]. The PMCT assessment may therefore focus on correlating a known history of trauma with the relevant findings, on the balance of probabilities.

Spinal Cord Injury

As might be predicted, intrinsic cord lesions, cord haemorrhage, complete and partial transections are more clearly appreciated at open autopsy with histology sampling, compared to PMCT, although this autopsy protocol involves complicated and extensive dissection. Open autopsy consideration of the spinal cord tissues is not routinely undertaken, unless specifically indicated by the case data.

PMCT cannot usually directly assess spinal cord injury [6], although it can be inferred through injury patterns (Fig. 10.29 and see Chap. 5). If cord injury can be confidently predicted from the available history and correlative imaging, then a cause of death may be given without the need for open autopsy dissection.

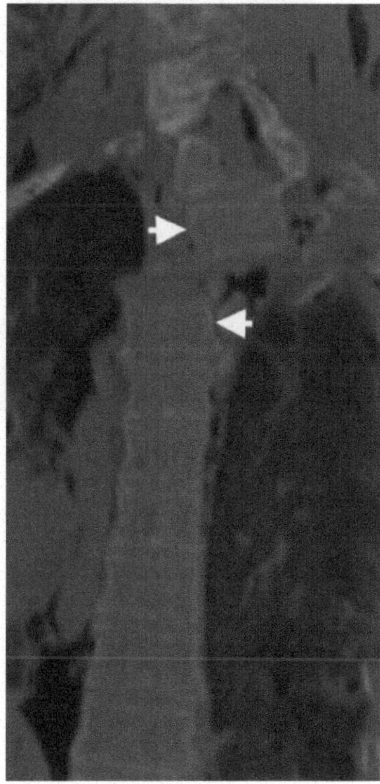

Fig. 10.29 Coronal view of the thoracic spine on bone windows showing a significant lateral fracture dislocation at T2–3 (arrows) and inferred spinal cord injury/transection, following a road traffic collision

Soft Tissue Injury

Large peripheral lacerations and soft tissue haematomas can be visualised on PMCT (Fig. 10.30), although minor soft tissue injuries are better demonstrated at direct external examination and/or open autopsy [7]. These lesser bleeds and injuries are unlikely to be of significance in the non-suspicious setting yet, if seen, should always be suitably explained by the history and circumstances. Unexpected and/or atypical bruising of the limbs and neck may be signs of neglect or criminality, which could merit forensic assessment. Many of the specific soft tissue injuries of the various body cavities are otherwise considered in their relevant chapters earlier in the book.

In trauma, angiography has been shown to be helpful in the depiction of traumatic lacerations [8]. As isolated injuries of the extremities are not usually the primary cause of death (unless catastrophic and therefore clearly visualised), it is difficult to justify the extra cost and resource in undertaking non-targeted/peripheral angiography in our practice.

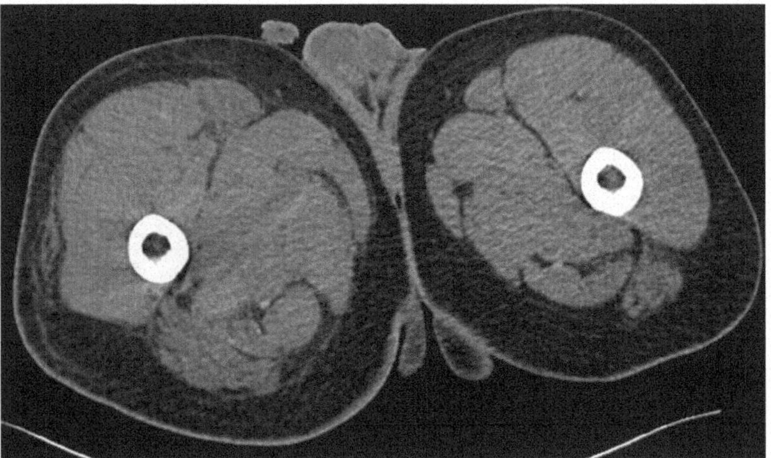

Fig. 10.30 Axial view of both upper thighs on soft tissue windows showing asymmetric right leg swelling due to intramuscular haematoma, evidenced by slightly hyperdense swelling and stranding. This resulted from a fall 1 week prior, on a background history of alcohol misuse with liver failure and clotting dysfunction

Musculoskeletal Infections

While unusual to come across unexpectedly, the reporter should generally be mindful of infections being present, in case one needs to take measures to protect anyone that may come into contact with the body. Infective pathology may relate to notifiable organisms (e.g. mycobacteria) although confirmation requires microbiology sampling techniques (potentially via a targeted needle biopsy).

In relation to a potential cause of death, PMCT may reveal established infective bony pathology, such as osteomyelitis, or vertebral destruction and/or collapse from spondylo-discitis, which may otherwise have been missed at routine open autopsy [9]. Yet, as with clinical CT, it cannot reliably *exclude* such infections. Spread of infection may also be a cause of death, such as from a systemic bacteraemic sepsis. Furthermore, one should always consider the possibility of infection in relation to recent medical/surgical procedures or implanted prostheses, although, just as it is with clinical imaging, it can be difficult to find imaging evidence of such infective processes and, for example, to separate a sterile joint effusion from a septic joint.

In the peripheral skeleton, a soft tissue abscess may be appreciated if it is sizeable or if there is associated bone destruction. Chronic ulceration with associated infection, particularly of the lower limbs, can be identified, commonly seen in the setting of diabetes and/or peripheral neurovascular disease (Figs. 10.31, 10.32, 10.33, and 10.34). This requires correlation with the clinical history and/or external findings.

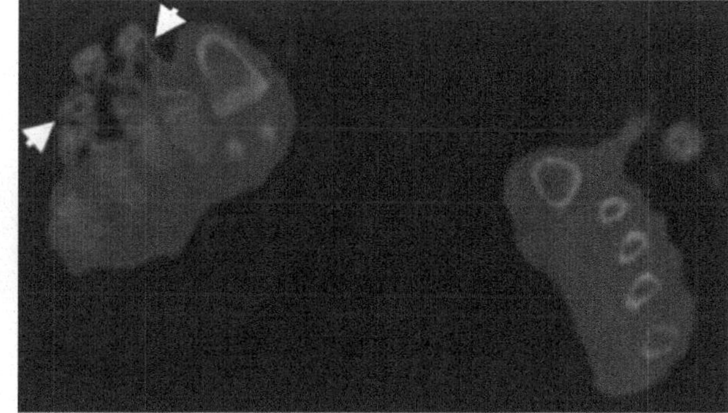

Fig. 10.31 Axial view of both feet on bone windows showing soft tissue loss and ulceration of the right toes (arrows) in the setting of severe peripheral vascular disease

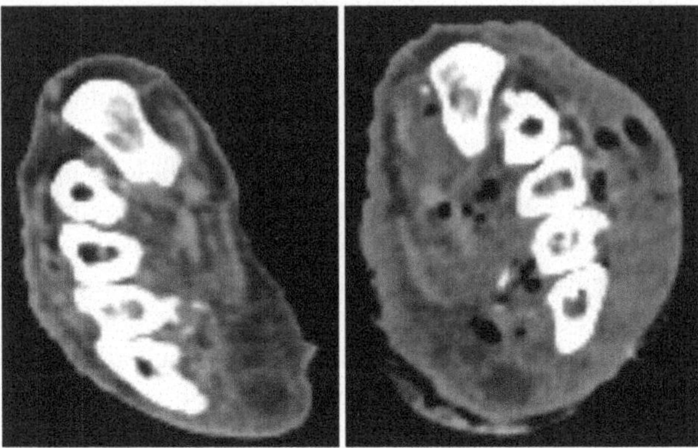

Fig. 10.32 Axial view of the forefeet on soft tissue windows showing asymmetric left-side subcutaneous soft tissue thickening with multiple locules of gas in the tissues, consistent with localised infection and abscess, correlated with the clinical details

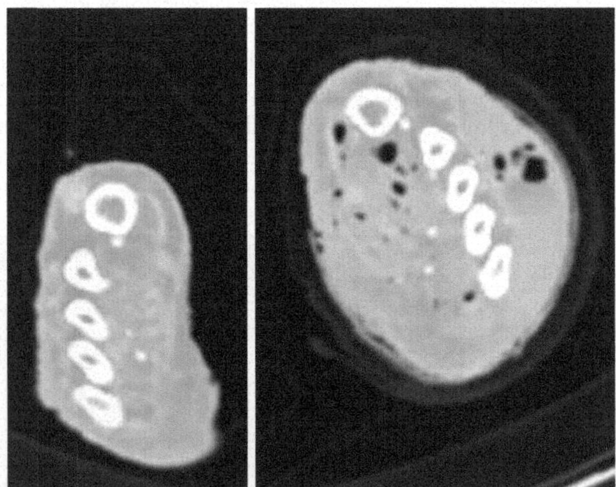

Fig. 10.33 Same case as Fig. 10.32, lung windows show the gas more clearly, and the relative absence of these changes in the right lower limb

Peripheral Vascular Disease

Vessel wall calcification is easily observed on PMCT (Fig. 10.35) and correlates with established peripheral vascular disease. Whilst a formal limb angiogram might better assess luminal patency, it is not essential here, as calcification indicates chronic arterial disease and is usually reflected in the past medical history. Other vascular findings relevant to significant underlying medical disease include bypass grafts and haemodialysis fistulae (Fig. 10.36), again usually reflected in the history.

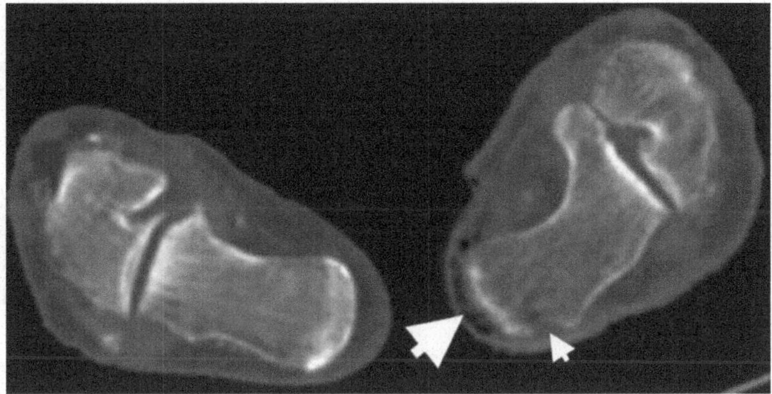

Fig. 10.34 Axial view of both hindfeet on bone windows shows thinned soft tissue with subcutaneous gas (infection/localised accelerated decomposition) over the posterior left heel tip (large arrow). There is cortical bone destruction consistent with osteomyelitis at a clinical site of ulceration laterally (small arrow)

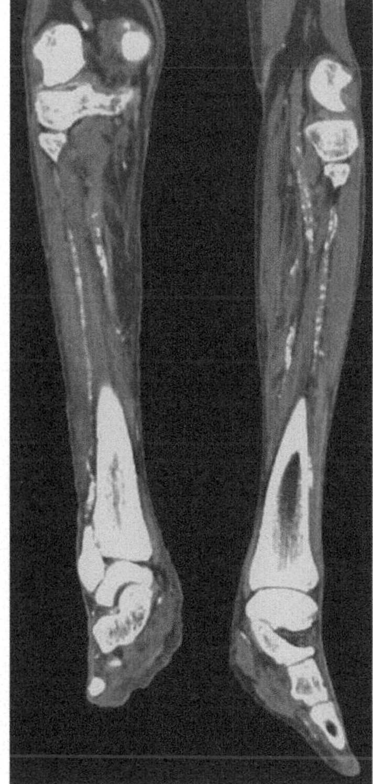

Fig. 10.35 Coronal view of the lower legs on soft tissue windows showing heavily calcified 3-vessel infra-popliteal peripheral vascular disease

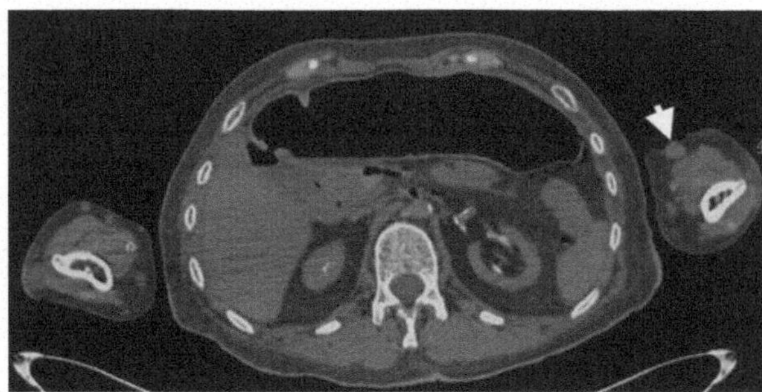

Fig. 10.36 Axial view at the level of the upper abdomen, scanned with 'arms by sides' on soft tissue windows shows a left antecubital fossa brachiocephalic fistula for dialysis (arrow). Note also atrophic left kidney with vascular calcification

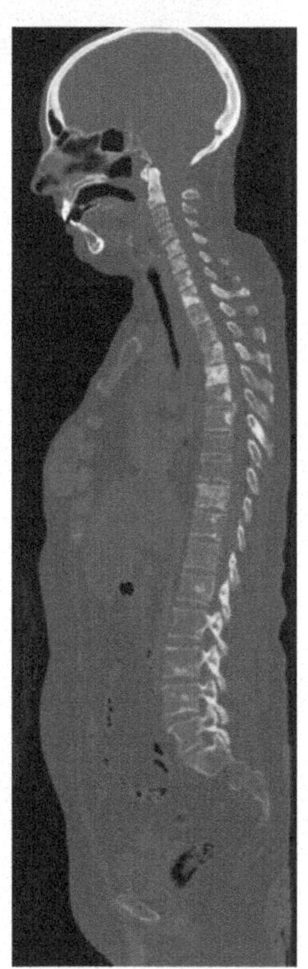

Fig. 10.37 Sagittal view of the spine on bone windows showing multiple sclerotic metastases (but no vertebral collapse) from known breast cancer (Note breast prosthesis in situ)

Musculoskeletal Neoplasia

The diagnosis and characterisation of soft tissue or bone tumour pathology is generally considered to be limited on clinical CT when compared to MRI. However, PMCT remains an appropriate, realistic solution for the assessment of primary and metastatic tumours after death, where the appearances (and limitations) are similar to clinical CT (Figs. 10.37 and 10.38). A known history of malignancy assists interpretation greatly, but, if this is not given, a broad search for the likely primary should be undertaken.

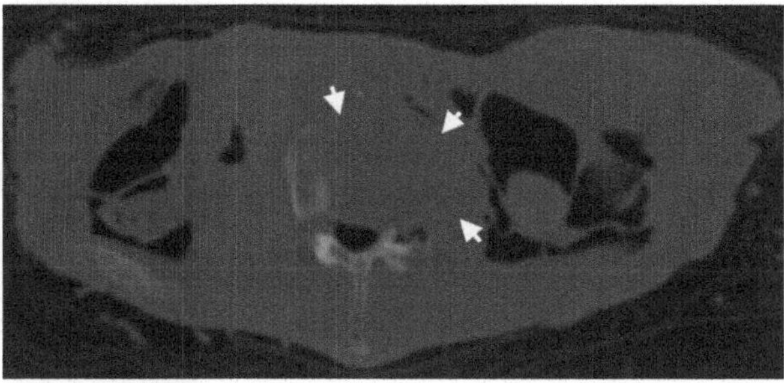

Fig. 10.38 Axial view of the lumbar spine on bone windows shows a large, destructive lesion partially replacing a vertebral body (arrows) with no known history of malignancy. Extensive gas in soft tissues from decomposition prevented the identification of a primary malignancy on PMCT

Special Circumstances: Fatal Major Trauma

PMCT offers a comprehensive examination of a body that has been subject to catastrophic multiple injuries. These may result from circumstances such as a vehicle (car/train etc.) collision (Figs. 10.39, 10.40, 10.41, and 10.42), a significant fall (Figs. 10.43 and 10.44) or extensive burns (Figs. 10.45, 10.46, and 10.47). In non-suspicious (but clearly unnatural) settings, these are likely to relate to suicide or be witnessed accidents.

Imaging is recognised as a useful adjunct to the post mortem trauma case evaluation [7, 10] but is increasingly being used to replace open autopsy in circumstances such as this. It provides a permanent and reviewable record of the injuries sustained.

Despite these possibilities, since a pathological external inspection has to occur in each case (and is necessary for toxicology samples to be obtained), the additional value of imaging when a body is *severely* fragmented is questionable in terms of adding meaningful information to the external assessment.

Interpretation of Fatal Trauma

For the radiologist encountering multiple severe injuries, there can be an overwhelming assortment of findings to describe, interpret and record, especially if approached from a clinical perspective. Occasionally, disarticulated body parts may be placed alongside a body in a body bag (Figs. 10.48 and 10.49), not necessarily in their correct anatomic location, and so review of the scout studies or volume-rendered imaging is helpful to provide an overview.

The key is to identify the injury/injuries which, on the balance of probability, caused death. This may be externally obvious, for example decapitation. Alternatively, the fatal injury may be internal, such as an aortic transection. When there are multiple and substantial injuries, it may be difficult to ascertain a single, overarching cause of death. In such cases, following listing of the contributing findings, a summation of 'multiple traumatic injuries' may be the best solution.

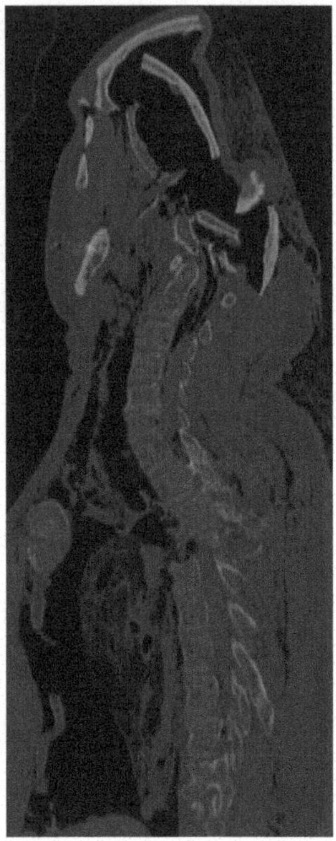

Fig. 10.39 Sagittal view of the head and cervico-thoracic spine on bone windows showing multiple severe traumatic injuries which are incompatible with life. These resulted from a road traffic collision

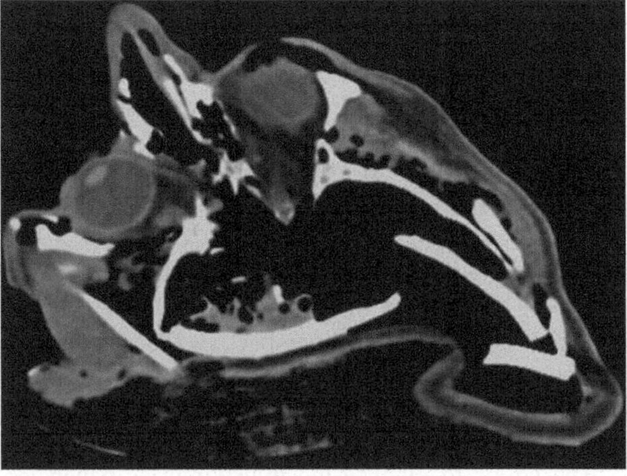

Fig. 10.40 Axial view of the head on soft tissue windows shows catastrophic traumatic head injury with multiple fractures and loss of brain tissues following a road traffic collision

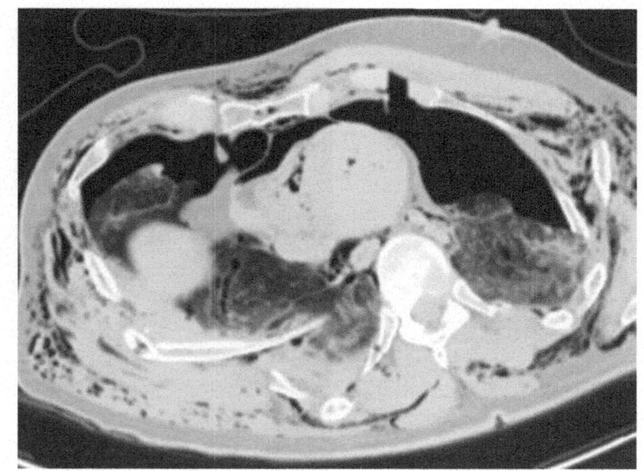

Fig. 10.41 Axial view of the chest on lung windows showing multiple, extensive crush injuries to the chest, incompatible with life, following a road traffic collision

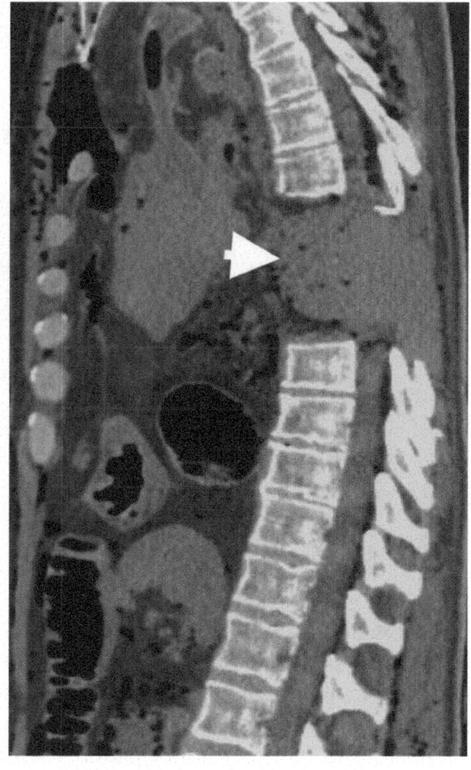

Fig. 10.42 Sagittal view of the thoracolumbar spine on soft tissue windows showing a severely distracted intervertebral fracture (with inferred spinal cord transection) and herniation of the liver through the defect (arrow), following a road traffic collision

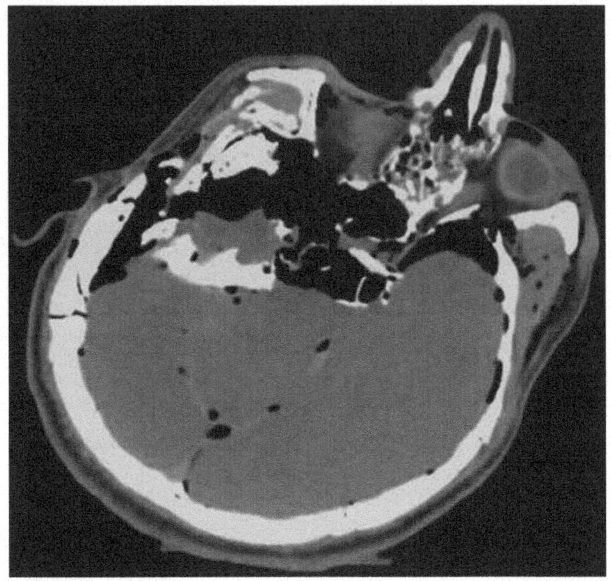

Fig. 10.43 Axial view of the head on soft tissue windows showing extensive, unsurvivable cranio-facial injuries following a fall from a high-rise building

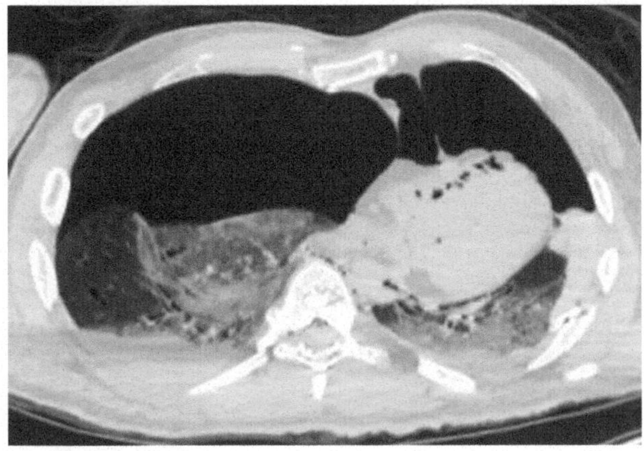

Fig. 10.44 Axial view of the chest on lung windows shows large bilateral pneumothoraces secondary to multiple rib fractures following a fall from a high-rise building

The scanned injuries should undoubtedly correlate with the mechanism of injury. In a non-suspicious case, these data will almost certainly be known and the focus of the PMCT investigation is to document injuries, seek underlying pathology if possible, and to confirm trauma as the cause of death.

Seeking to interpret injury patterns without a known mechanism is beyond the scope of this book, implying a suspicion of criminality and therefore forensic

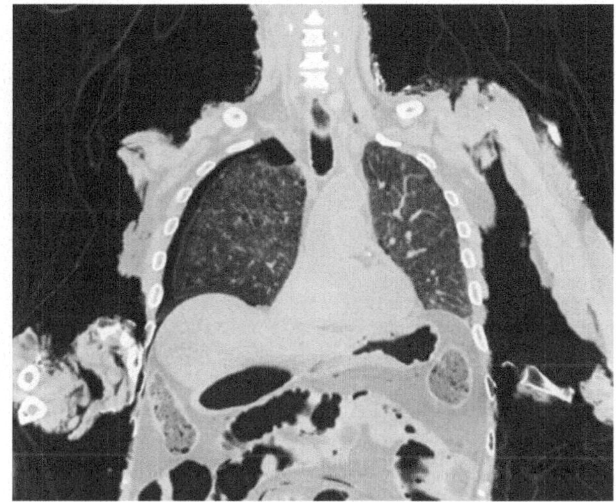

Fig. 10.45 Coronal view of the chest and arms on lung windows showing extensive superficial soft tissue loss and a right-side pneumothorax due to severe burn injury

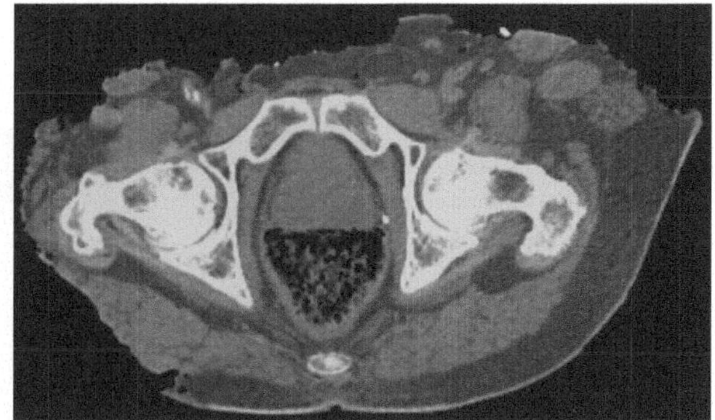

Fig. 10.46 Same case as Fig. 10.45, axial view of the pelvis on soft tissue windows shows extensive anterolateral superficial soft tissue loss due to burn injury

investigation. This is detailed in other texts [5, 11]. This pattern interpretation is more concerned with understanding the events surrounding the death, rather than identify the cause of death itself.

Undoubtedly PMCT can depict skeletal injuries with more ease and accuracy than a non-forensic open autopsy, but it clearly also has a role in enhancing and directing forensic skeletal assessment. PMCT can demonstrate a wide range of major injuries but is reported to be generally less useful for abdominal findings [6], minor soft tissue and aortic injuries [7]. As such, PMCT is unlikely to be sufficient alone for forensic cases, as even minor findings may be of critical relevance to the investigation.

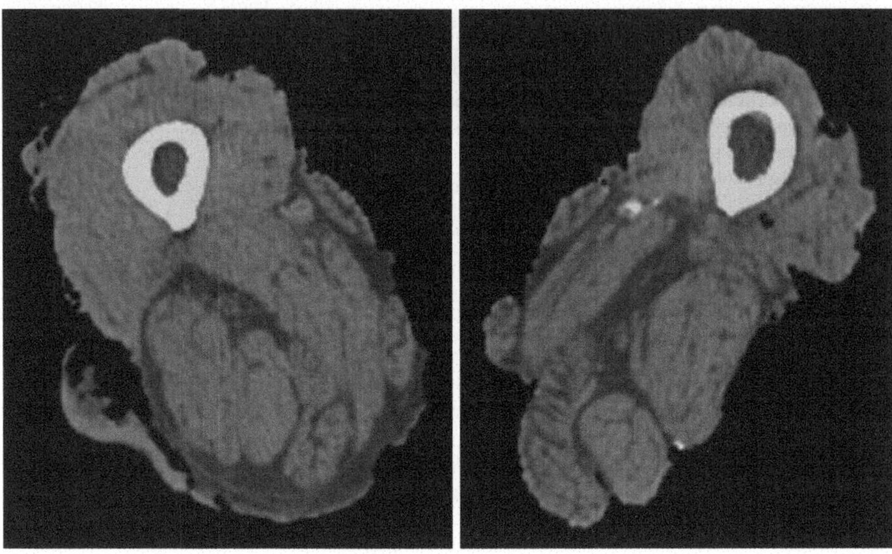

Fig. 10.47 Same case as Fig. 10.45, axial view of both thighs on soft tissue windows shows extensive superficial soft tissue loss due to burn injury

Fig. 10.48 Non-orthogonal view of an amputated foot (which was also placed in the body bag) on bone windows showing multiple fractures and severe soft tissue injury following a road traffic crush injury

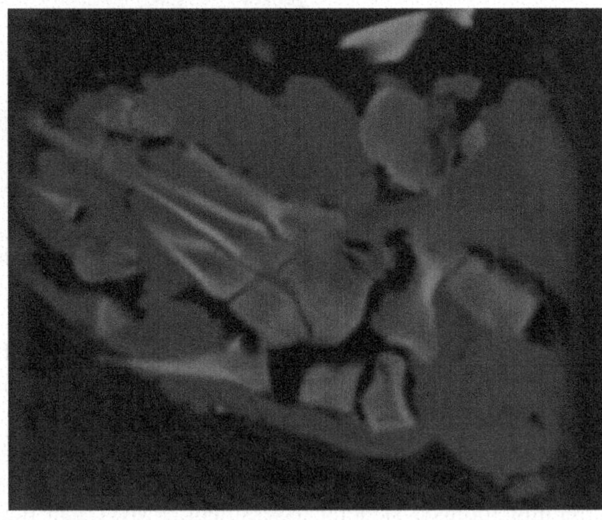

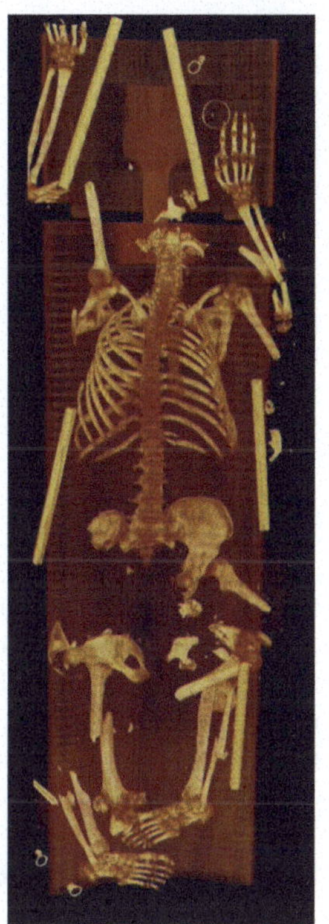

Fig. 10.49 Volume rendered image of multiple skeletal fractures and disarticulated body parts scanned within a body bag after a train collision

Fatal Haemorrhage as a Consequence of Injury

Determining haemorrhage/exsanguination as a cause of death can be difficult at both open autopsy and PMCT. This diagnosis may be considered when trauma is less extensive than some of the examples described earlier, yet where there has been critical injury to a vascular structure. Factors to consider include the history, documentation a large volume of haemorrhage at the scene or presence of profuse internal haemorrhage. Police and paramedic reports may occasionally offer this detail, although the descriptions vary in completeness (and accuracy) in the non-suspicious setting.

In terms of imaging findings, as expected, haemorrhage is generally hyperdense, although the blood can separate with hypostasis, resulting in a layered 'fluid–fluid' level (Fig. 10.50). One should appreciate that, with such appearances, it is the whole volume of fluid that is 'blood', not just the dependent hyperdense component which only represents the sedimented cell fraction. Most patients who die of fatal haemorrhage will show a general collapse of their vessels [12]. This feature will support the diagnosis but is unfortunately both non-specific and common on PMCT.

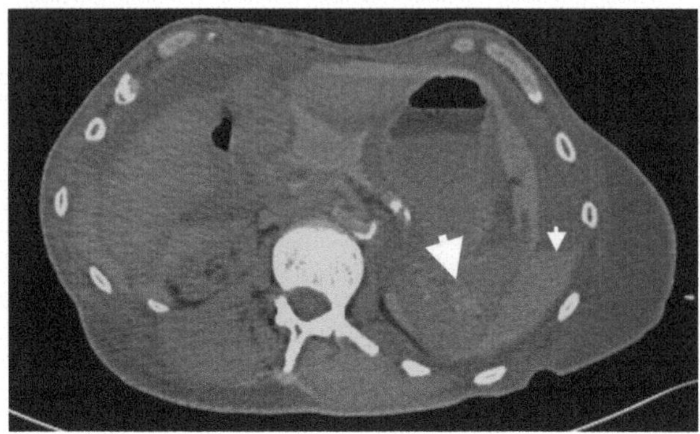

Fig. 10.50 Axial view of the upper abdomen on soft tissue windows showing extensive intra-abdominal haemorrhage with layered separation (small arrow) possibly secondary to the splenic laceration (large arrow), although potentially further parenchymal and vascular injury may be obscured

Adding to the difficulty, when a large volume of internal haemorrhage is present, the origin may be speculative as haematoma can obscure the underlying vascular anatomy. Interpretation of the history and 'central' or 'maximal' location of blood may reveal the most likely site. Where available, post mortem angiography (PMCTA) may permit a more specific localisation [8], but it should be understood that this adds significantly to the complexity and cost of the PMCT.

Reporting Bone and Soft Tissue Findings: Pearls and Pitfalls

The role of the radiologist (in a non-suspicious trauma case) is to interpret and document the injuries and thereby deduce a likely medical cause of death. This may be a single directly fatal injury, a summation of multiple injuries or a related cause such as exsanguination.

In general, any fractures, soft tissue asymmetry/pathology, significant vascular calcification, degenerative changes, joint replacements and implants should be mentioned and be correlated with clinical data and/or external findings.

Commentary of osteopenia may be of relevance in considering fractures.

It is also suggested to routinely document the *absence* of fractures, as this bony assessment is a key advantage of PMCT over routine open autopsy. This also obviates the need for speculative extensive body dissection should an invasive examination proceed.

Example PMCT report phrases:

- No acute fractures demonstrated.
- No destructive or sinister bone lesions.
- No soft tissue mass, swelling or secondary signs of deep venous thrombosis in the lower extremities.

- There are multiple catastrophic, unsurvivable cranial and vertebral injuries.
- Destructive lucency of the bone is seen with associated acute fracture, suspicious of pathological fracture.
- Age indeterminate vertebral wedge fractures are seen with diffuse osteopenia (likely osteoporosis).
- Mid thoracic vertebral fracture, in the absence of a traumatic history, is judged to be injury from attempted cardiopulmonary resuscitation.

References

1. Kudo S, Kawasumi Y, Usui A, Arakawa M, Yamagishi N, Igari Y, et al. Post-mortem computed tomography of cervical intervertebral separation: Retrospective review and comparison of the autopsy results of 57 separations. J Forensic Radiol Imaging [Internet]. 2018;12:57–63. https://linkinghub.elsevier.com/retrieve/pii/S2212478017300862.
2. Kawasumi Y, Usui A, Hosokai Y, Sato M, Hayashizaki Y, Saito H, et al. PMCT findings of intervertebral separation. J Forensic Radiol Imaging [Internet]. 2014;2(4):182–7. https://linkinghub.elsevier.com/retrieve/pii/S2212478014001051.
3. Iwase H, Yamamoto S, Yajima D, Hayakawa M, Kobayashi K, Otsuka K, et al. Can cervical spine injury be correctly diagnosed by postmortem computed tomography? Leg Med [Internet]. 2009;11(4):168–74. https://linkinghub.elsevier.com/retrieve/pii/S1344622309001679.
4. Makino Y, Yokota H, Hayakawa M, Yajima D, Inokuchi G, Nakatani E, et al. Spinal cord injuries with normal postmortem CT findings: a pitfall of virtual autopsy for detecting traumatic death. Am J Roentgenol [Internet]. 2014;203(2):240–4. http://www.ajronline.org/doi/10.2214/AJR.13.11775.
5. Saukko P, Knight B. Knight's forensic pathology [Internet]. 4th ed. Boca Raton: CRC Press; 2015. https://www.routledge.com/Knights-Forensic-Pathology/Saukko-Knight/p/book/9780340972533.
6. Panda A, Kumar A, Gamanagatti S, Mishra B. Virtopsy computed tomography in trauma: Normal postmortem changes and pathologic Spectrum of findings. Curr Probl Diagn Radiol [Internet]. 2015;44(5):391–406. https://linkinghub.elsevier.com/retrieve/pii/S0363018815000420.
7. Jalalzadeh H, Giannakopoulos GF, Berger FH, Fronczek J, van de Goot FRW, Reijnders UJ, et al. Post-mortem imaging compared with autopsy in trauma victims—a systematic review. Forensic Sci Int [Internet]. 2015;257:29–48. https://linkinghub.elsevier.com/retrieve/pii/S0379073815003047.
8. Ross SG, Bolliger SA, Ampanozi G, Oesterhelweg L, Thali MJ, Flach PM. Postmortem CT angiography: capabilities and limitations in traumatic and natural causes of death. Radiographics [Internet]. 2014;34(3):830–46. http://pubs.rsna.org/doi/10.1148/rg.343115169.
9. Clarke M, McGregor A, Robinson C, Amoroso J, Morgan B, Rutty GN. Identifying the correct cause of death: the role of post-mortem computed tomography in sudden unexplained death. J Forensic Radiol Imaging [Internet]. 2014;2(4):210–2. https://linkinghub.elsevier.com/retrieve/pii/S2212478014001075.
10. Scholing M, Saltzherr TP, Fung Kon Jin PHP, Ponsen KJ, Reitsma JB, Lameris JS, et al. The value of postmortem computed tomography as an alternative for autopsy in trauma victims: a systematic review. Eur Radiol [Internet]. 2009;19(10):2333–41. http://link.springer.com/10.1007/s00330-009-1440-4.
11. Levy AD, Harcke HT. Essentials of forensic imaging [Internet]. Boca Raton: CRC Press; 2010. https://www.taylorfrancis.com/books/9781420091120.
12. Aghayev E, Sonnenschein M, Jackowski C, Thali M, Buck U, Yen K, et al. Postmortem radiology of fatal hemorrhage: measurements of cross-sectional areas of major blood vessels and volumes of aorta and spleen on MDCT and volumes of heart chambers on MRI. Am J Roentgenol [Internet]. 2006;187(1):209–15. http://www.ajronline.org/doi/10.2214/AJR.05.0222.

Findings Related to Attempted Cardiopulmonary Resuscitation on Post Mortem Computed Tomography

11

Introduction

As indicated throughout this book, there are certain findings on post mortem computed tomography (PMCT) which are commonly seen after attempted cardiopulmonary resuscitation (CPR). It is important to appreciate that CPR itself is a form of trauma and so findings could significantly overlap with trauma from other causes.

This range of features, particularly those found in the thorax, are important to recognise in order to avoid misinterpretations that might lead to an incorrect cause of death or misidentification of pre-existing disease [1, 2]. It is understood that, even with experienced radiological interpretation, it may not be possible to completely differentiate the possible aetiologies of the features seen.

In addition to the investigation of cause of death, PMCT can also be used to provide post-resuscitation feedback (often in terms of case audit) to the paramedic and medical teams involved in order to aid learning [3, 4]. Rarely, errors identified by PMCT can be instrumental in pointing to training needs, for example practitioners failing to correctly intubate the airway. On occasion, despite history of attempted CPR (often bystander), there are no appreciable imaging findings related to the efforts.

In many circumstances, however, it is of some reassurance to the CPR practitioners and families to document that vigorous efforts were made to render assistance to the deceased.

Autopsy Following CPR: The Pathologist's Perspective

It would be fair to state that many of the cases that require open autopsy have had variable resuscitation measures, including assisted ventilation and chest compressions, alongside other medical strategies. The assessment of such cases deals with the background to the cardiorespiratory arrest and death with its underlying

A. Shenton et al., *Post Mortem CT for Non-Suspicious Adult Deaths*,
https://doi.org/10.1007/978-3-030-70829-0_11

pathologies, but also has to address the impact and adequacy of any resuscitation efforts. This is covered in greater detail in other autopsy reference texts [5].

Open autopsy on the body starts with the external perspective, noting the presence of lines, drains, artificial airways, etc. It is generally recommended that no devices or lines are removed from the body following failed resuscitation, before autopsy, as these items may be of material significance in assessment the case, along with medicolegal impact.

Any device entering the body needs to be checked for position and local complication. The pathologist may cut such lines flush with the body, perhaps pushing inward slightly in order to avoid displacement during the body handling. This process is particularly important for any item that enters the thoracic or abdominal cavity, with the need to check for associated trauma and/or infection.

The autopsy approach is standard for all cases [5]. In post-resuscitation cases, most interest focuses on the chest and to a degree the abdomen/retroperitoneum. The general access point for the chest, abdomen and related tissues is through a Y-shaped incision around the upper neck with a longitudinal incision from the sternum down to the pubis allowing reflection of skin, soft tissue, muscle and removal of the rib plate (sternum and anterior ribs). This process allows good inspection of the cavities and immediate evaluation of issues that are pertinent to the resuscitation—or the cause of the cardiorespiratory arrest.

Rib fractures are common in resuscitation cases and generally not considered in detail unless there is underlying mediastinal, cardiac or lung injury. On occasion, some rib (or other bone) may be retained for histology, in order to consider osteoporosis or underlying metabolic bone disease. However, this investigation is very rare.

Macroscopic photographs are vital in cases of perceived complications from resuscitation, such as liver tears and haemorrhage or misplacement of airways/chest drains. There should be a low threshold for autopsy histology in this scenario.

Cardiopulmonary Resuscitation

This broad term is used to describe a variety of emergency, potentially lifesaving, activities that centre on chest compressions and artificial/assisted ventilation. With medical (rather than bystander) intervention, there may also be the placement of airway adjuncts and vascular access lines, administration of drugs and/or fluids and occasionally cavity drain insertions. It is to be remembered that cardiac defibrillation is variably available in the community but is standard in hospital/medical settings.

As always, the background case data are vital, including the prior medical history supplemented by ambulance or hospital notes. One particular piece of information needed for the correlation of findings on PMCT is whether chest compressions took place, although this is usually assumed when the abbreviation term 'CPR' is used.

Some of the CPR interventions will be physically evident (e.g. when defibrillator pads, intraosseous/vascular lines or artificial airways are left in place, Figs. 11.1 and 11.2, see also Chap. 4). Other interventions leave secondary evidence (such as fractures resulting from chest compressions, Fig. 11.3) and are further discussed in this chapter.

During CPR, the correct placement and position of relevant tubes and devices is crucial to ensure effectiveness. By the time of PMCT, their positions may have altered and may no longer be the same as when CPR was in progress (for example artificial airways may be pushed further inwards, Fig. 11.4). Considerable caution is advised when the radiologist is tempted to use the term 'misplaced' with respect to any medical device, especially if this was unlikely to have changed the final outcome. Such comment might be misunderstood as indicating imperfect medical treatment and cause unnecessary distress to relatives.

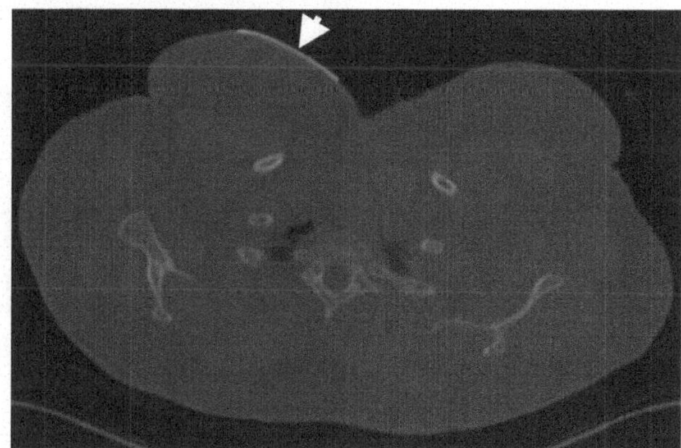

Fig. 11.1 Axial view of the upper chest on bone windows shows a thin, radio-dense defibrillator pad on the skin of the right anterior chest wall (arrow)

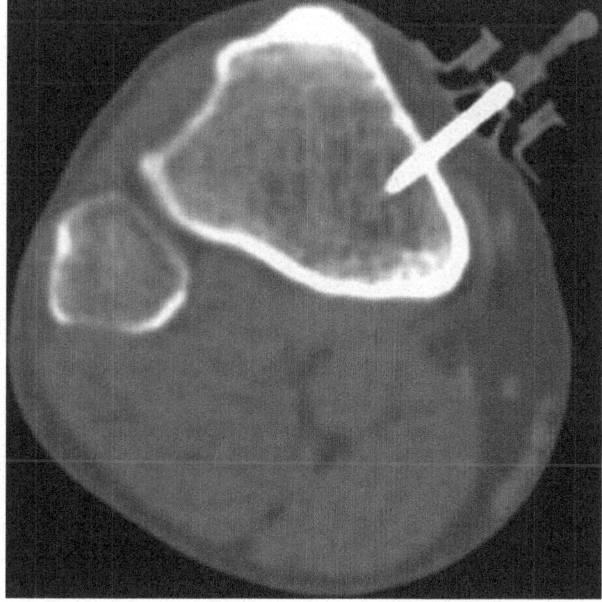

Fig. 11.2 Axial view of the right proximal tibia, windowed to show an intra-osseous needle with its tip in the marrow cavity

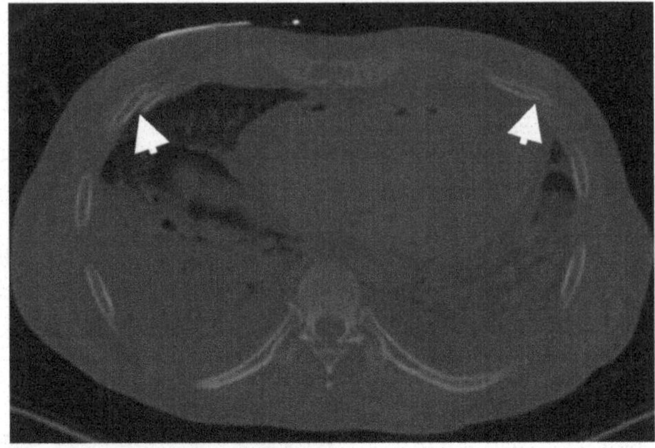

Fig. 11.3 Axial view of the chest on bone windows shows a defibrillator pad over the right anterior chest wall, bilateral rib fractures (arrows), tiny volume of intra-cardiac gas and extensive lung opacity following CPR attempts for 1 hour

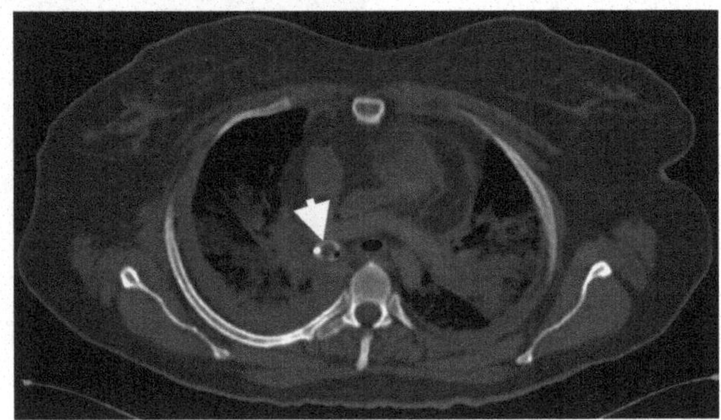

Fig. 11.4 Axial view of the chest on soft tissue windows following CPR attempts shows an endotracheal tube in the right main bronchus (arrow)

Skeletal Findings on PMCT

Rib and Cartilage Fractures

A very common finding after CPR attempts with chest compressions is of multiple rib fractures. These are usually bilateral, anterior or anterolateral and involve the second to seventh ribs [3] or more commonly the third to sixth ribs [6].

These rib fractures may be 'complete' (Figs. 11.5 and 11.6) or 'incomplete' (often buckle type), usually involving the inner cortex, as this side is compressed, (Figs. 11.7 and 11.8). Occasionally, a combination of types may be seen (Figs. 11.3, 11.9, and 11.10). In addition, or sometimes instead of fractured ribs, fractures of the costal cartilages may be seen (Figs. 11.11, 11.12, and 11.13).

When fractures are complete there may be displacement of the bone/cartilage ends, relating to a combination of the intensity of the resuscitation, the pre-existing bone quality and the background chest compliance. Yet, the ribs do not have to be visibly displaced on the scan to have caused underlying injuries to the mediastinum, lungs or upper abdomen. During the multiple, rapid physical compressions of the

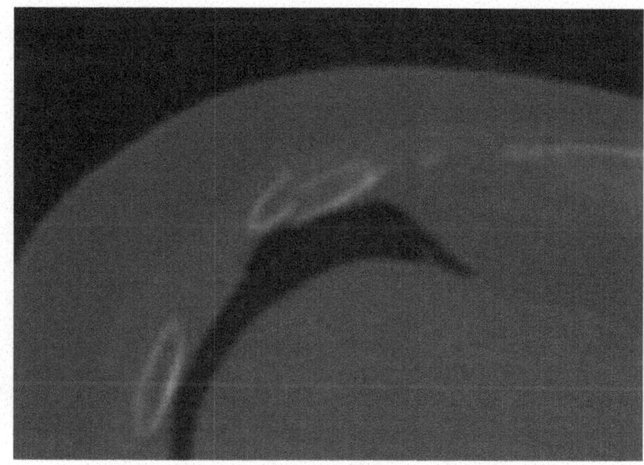

Fig. 11.5 Axial view of a right anterior rib on bone windows shows a complete rib fracture following CPR attempts

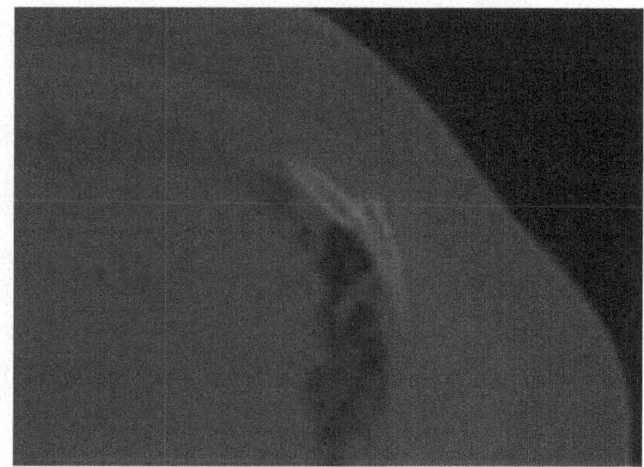

Fig. 11.6 Axial view of a left anterior rib on bone windows shows a complete rib fracture following CPR attempts

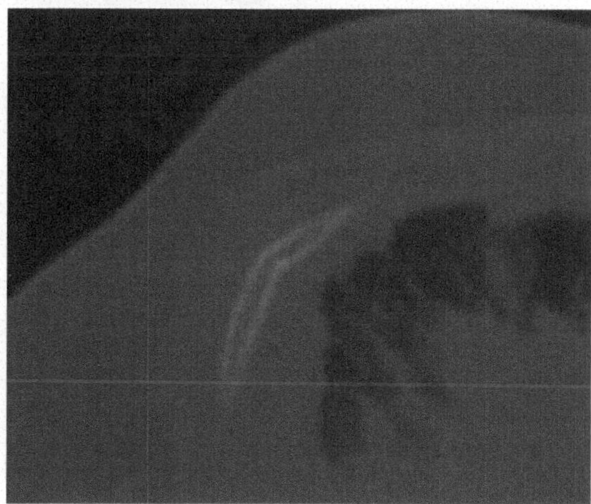

Fig. 11.7 Axial view of a right anterior rib on bone windows shows an incomplete buckle fracture of the inner cortex following CPR attempts

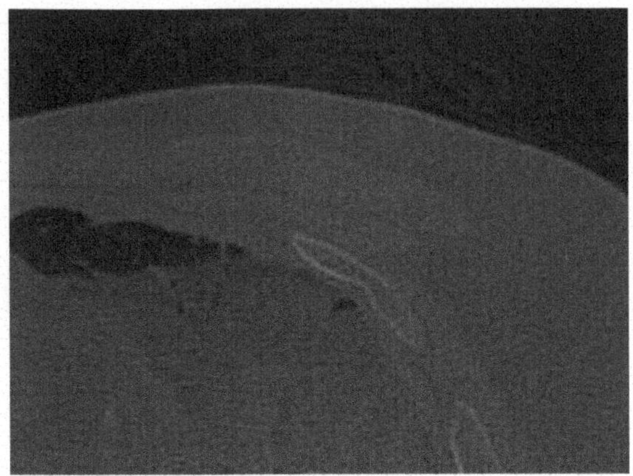

Fig. 11.8 Axial view of a left anterior rib on bone windows shows an incomplete buckle fracture of the inner cortex following CPR attempts

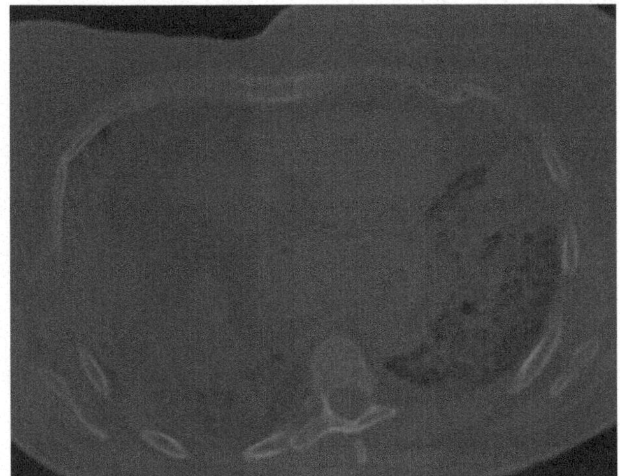

Fig. 11.9 Axial view of the chest on bone windows showing bilateral anterior rib fractures resulting from CPR attempts, buckle type on the right and displaced, complete on the left

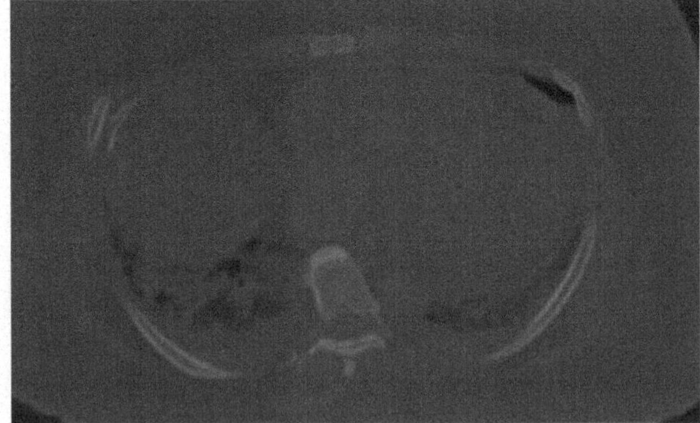

Fig. 11.10 Axial view of the chest on bone windows showing bilateral anterior rib fractures resulting from CPR attempts, complete with displacement on the right and buckle on the left with small underlying pneumothorax

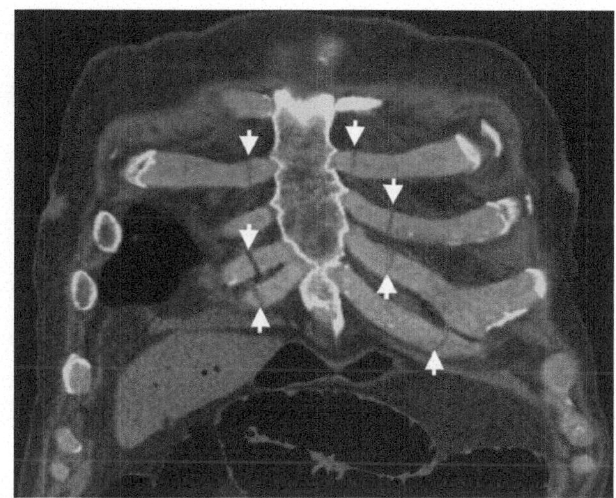

Fig. 11.11 Coronal view of the anterior chest wall on soft tissue windows shows multiple, bilateral, vertically orientated costal cartilage fractures resulting from CPR attempts

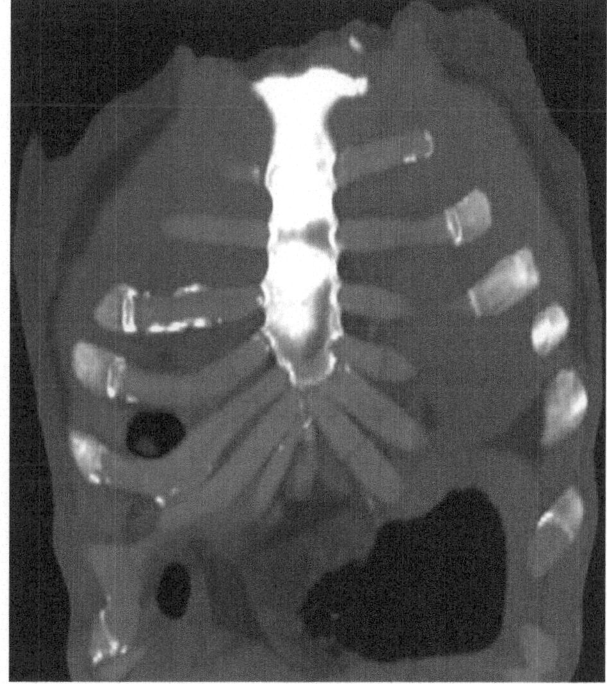

Fig. 11.12 Coronal maximum intensity projection of the anterior chest wall shows multiple, undisplaced bilateral costal cartilage fractures resulting from CPR attempts

chest, their displacement may have been more considerable. Occasionally, there are many displaced fractures that do not return to a normal chest architecture. This results in a residual deformity, such as a depressed sternum and/or anterior chest wall (Figs. 11.13, 11.14, and 11.15).

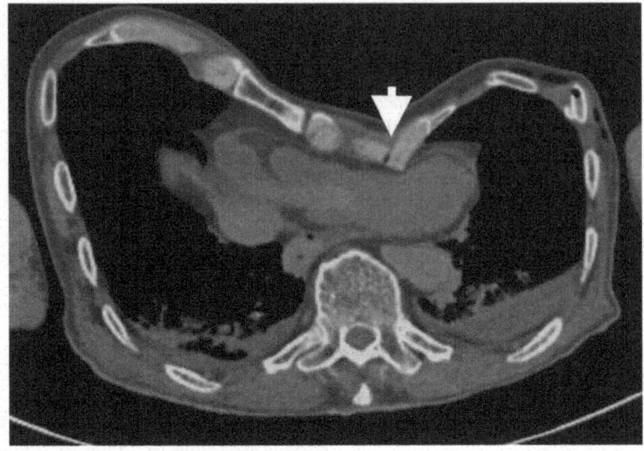

Fig. 11.13 Axial view of the chest on soft tissue windows shows a depressed left parasternal costal cartilage fracture (arrow) resulting in chest wall deformity and compression of mediastinal structures

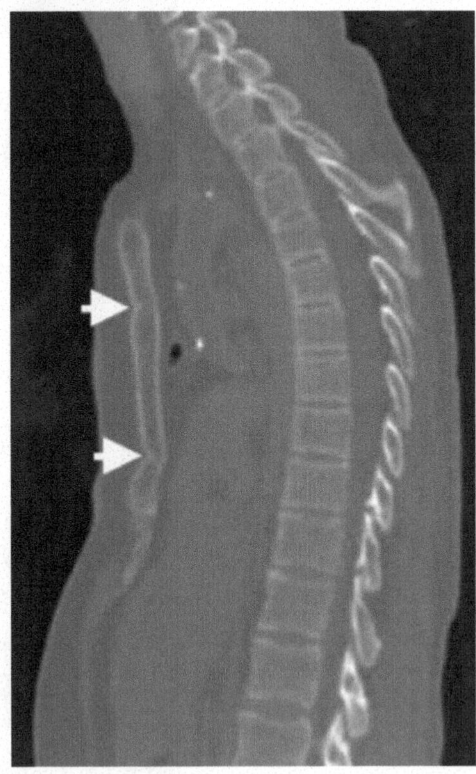

Fig. 11.14 Sagittal view of the chest on bone windows showing multiple sternal fractures (arrows) and depression of the sternum

By contrast, and important to bear in mind, posterior rib fractures are generally considered to be inconsistent with CPR (Fig. 11.16), although these might be attributed to resuscitation attempts if an external mechanical chest compression device has been used [6]. With use of such devices, the number of fractures demonstrated may also generally be higher [6].

It has been reported that PMCT has a low sensitivity for rib fractures compared to a forensic autopsy where ribs are individually dissected [7] and potentially

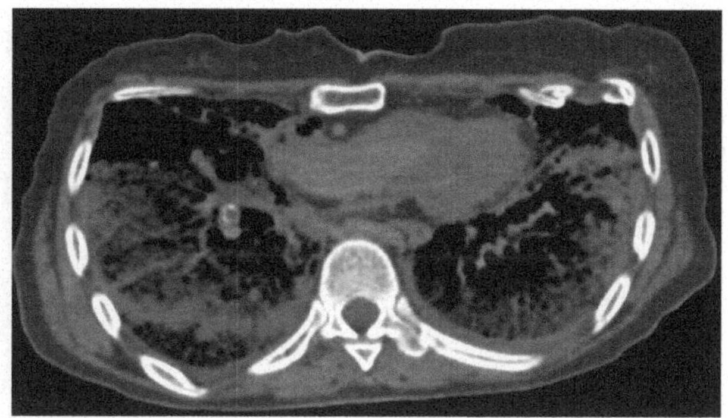

Fig. 11.15 Same case as Fig. 11.14, axial view of the chest on soft tissue windows showing sternal depression secondary to bilateral rib fractures and flattening of the anterior chest wall

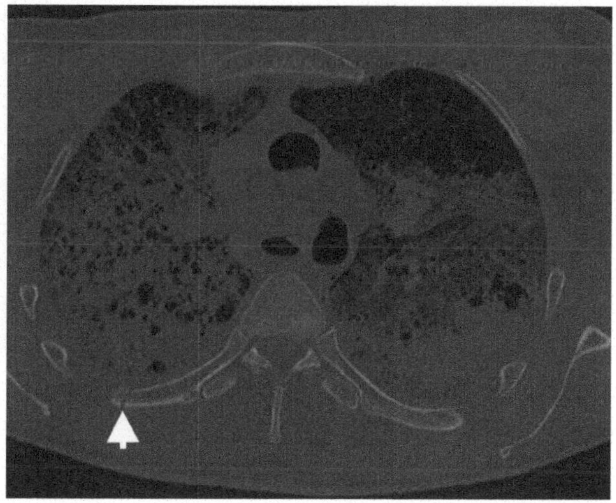

Fig. 11.16 Axial view of the chest on bone windows showing an acute right posterior rib fracture (arrow) following a road traffic collision

subject to histology. However, this is not considered to be the case when compared to a routine coronial autopsy—where the skeleton is only minimally reviewed and dissected. PMCT also offers a record of skeletal appearances prior to removal of the chest plate or other dissection at open autopsy. This can be reviewed later, potentially days and weeks (or years!) following the autopsy for correlation.

Sternal Fractures

Sternal fractures are also sometimes seen following CPR attempts. These are usually of the mid-sternum and can either be complete (Figs. 11.17 and 11.18) or incomplete (Figs. 11.19, 11.20, and 11.21). The PMCT report should describe such fractures and the residual degree of displacement (which, just as for the ribs, may have been significantly more during chest compressions) to correlate with any associated mediastinal injury.

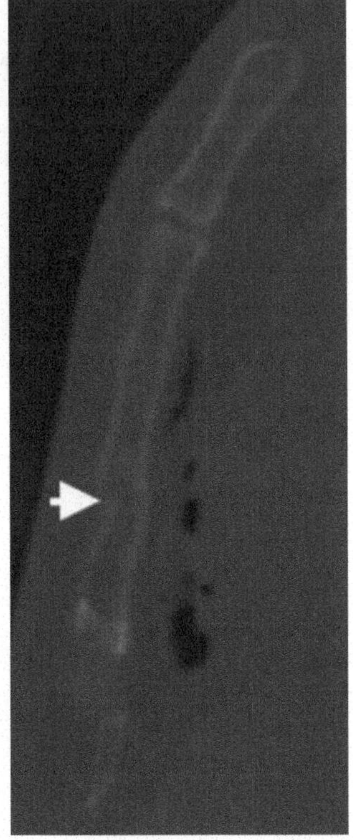

Fig. 11.17 Sagittal view of the sternum on bone windows showing a complete but minimally displaced sternal fracture (arrow) following CPR attempts

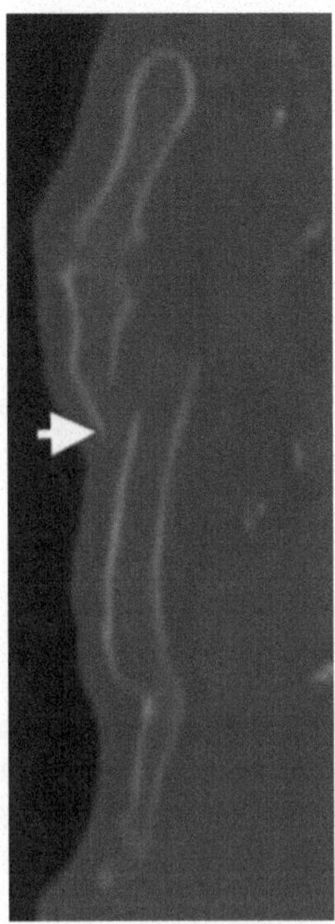

Fig. 11.18 Sagittal view of the sternum on bone windows showing a displaced mid-sternal fracture (arrow) following CPR attempts

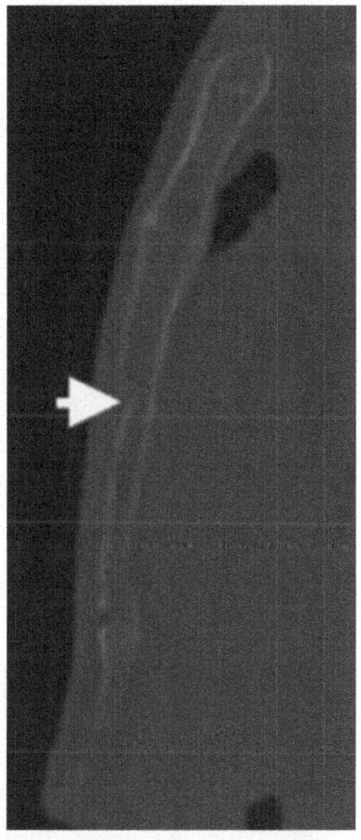

Fig. 11.19 Sagittal view of the sternum on bone windows showing an incomplete, anterior cortex sternal fracture (arrow) following CPR attempts

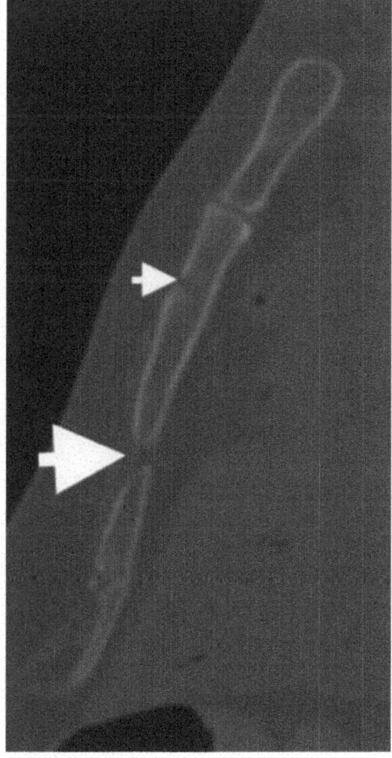

Fig. 11.20 Sagittal view of the sternum on bone windows showing an incomplete, anterior cortex sternal fracture (small arrow) following CPR attempts and an incidental, well-corticated sternal foramen inferiorly (large arrow)

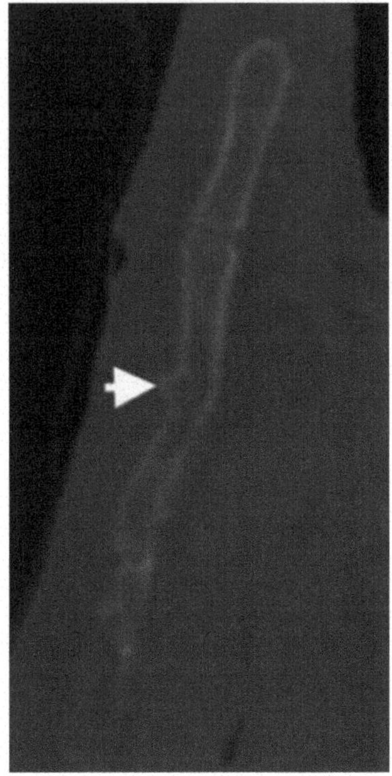

Fig. 11.21 Sagittal view of the sternum on bone windows showing a buckled but incomplete sternal fracture (arrow) following CPR attempts

Vertebral Fractures

More unusually, fractures of the mid thoracic spine (often around the T6 level) have also been reported following CPR [8]. The incidence appears higher with the use of mechanical CPR devices and more likely if there is osteopenia/osteoporosis, rigidity of the spine or existing kyphosis (Figs. 11.22 and 11.23). To make the interpretation of CPR-related vertebral fractures, one will need verification of the absence of trauma before the cardio-respiratory arrest and exclusion of a post mortem handling or transport-related injury. This means that cases that sustained trauma before death are more difficult to interpret (Fig. 11.24). One may consider that the absence of significant haematoma around a vertebral fracture supports the interpretation of a post mortem nature.

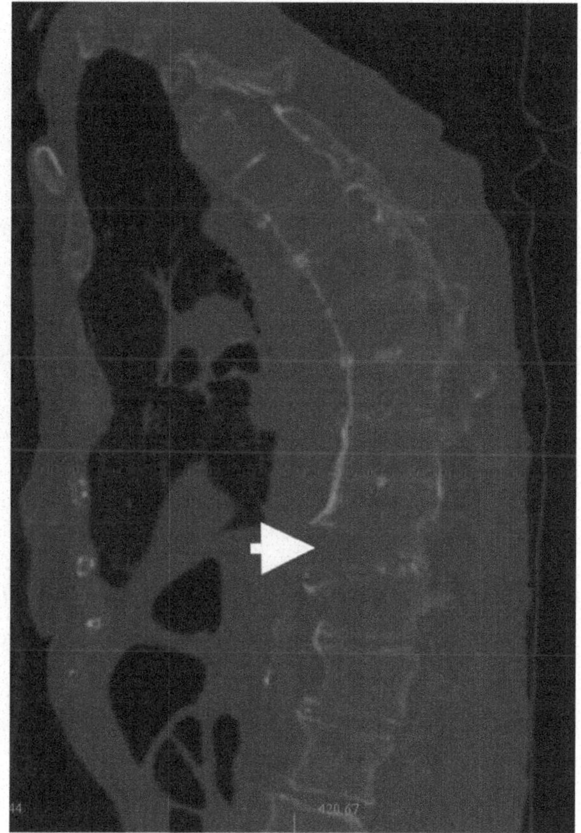

Fig. 11.22 Sagittal view of the thoracic spine on bone windows showing a fracture of an intervertebral disc space (arrow) in the setting of ankylosis and kyphosis. There was no known history of trauma other than chest compressions performed during CPR attempts

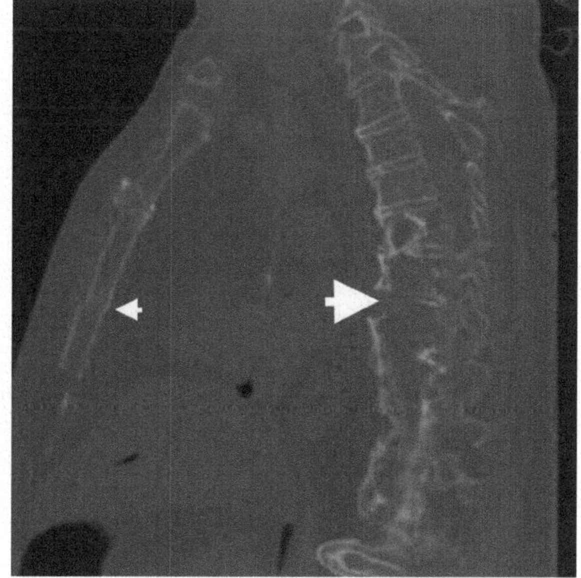

Fig. 11.23 Sagittal view of the chest on bone windows showing a sternal fracture (small arrow) and a corresponding level fracture through the intervertebral disc space (large arrow), both sustained following chest compressions in the setting of a degenerate, partially rigid spine and background of osteopaenia

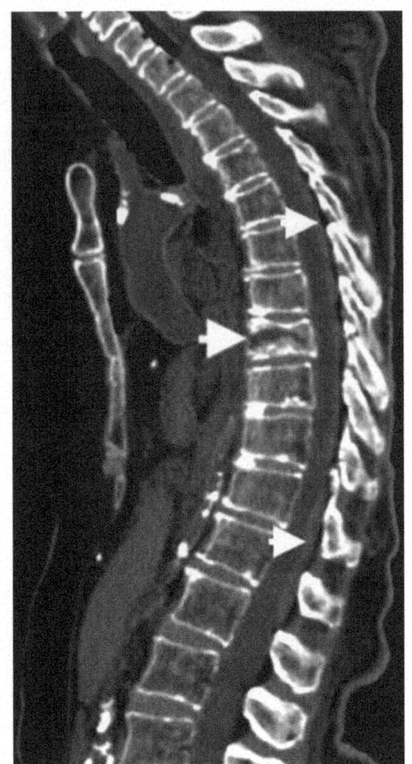

Fig. 11.24 Sagittal view of the thoracic spine windowed to show a vertebral canal haematoma (small arrows) centred around an acute, transverse T7 fracture (large arrow), involving the posterior elements. The patient was found unresponsive at the bottom of the stairs (presumed fall) and cardiopulmonary resuscitation was attempted. Note also a sternal fracture at the same level of the vertebral fracture. In this case it is difficult to determine whether the vertebral fracture and/or haematoma are related to the initial trauma or chest compressions

Soft Tissue Findings on PMCT

Soft tissue findings relating to CPR are commonly secondary to the chest wall fractures described earlier, although it is possible to have isolated soft tissue injury resulting from CPR attempts, especially in the younger population.

Small haemo/pneumothoraces, pneumomediastinum, lung contusions or lacerations, small haemopericardium and even peri-hepatic, peri-splenic and retro-peritoneal haemorrhages have all been reported to potentially be secondary to CPR-related soft tissue injury [9].

It can be difficult to distinguish between CPR-related lung contusion and other pathology such as pulmonary oedema, infection or post mortem atelectasis. Fluid resuscitation may also complicate the picture. Often, following CPR, the lungs appear very congested (Fig. 11.25) with non-specific diffuse ground-glass opacity and areas of collapse and consolidation. These broad, overlapping differential diagnoses often limit PMCT diagnostic interpretation.

Haemothorax and Pneumothorax

PMCT is sensitive to even tiny pneumothoraces (Fig. 11.25), more so than traditional autopsy methods that require time-consuming, special techniques to accurately demonstrate gas in the chest cavities. When reporting a pneumothorax, it is imperative that one must also consider the level of decomposition, so as not to falsely attribute autolytic gas production to that indicative of trauma/pathology (see Chap. 3).

The volume of a CPR-related post mortem haemo/pneumothorax is variable and dependent on multiple factors such as the manual or mechanical vigour of CPR and the length of resuscitation attempts. Any underlying coagulopathy may have bearing on local blood loss. Resuscitation-linked blood and air collections (Fig. 11.26), however, tend to be smaller in volume when compared to those resulting directly from fatal pathologies.

That being said, it is important to appreciate that a pneumothorax may be exacerbated by artificial ventilation devices. The use of external mechanical chest compression devices is generally associated with greater soft tissue injury and haemorrhage [6] (Figs. 11.27 and 11.28).

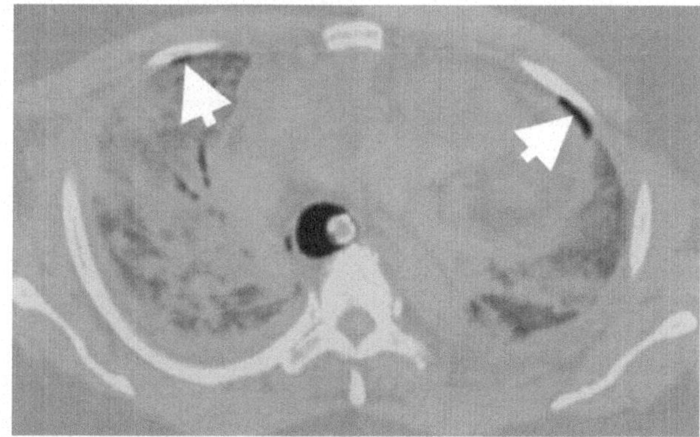

Fig. 11.25 Axial view of the chest on lung windows showing tiny bilateral pneumothoraces (arrows) resulting from rib fractures sustained during attempted CPR. The lungs are opacified with mixed ground glass density and patchy consolidation and there is also an endotracheal tube with cuff inflated in the trachea

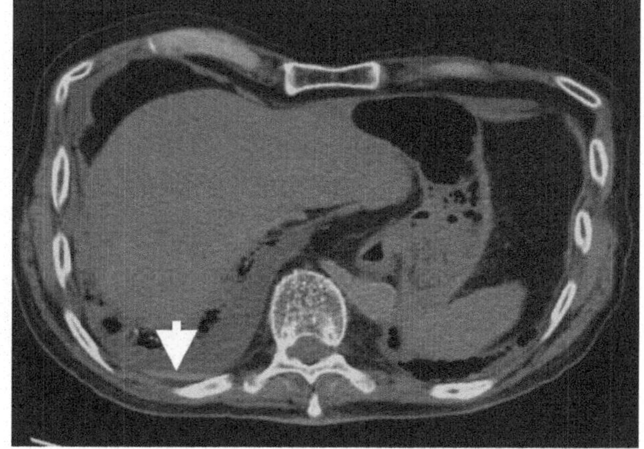

Fig. 11.26 Axial view of the lower chest on soft tissue windows shows a small layered density in the right pleural space, indicative of separated blood products/ haemothorax and judged to be secondary to CPR related injury. Note the right anterolateral buckled rib fracture and asymmetric chest wall

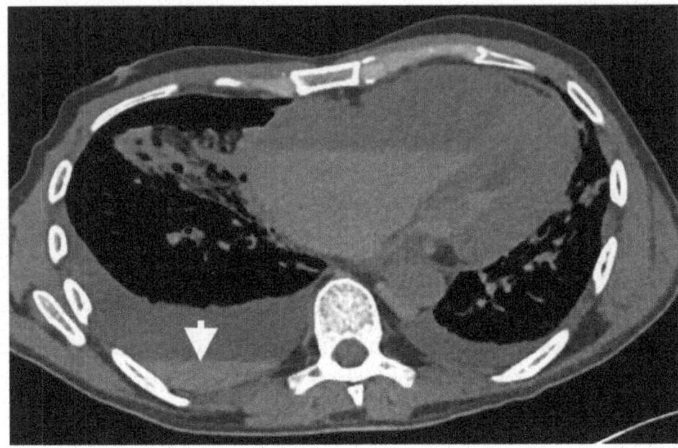

Fig. 11.27 Axial view of the chest on soft tissue windows shows a moderate size, right side layered haemothorax (arrow) after prolonged cardiopulmonary resuscitation attempts using an external mechanical chest compression device. The right atrium is dilated and contains a similar layered separation of blood products

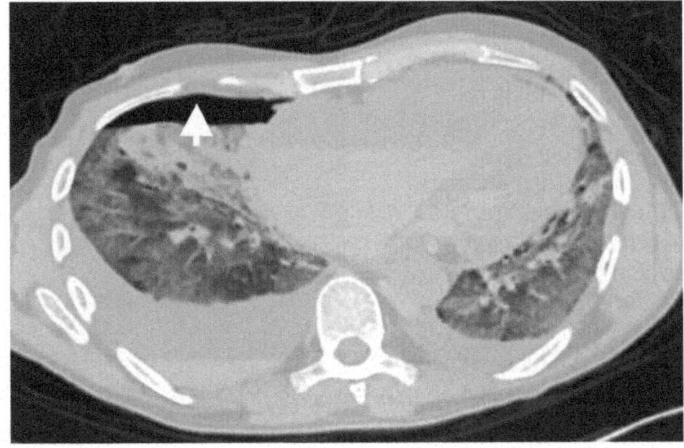

Fig. 11.28 Same case as Fig. 11.27, axial view of the chest on lung windows shows a right anterior pneumothorax after prolonged cardiopulmonary resuscitation attempts using an external mechanical chest compression device and ventilation via endotracheal intubation (not seen on this image)

It is emphasised that rib fractures after CPR are extremely unlikely to cause a post mortem aortic rupture, leading to massive haemothoraces. Aortic injury is by far more in keeping with true pathology, suggested by massive trauma/penetrating chest injury or primary rupture in the setting of chest pain with sudden collapse.

Pre-Sternal Haematoma

If an external mechanical chest compression device has been used during CPR, there is a higher incidence of subcutaneous pre-sternal haematoma formation [9] (Figs. 11.29 and 11.30). Otherwise, these are rarely seen.

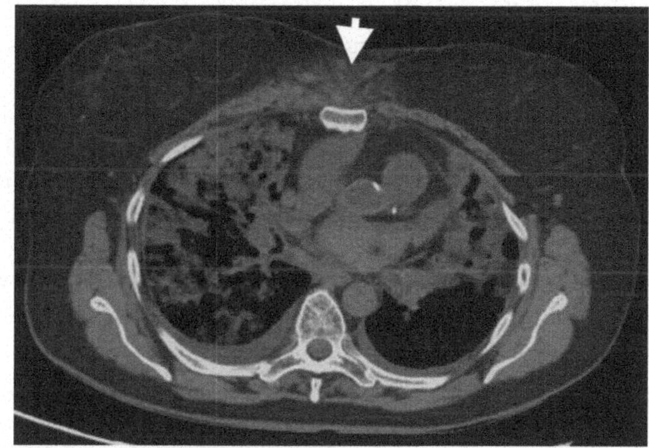

Fig. 11.29 Axial view of the chest on soft tissue windows shows a pre-sternal soft tissue haematoma (arrow) following CPR attempts using an external mechanical chest compression device

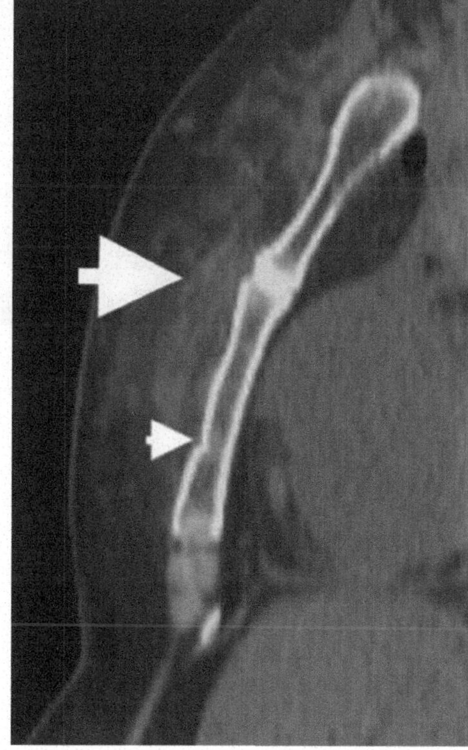

Fig. 11.30 Same case as Fig. 11.29, sagittal view of the sternum shows a pre-sternal haematoma (large arrow) and a fracture of the anterior cortex of the sternum (small arrow) after CPR attempts using an external mechanical chest compression device

Intravascular Gas and Dilated Right Atrium

Theories to explain gas in the vasculature following CPR (outside the setting of fatal trauma) include that it results from intravenous catheterisation, pulmonary injury from chest compressions or possibly pneumatisation of gas that was dissolved in the blood. This gas can be seen particularly in the cardiac chambers (Figs. 11.3 and 11.31) and liver [1, 2]. The differential is commonly seen decomposition gas, yet both of these origins should be distinguished from gas relating to pathology, for example in the abdomen.

Dilatation of the right atrium is also a feature seen on PMCT after CPR attempts, possibly due to right heart 'congestion' and/or increased intravascular fluid administered during resuscitation (Figs. 11.27 and 11.31). Fluid shifts within the circulation (realignment of blood) may also reflect the equalisation of pressures in the various vascular compartments after death. This finding is variable and difficult to quantify against potentially pre-existing atrial dilatation without comparative imaging [1, 10].

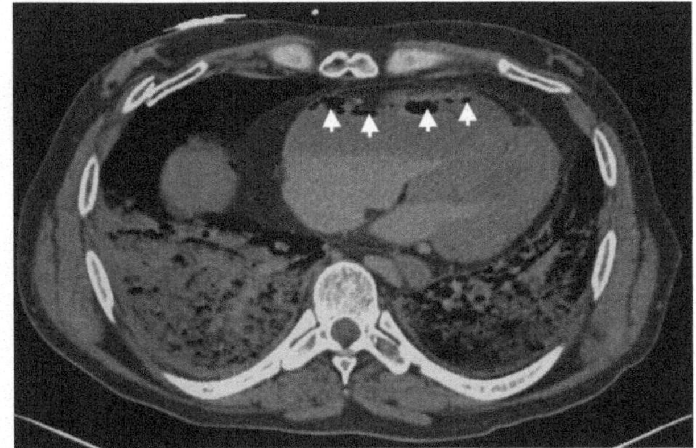

Fig. 11.31 Axial view of the chest on soft tissue windows showing multiple locules of intracardiac gas (arrows), dilated right atrium, right anterolateral rib fracture and extensive lung congestion seen after 1 hour of in-hospital CPR following a suicide by hanging

Abdominal Findings Following CPR

Small to moderate volumes of intra-peritoneal haemorrhage (Fig. 11.32) and retroperitoneal haemorrhage (Figs. 11.33 and 11.34) may be seen following CPR attempts, when no other explanation (such as abdominal trauma or a ruptured aorta) is found. Such collections are presumed to reflect tiny visceral lacerations of the liver and/or spleen although these may not be clearly appreciated on routine PMCT.

In hospital, when resuscitation attempts follow radiological investigations or procedures involving iodinated contrast, haemorrhage may be even more hyperdense than usual owing to contrast material held in the circulation prior to cardiorespiratory arrest (Fig. 11.35).

Distension of the stomach and gastrointestinal (GI) tract can be seen following CPR with artificial respiration using a facemask or poorly fitting laryngeal mask (often used prior to intubation), as gas passes into both the trachea and the oesophagus (Fig. 11.36). CPR is also reported to cause intra-mural GI tract or intra-hepatic gas [10] although, to confidently report this finding, it would have to be seen as out of proportion to decomposition gas elsewhere and without any prior abdominal symptoms that might suggest acute GI pathology.

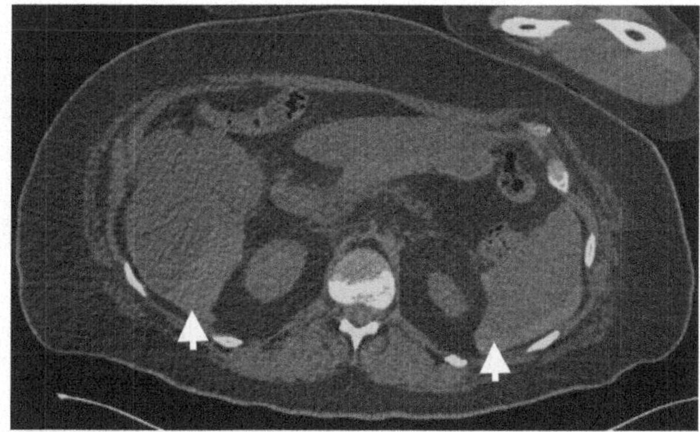

Fig. 11.32 Axial view of the upper abdomen on soft tissue windows showing a small volume of high-density fluid dependently around the liver and spleen (arrows) judged to be intraperitoneal haemorrhage following CPR attempts

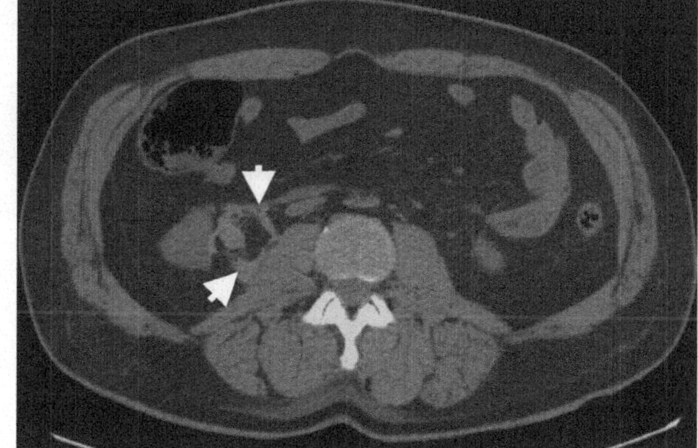

Fig. 11.33 Axial view of the mid abdomen on soft tissue windows shows a small volume of streaky high-density fluid in the right retroperitoneal space (arrows) judged to be haemorrhage following CPR attempts. There was no history of abdominal trauma and no haemorrhage around the collapsed aorta

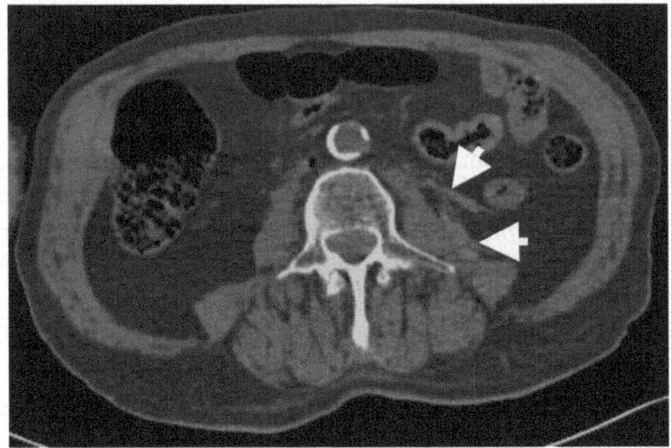

Fig. 11.34 Axial view of the mid abdomen on soft tissue windows shows a small volume of streaky high-density fluid in the left retroperitoneal space (arrows) judged to be haemorrhage following CPR attempts. There is no haemorrhage around the non-aneurysmal aorta

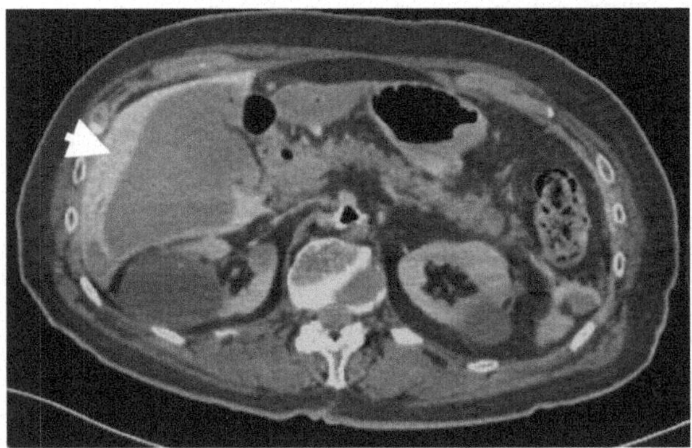

Fig. 11.35 Axial view of the upper abdomen on soft tissue windows showing peri-hepatic haemorrhage (arrow) judged to be secondary to liver injury during in-hospital CPR. This appears more dense than expected due to the presence of iodinated contrast from preceding radiological intervention. Contrast also 'enhances' the kidneys to reveal several simple cysts

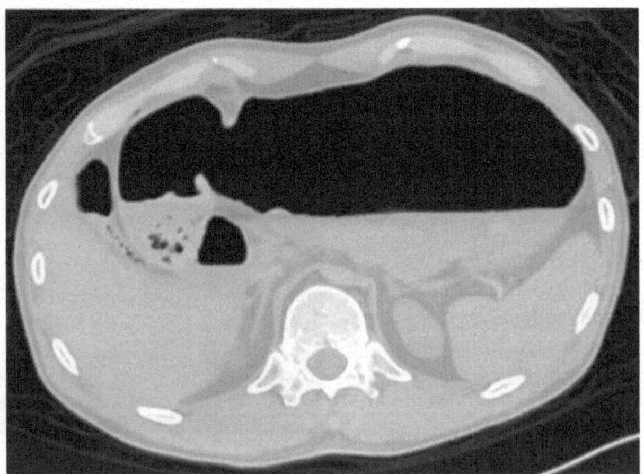

Fig. 11.36 Axial view of the upper abdomen on lung windows shows a markedly distended, gas filled stomach following prolonged resuscitation attempts with multiple airway interventions

Reporting CPR-Related Findings: Pearls and Pitfalls

A history of whether CPR was attempted (and specifically chest compressions) should be available, or sought, when considering PMCT. If these data are not available, then caution should be taken when interpreting the scan findings.

A description of the positions of lines/tubes etc. may be given in the understanding that their position may have altered after death.

Posterior rib fractures are generally considered inconsistent with CPR.

Knowledge of the use of external chest compression devices is important, as this may result in more CPR-associated injury.

When CPR has been performed, a description of the findings can be made with a statement to suggest these are 'in keeping' or 'consistent with' injury from attempted CPR.

Example PMCT report phrases:

- It is noted from the supporting information that cardiopulmonary resuscitation (CPR) including chest compressions was attempted.
- Endotracheal tube with tip located just above the carina at the time of scanning.
- Bilateral anterior rib buckle fractures / sternal fractures in keeping with attempted CPR.
- Small haemothorax/pneumothorax is in keeping with CPR related injury.
- Small volume of upper abdominal haemorrhage judged most likely to have resulted from the prolonged CPR attempts.

References

1. Murakami T, Uetani M, Ikematsu K. Postmortem CT in emergency department: influence of cardiopulmonary resuscitation. Poster session presented at: European Congress of Radiology; 2012 March 1–5; Vienna, Austria. [Internet]. https://doi.org/10.1594/ecr2012/C-1440.
2. Offiah CE, Dean J. Post-mortem CT and MRI: appropriate post-mortem imaging appearances and changes related to cardiopulmonary resuscitation. Br J Radiol [Internet]. 2016;89(1058):20150851. http://www.birpublications.org/doi/10.1259/bjr.20150851.
3. Bolster F, Ali Z, Fowler D, Daly B. Imaging of resuscitation and emergency resuscitation devices—Lessons learned from post mortem computed tomography. J Forensic Radiol Imaging [Internet]. 2019;17:23–30. https://linkinghub.elsevier.com/retrieve/pii/S2212478019300383.
4. Lotan E, Portnoy O, Konen E, Simon D, Guranda L. The role of early postmortem CT in the evaluation of support-line misplacement in patients with severe trauma. Am J Roentgenol [Internet]. 2015;204(1):3–7. http://www.ajronline.org/doi/10.2214/AJR.14.12796.
5. Suvarna SK, editor. Atlas of adult autopsy [Internet]. 1st ed. Cham: Springer International Publishing; 2016. http://link.springer.com/10.1007/978-3-319-27022-7.
6. Koga Y, Fujita M, Yagi T, Nakahara T, Miyauchi T, Kaneda K, et al. Effects of mechanical chest compression device with a load-distributing band on post-resuscitation injuries identified

by post-mortem computed tomography. Resuscitation [Internet]. 2015;96:226–31. https://linkinghub.elsevier.com/retrieve/pii/S030095721500386X.

7. Schulze C, Hoppe H, Schweitzer W, Schwendener N, Grabherr S, Jackowski C. Rib fractures at postmortem computed tomography (PMCT) validated against the autopsy. Forensic Sci Int [Internet]. 2013;233(1–3):90–8. https://linkinghub.elsevier.com/retrieve/pii/S0379073813004027.
8. Bohara M, Ohara Y, Mizuno J, Matsuoka H, Hattori N, Arita K. Cardiopulmonary resuscitation-induced thoracic vertebral fracture: a case report. NMC Case Rep J [Internet]. 2014;2(3):106–8. https://www.jstage.jst.go.jp/article/nmccrj/2/3/2_cr.2014-0383/_article.
9. Baumeister R, Held U, Thali MJ, Flach PM, Ross S. Forensic imaging findings by post-mortem computed tomography after manual versus mechanical chest compression. J Forensic Radiol Imaging [Internet]. 2015;3(3):167–73. https://linkinghub.elsevier.com/retrieve/pii/S2212478015300095.
10. Ishida M, Gonoi W, Okuma H, Shirota G, Shintani Y, Abe H, et al. Common postmortem computed tomography findings following atraumatic death: differentiation between normal postmortem changes and pathologic lesions. Korean J Radiol [Internet]. 2015;16(4):798. https://www.kjronline.org/DOIx.php?id=10.3348/kjr.2015.16.4.798.

The manufacturer's authorised representative in the EU is Springer Nature Customer Service Centre GmbH, Europaplatz 3, 69115 Heidelberg, Germany. If you have any concerns regarding our products, please contact ProductSafety@springernature.com

Printed and bound by CPI Group (UK) Ltd, Croydon, CR0 4YY
17/07/2026
02170250-0002